s

CLINICAL STUDIES IN NEUROLOGY

Oh that one would hear me! behold, my desire is, that the Almighty would answer me, and that mine adversary had written a book.

—JOB, CHAPTER 31.

R Denis Giblin

New York
April '71

Clinical Studies
in NEUROLOGY

By

HARRY LEE PARKER, M.S., M.D., F.R.C.P.I.

Professor of Neurology
Mayo Foundation, Graduate School, University of Minnesota
Senior Consultant, Section of Neurology
Mayo Clinic, Rochester, Minnesota

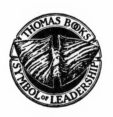

Second Printing

CHARLES C THOMAS · PUBLISHER
Springfield · Illinois · U.S.A.

Published and Distributed Throughout the World by
CHARLES C THOMAS • PUBLISHER
BANNERSTONE HOUSE
301–327 East Lawrence Avenue, Springfield, Illinois, U.S.A.
NATCHEZ PLANTATION HOUSE
735 North Atlantic Boulevard, Fort Lauderdale, Florida, U.S.A.

© *1956, by* CHARLES C THOMAS • PUBLISHER
Library of Congress Catalog Card Number: 55–11244

First Printing, 1956
Second Printing, 1969

With THOMAS BOOKS *careful attention is given to all details of
manufacturing and design. It is the Publisher's desire to present books
that are satisfactory as to their physical qualities and artistic possibilities
and appropriate for their particular use.* THOMAS BOOKS *will be true
to those laws of quality that assure a good name and good will.*

Printed in the United States of America

BB-14

DEDICATION

To the eternal medical student, who, during his first close acquaintance with patients in hospital wards, acquires to himself, besides clinical instruction, every disease in the calendar.

He first has in his mind that he has tuberculosis of the lungs, in a hopeless stage. Endless cigarettes and a smoker's cough help out this conviction. Carcinoma of the stomach follows, as a result of late hours and copious draughts of cheap beer. But why does he have sarcoma of the jaw? "Elementary, my dear Watson. He is erupting his wisdom teeth!"

—PARAPHRASED FROM THE WORKS
OF SIR ARTHUR CONAN DOYLE.

FOREWORD

IT IS RIGHT and proper that a strong interest be cultivated in a student of medicine in his senior years. Less just and good is it that he be forced to swallow indigestible theory and dogma. The former principle he will remember forever after; the latter, at a later date, he will gleefully discard as the snake, wriggling with pleasure, gets rid of his own skin.

For fifteen years, I had taught postgraduate students at the Mayo Clinic. It was a labor of love since these young men are carefully selected as being of high intelligence and of a previous faultless career. They absorbed information with an unparalleled gusto, and could ask and answer questions in neurology that were controversial topics. They could go further and discuss modernities of which I was ignorant, much to my own embarrassment. Apart from that, it was in a pleasant and an easy milieu of teacher and student with advantages, I hope, to both.

In 1934, I was invited to take the chair of neurology at my parent university, Trinity College, Dublin. Also, I was elected to take the position of senior staff physician at the Richmond Hospital, one of the oldest and largest institutions in the Irish capital. My task there was to care for the indigent sick. More important was it that there was an active system in that hospital of the bedside teaching of undergraduate students.

The system in the Dublin hospitals, as far as teaching was concerned, was an eclectic one. The medical student paid his fees to the hospital he joined, but thereafter he could roam as he wished to other hospitals for bedside lectures, and, of course, to wherever he thought he got the best value. Ultimately, he served his internship in his own hospital, but even then he could go where he pleased for those morning classes which seemed the most attractive. There was no discrimination shown in the Richmond Hospital against these roving students; regardless of their school, hospital or anything else, we felt that these men honored us by attending our classes. The bulk of the crowd present was an index of our educational appeal.

The hospital itself was a conglomerate pile of hardcut stone of over two hundred years agrowing. By the twentieth century, the surgeons grabbed the newer red brick buildings, more cheerful and more in keeping with the motto: "Cut well, sew well, and get well," and so it was that the humble physician-healers were allocated to the older part of the building. The wards therein were rat-ridden, cold, bleak and sinister. There were no carpets, window curtains or decorations of any kind. There was nothing to make dying a final act of happiness except in so far as members of the skull-capped, monk-robed Capuchin order, with sandals on their feet, who lived near by, could do the necessary facilitated exitus from this drear world to a hopefully better one in the next.

Clinical instruction for me was on a Tuesday morning, and, for some reason or another, the weather was usually damp, cold and forbidding. In phantasy, I likened myself to Charcot at the Salpêtrière with his "Leçons sur mardi." Alas, there was not forthcoming his histrionic ability, his genius for research, or his aptitude for correlating new facts. There was no audience such as he had, in the form of journalists, celebrities, demimondaines or even prostitutes. All I had in the beginning was a group of callow neophytes, trying to hide their dread of neurology and floundering in a spirit of complete frustration. In their white coats, with dumb, bleak, tallow-colored faces, I likened them in earlier years to a flock of sheep who had lost their bellwether.

It was a challenge, however, and from a corporal's guard of a few lost souls, who knew nowhere else to go, a change occurred within a scant few years. The dreary hospital wards on these Tuesday mornings soon became packed with a jostling, pushing, vibrant throng of youngsters, forcing their way to the bedside. The back rows stood on chairs and the rest figuratively hung from the light fixtures. Some, weary from misspent nights, sank on the torso of a patient nearby; some carried on a discussion at the back of the ward with loud voices. It was not good for teaching, but even with a lecture room, as was available, I could not see submissive row-on-row listening to the anathemas of anathemas, as embodied in a formal lecture. We carried on the effort to teach.

The patients were carefully selected. Some we had as real property, inmates of the hospital. Some were abducted slyly from elsewhere, and some were simply and sordidly bribed with shining silver pieces of money. At any cost, a fresh case was shown to the class each week and they received it eagerly. A new and pure victim was sacrificed to the God of Knowledge! Each problem was a clear-cut example of classic disease involving the nervous system. Occasionally and when possible, follow-up studies of the same patient were made.

From early October to June, the students saw, felt, smelled and listened to patients representing many of the more common diseases of the nervous system and a few of the rare. It was thought better to gain a sound knowledge of a few basic problems rather than a scattering knowledge of everything leading to nothing. There was no possible attempt at systemization.

And so, coming to this book. There is herein recorded the notes of these morning talks as they were given. Needless to say, the clinical material had been well studied during earlier weeks, and the presentation had to be scientifically word-perfect, lest confusion fall on teacher and students alike. The talks as recorded here were simple, personal and practical. They are now presented in written form, with a hope that they may help future generations of medical students and newly fledged postgraduates. Recent advances in neurologic fields have been added. The book is nevertheless not one that contains all things for all men. Better writers than I have done that and successfully. An accusation may be made here of oversimplification. A truth, simple as it may be, is none the less complex. As Hughlings Jackson said: "Never forget that we may run the risk of being over-educated and yet under-cultivated."

Medical books, on the whole, are dull reading. To be precise is to lose a latitude of romantic expression. Illustrations, plain and colored, help a great deal but yet are prohibitively expensive. They can not show all the nuances of ever-changing disease of the nervous system unless reproduced more times than the text can carry.

From time immemorial, the written sentence has been used to teach, to record observations and to illuminate in centuries-old manuscripts a passing impression, a long-forgotten feeling of someone who was faced with mortality and tried to reach beyond it. What matters the nature of his scribbles if he got all his facts in solemn array, as were pleasing to himself?

Here in this book is an echo of what went on in my wards during those twelve years. Students were taught to see, to hear, to feel and even, as young puppies, to rub their noses in the foul odor of disease. One can not altogether reproduce this with an inhibited pen and a frustratingly bleak, mocking, white, empty page of paper. It is a verity, however, that if a certain imagination is used by the writer, coupled with an appeal to the reader to stand by at all costs, the two—reader and writer—may get together for their personal and mutual satisfaction.

H. L. P.

CONTENTS

April

May

June

CLINICAL STUDIES IN NEUROLOGY

OCTOBER

I'll be suppos'd upon a book, his face is the worst thing about him.

—SHAKESPEARE: *Measure for Measure.*

1

Good morning! I welcome you to these wards wherein Sir Dominic Corrigan at one time worked and taught. You know by now of his observations on disease of the heart and its vessels and the so-called water-hammer pulse for which his name is remembered. I passed his house this morning on Merrion Square. The trees in front had their sullen leaves soaked by rain and drooped listlessly. There were none of the flamboyant golden yellows and fiery reds as seen in the farewell from summer of an American fall.

Two patients will be presented today and on every following Tuesday of this academic year. To a patient, there is nothing of a minor nature in his illness. Disease is hated and dreaded by all. However, for our purpose, there will be one patient who is the more seriously ill, as contrasted with a minor illness more easily described and taking up a shorter time in the morning demonstration.

Here in this bed is a rugged, powerful man aged forty-eight. He looks miserable and haggard, and he has every reason to be so, for he has such a pain in his face that all the devils out of Hell might be tearing at it. The pain is in his forehead, his eye, his cheek and in his lower jaw. Anatomically, it is confined to the area supplied by the fifth cranial nerve. This pain is sharp, lancinating, burning, and of a shocklike character. It is unbearable, and relieved by no simple medication.

He is asked to shake my hand, and as he rises from his bed the agony strikes him. You may see that his face reddens, his eyes gush tears, and the friendly handclasp is not completed. His face

5

is now contorted in pain, but following its few seconds or minutes of duration there is replaced a masklike expression of facial immobility. There is in this expression the hope of avoidance and dread of recurrence.

Any movement of his face, jaws or tongue produces immediate paroxysms. He can not eat, talk, spit or curse. He can not even pray to God to relieve him. Washing his face is impossible. The side involved here is the right, and it is covered with grime; it is greasy and unshaven. He points to areas where these paroxysms are more likely to arise, but does not dare touch them. We call these areas "trigger zones." The alae of his nose, his upper lip and his eyebrows are mostly concerned. Even touching one hair on his face will institute a paroxysm.

This facial pain has been with him for nearly five years. At first it was only in his cheek; later it spread to his lower jaw and finally to his forehead. There have been remissions of months with weeks of pain in between, but gradually the pain-free intervals are getting shorter and the area of face involved is becoming larger. All divisions of the fifth cranial nerve are now involved.

During a pain-free period he can do what he likes with his face, but sooner or later he feels his face, as he calls it, "alive," and then he has to respect it greatly. Even during painful periods his pain is never the same from one day, hour or minute to the next similar period. The suffering is unpredictable when the pain is on a rampage; his worst time is the morning when he is accustomed to yawn, spit, brush his teeth, shave and wash his face, and finally start but not always finish his breakfast. Strangely enough, his pain sometimes tires of torturing him, for on beginning to eat a meal he will be struck by the pain a few times, and then as he persists frantically in shoveling his food down, grudgingly the pain remits and he finishes his meal. Occasionally he gets a few warning little jabs of pain while he is quiet and doing nothing, and then all Hell is let loose in one paroxysm after another. Between his pains there is often a burning sensation over the area involved.

Persons with this trouble are a very reasonable and sensible group. They are so happy to be free of pain in the free intervals that they are inordinately thankful to the powers that be. They are not neurotic. For this reason even during a pain-free interval the diagnosis is seldom in doubt. And yet all we have then is their own description, and no leading questions are allowed. As St. Paul has said, "There are so many kinds of voices in the world and none of them is without significance. Therefore, if I know not the meaning of the voice I shall be unto him that speaks a barbarian and he that speaks shall be a barbarian unto me." I present this sufferer from *tic douloureux* or *paroxysmal trigeminal neuralgia* during an attack, but yet, in a free interval, with a little encouragement, he can tell you all you need to know.

The cause of tic douloureux is as yet unknown. Dr. Henry Head of London took a ganglion extirpated by Sir Victor Horsley for the treatment of the disease and spent many months sectioning and examining it under the microscope. Finally, his preparations were used by a medical school as normal histologic sections of the fifth nerve apparatus to teach students of anatomy!

In the differential diagnosis of trigeminal neuralgia, there are two diseases which produce, though rarely, an identical pain syndrome. The first is an acoustic neurofibromatous tumor arising from the eighth nerve, and the second is multiple sclerosis. A careful neurologic examination is therefore always essential in trigeminal neuralgia.

Diagnosis and treatment here go hand in hand. For adequate diagnosis, it is essential that during the "live" periods all incoming stimuli provoke the pain. There are many different pains in the face, but only in this disease does facial activity of one sort or another count; movement of any muscle invokes all muscles in the body—hence the paroxysm of pain when the patient greeted me. Closer yet to the point is touching or moving the face. Without these factors the diagnosis is not possible.

Treatment up to date is the abolition of all incoming stimuli. The sensory root of the fifth nerve must be sacrificed. It can be done by chemical means, injection of the fifth nerve trunks with alcohol, or intracranial section of the posterior root. A bargain must be struck agreeable to both physician and patient. It is a hard one, and permits of no breach of contract thereafter; more so, the contract must be accepted willingly and after all cards are on the table. Granted it is that treatment is unsatisfactory, for it means destruction of the fifth nerve, the sensory nerve of the face. This may be done temporarily and with injection of alcohol into the three branches of the nerve, or permanently by cutting the posterior root after it has left the ganglion and just before it enters the brain stem. In the first case there is a numbness of the area served by the fifth nerve lasting for an average of nine months, but as feeling returns so does the pain. In the second case the numbness and relief of pain are permanent. His pain is cured but his face is anesthetic! There is no going back to the period of a normally feeling face—but the old intense and ever-dreaded pain is gone.

All this seems easy and can be reduced to the syllogism: normal sensation—pain; numb face—no pain. It does not take into consideration the human psychology of pain, particularly the woman-baby complex wherein the mother forgets the pains of labor after her child is born. Or in another light, the Devil was sick: a saint would be; the Devil was well: the *Devil* a saint was he.

Accordingly, patients are carefully selected. In early stages of the disease one, two, three or more injections of alcohol are advised. Each time, a temporary relief with an education into what a numb face is like; and each time, *pari passu*, the sensation returns and so does the pain. This latter dominates the picture and brutalizes the patient, so that finally at an older and wiser period he elects to have done the radical and final severance of his consciousness from pain and of course normal sensation in the area of the face and head supplied by the fifth nerve. These folks are in the end very happy and satisfied persons.

The complications of the radical operation need not be entered into. Earlier surgeons dreaded an associated facial paralysis due to what was assumed to be interference with the greater superficial petrosal nerve. Seldom is this seen now, nor is the equally dreaded neuroparalytic keratitis. The cornea is anesthetic after the operation, and every fragment of dust, especially in those trades involving exposure to dust, may lead to loss of an eye. This is guarded against by covering up the eye with a glass shield or by the wearing of a set of eyeglasses with a plastic cup around the eye, a much more practical and cosmetic arrangement.

Any destruction of living nervous tissue is a gross procedure and is not ideal. The patient exchanges a numbness of his face for banishment of a pain. When the pain has thoroughly brutalized him, he is well satisfied in even measure for such a procedure. More recently, a surgical operation has been devised to release the dural envelope supposedly compressing the gasserian ganglion and the posterior root. The pathways of sensations are not cut and the patient's milieu is unchanged by the operation. May it fulfill the hopes and prayers that attend its inauguration.

2

SIR CHARLES BELL, Edinburgh and London surgeon of the nineteenth century, was somewhat of a dandy. Portraits show him as a dapper smiling little man. He danced a full measure at the ball given in Brussels on the eve of Waterloo, and spent the next few days lopping off shot-riddled arms and legs. He is best remembered by his studies of the face, both human and animal, and in his numberless exquisite drawings. It is consistent that he also wrote on expression by movements of the hands, a thing on which every shrewd legal attorney counts in cross-examination of a slippery witness.

This patient, a girl aged twenty-three, is now free of pain, and her facial problem is entirely motor and concerned with damage to the seventh cranial nerve as contrasted with what we saw earlier, which involves the fifth. Although there is now no suffering, it is a serious affliction in a single girl of marriageable age.

Ten days ago, she alleges, she slept with a window open and subject to the blast of a cold autumn morning. At any rate, she awoke with a dull nagging pain over her mastoid area and in the ear. She hopped out of bed to perform her morning ablutions. To her horror, she found on looking in the mirror that she had not the same face as she retired with. It was the very opposite of "God has given you one face and you make yourselves another." This fair Ophelia had no hand in her disfigurement. Her face was distorted and pulled to one side. Her right eye looked stonily on as she tried to close its lids. Brushing her teeth, she found that she could not spit straight, and later at breakfast, the food lodged between her cheek and teeth and had to be hooked out with her index finger. On leaving home, she found her right eye watering so that tears ran ceaselessly down her cheek.

And now you see her with a fully developed *Bell's palsy*: paralysis of the seventh cranial nerve. Even in repose the normal side pulls the face over to itself. She can not, on the right side, wrinkle her forehead, frown, close her eye, whistle, sneer, or blow out her cheeks, and if she ever had control of her platysma muscles, this movement on the right is gone. The eye is reddened from exposure to dust. If she laughs or cries, it is all on the left side, and a grotesque deformity results. The muscles on the right do not react to galvanic or faradic electric stimulation at this stage. She is not happy with this misfortune—perhaps the only thing worse for a woman of her age would be to lose her crowning glory—her hair!

The pain in the mastoid area has now gone, but the facial paralysis remains, and the question of treatment and prognosis comes up. It is gratifying that in nearly all cases of Bell's palsy the patients recover within weeks or months, no matter what is done. Spring and fall are common periods of occurrence, and it is probable that some infection attacks the mucous membrane of the fallopian canal, and it swells. Since in this intricate bony tunnel it can not swell outward, it must peradventure crush and bruise inward the seventh cranial nerve. If only a mere bruise has occurred, recovery within a few weeks is possible, but if the nerve is destroyed it is a matter of months before regeneration recurs. In the interim, the patient must be kept busy, lest despair and frustration lead to a nervous depression.

I am now asking this girl in succession to raise her eyebrows, to close her eyes and to show her teeth in front of a mirror. I have instructed her, once she is home again, to do these movements, to massage with some harmless medium her forehead, her cheek and her lower jaw, on the right side. She will do both for thirty minutes night and morning, at home, all before a mirror. She can therefore keep track of whatever recovery ensues, and once movement appears she will be all the more encouraged. Following her facial exercises and massage, she is to put hot compresses on her face for another ten minutes. Such simple procedures will give her content, although regeneration and recovery necessarily follow on their own path. Electric stimulation is painful and costly.

A cut skin heals in six days, a broken bone in six weeks, but a damaged nerve may take six months or more. In each case nature is more than kind; she overdoes repair. Keloid scar in the skin and a large hunk of callus in the bone are common reparative responses. In an old and slowly recovering Bell's palsy the face recovers and over-recovers. Movement is excessive on the formerly paralyzed side, and deeper creases appear in the nasolabial folds. Closing the eye will send the whole face into contraction, but this is to be expected and is a happier ending than a face that has on one side no human expression.

"Can you do Addition?" the White Queen asked.
"What's one and one and one and one and one and one
and one and one and one and one?"
"I don't know," said Alice, "I lost count."
                    —LEWIS CARROLL: *Through the Looking-Glass.*

3

Good morning! I passed Ely Place on my way here; it was raining
as usual. On impulse I stopped at the former dwelling place of
George Moore. Poor man—Dubliners always greedy for a catch
phrase said, "Many have kissed but never told—George never
kissed but always told!" Nevertheless, Moore rescued in the nineteenth century the English novel from the sickly Victorian
sentimentalities then in vogue. George was quite a man. He re-
counts, from his own imagination, the story of a Texas school-
marm who came as a virgin all the way here to have a child by
him and so create a dynasty of vigor and intellect. And as George
tells it, she did just that and no more.

In this bed here is a girl who, unlike her New World prototype,
is traveling hopefully but who will not arrive. She cannot walk
as well as she is accustomed to do. Further, her vision is affected,
in that all she sees is double. Let us get her out of bed and have
her walk for us. Her progression to the end of the ward is one
of a swaying measure; there is a certain rigidity of her lower
limbs, so that her feet hug the ground.

Talking to her when she is back in her bed, one appreciates
a tremendous sense of kindness and good will. Around the ward
in the afternoon she is neatly and pleasantly dressed, and I may
say no aid to beauty is neglected. The nurses in charge adore
her, for nothing is too hard for her to do in helping the sick.
Altogether this young woman, aged twenty-five, is a jewel

beyond price. She is everyone's friend and nobody's enemy, and there is ever an intense irradiation of optimism from her. She is, in short, Eleanor Porter's "Pollyanna," believing good in everybody and happy in everything. We have forgotten, however, that this girl is ill and patiently seeking help.

Looking at her eye movements, one sees that she has nystagmus, a vibration of her eyes in lateral and upward gaze; there is also a rotatory component. Movements of her eyes to either side are poor. Significant above all things is that the out-turning eye in this limited motion goes into nystagmus more than the other. The right optic disk is paler than the left.

All tendon reflexes are exaggerated. Hoffmann's sign in the flick of the second finger is present; the abdominal reflexes are absent, but Babinski's sign is easily shown and is present bilaterally. Vibration sense is diminished over the malleoli, but joint sensibility is preserved. There is an oscillating titubation in walking that makes for a jiggling up-and-down movement, and on turning suddenly the patient sways to one side and seems likely to fall.

Examination of the cerebrospinal fluid was done yesterday. There is an increase of small lymphocytes (15 per cubic millimeter), and the total protein estimation is 80 mg. per 100 cc. The colloidal-gold curve is 555554321.

At this stage of the demonstration, I would draw your attention to the fact that this girl's clinical picture can *not* be produced by one lesion. It is like the mathematics lesson in *Through the Looking-Glass,* a process of addition. No one sign constitutes the diagnosis; it is the sum of many over the years. There is manifest evidence of damage to the cerebrospinal motor pathways. If a preparation of the brain and spinal cord were nailed to a barn door and shot at with a spread of No. 6 shot, the pyramidal tracts could not in all verity escape. And seldom are there lacking signs of such involvement in this disease. It consists of multiple, disseminated plaques of hardening in the spinal cord. At first there is merely a process of destruction of the myelin sheaths; the axis cylinder remains intact. Later gliosis, the scar formation of the central nervous system, dominates the picture.

Earlier observers saw the late results of the disease and stressed the hardening process, so at that far-off time it was called disseminated "sclerosis."

And now may we discuss the history of this patient, the prognosis of the disease and what therapy is to be considered? To do so, with freedom from embarrassing the patient, we must move to another ward. Some of you, moreover, have become silent, stupid, broody and lost in rapt contemplation of your individual omphalos. Let us go elsewhere.

At the age of twenty this girl lost the vision in her right eye. Peculiarly enough, the loss was only for central objects. Looking at a picture, she saw that the perimeter was distinct but that the images in the center were gone. She could not read print. Her medical adviser blamed an infected tooth and it was removed. This monocular blindness cleared within a few days. The whole period of blindness was less than four weeks.

At the age of twenty-two she was working as a typist. That summer, and within one or two weeks, her hands became clumsy, awkward and numb, and she struck the wrong keys repeatedly. She had to resign, and spent the summer at home helping her mother as best as she could. By autumn the clumsiness cleared up, and she was again able to dress herself, to write and to type.

Now she is admitted to the hospital after being presumably well and without complaint for nearly two years. The present symptoms of ataxia in gait and dragging of her legs have been present for six months; they are getting slowly but steadily worse.

The history, findings and laboratory reports are so typical of *multiple sclerosis* that I am envenomed with suspicion. Such a diagnosis too often is a bottomless pit into which sundry and all diseases of the central nervous system are thrown. Tumor of the structures around the spinal cord in its upper cervical region must be considered and a cerebellar tumor may call under false signals. But by and large, the history and findings of this poor little one, if you know your job and apply yourself to it, can not lead you astray.

This girl has been here over a month. I have studied her case daily, and so have my assistants; we find no other possible diagnosis. We have assumed our original opinion to be incorrect and have had it called to the bar of justice, indicted, tried, and finally given to a jury of our peers. Grudgingly, we must admit that the diagnosis remains intrinsically the same.

If amongst you there are single men needing wives, for the love of God keep away from girls with multiple, disseminated sclerosis or sclérose en plaques. Should you marry, you will become a helpless microcosm in their clutches. You will want to succor, provide for and otherwise support them, regardless of what offspring appears, to be motherless and uncared for. Females with multiple sclerosis are very much the reverse of sterile —they are surprisingly fruitful, and their progeny suffer as one would expect, from neglect. On the male side, the economic situation is that being physically unfit, that is all that counts. No girls will marry them, such as they are.

And now I see the question trembling on every lip. What are we going to do for this charming and sprightly young lady to cure her of the foul disease that has entered into her? I can say to her, "We are going to treat you *secundum artem.* You will get medicine, physical therapy, and lots of loving-kindness, as you so truly desire and deserve. You will improve while here, but remember Robert Louis Stevenson's saying in one of his priceless essays, 'It is better to travel hopefully than to arrive.'" Some of the best scientific minds of today are working on this problem. These patients have remissions of months or years in which they become ostensibly normal, and why? We ought to find out that mechanism. Again, the life cycle of multiple sclerosis is not so short as the textbooks of previous years insisted. Some patients live out their life span, useful, active and happy. Is multiple sclerosis the same former fellow traveler with tabes dorsalis in relative frequency and chronicity; or is it also becoming a dead and dying disease? I hope so with all my heart.

4

MISTRESS X in bed No. 4 has a problem all her own. She has had two experiences: she has gained weight around her hips, and later she has gathered to herself a numbness around the outer part of her thigh. At the risk of bringing blushes to her face, I am asking the head nurse to uncover the part involved. The complaint is of a burning, stinging sensation sharply circumscribed and at the same time numb. There is an anesthesia—dolorosa!

My house officer, with pin, cotton wool and a hot bottle, has delineated on her right thigh the numb area, always working from the area of diminished sensibility to that area where feeling is normal. As a result, an area the size of the palm of a man's hand is mapped out on the lateral surface of this meaty and fatty thigh.

My earliest experience of this syndrome was when a physician-patient and I discussed this, his personal, problem. He did not know what was wrong with him, nor did I. We talked in terms of tumor and growths on the spinal cord, of grave situations such as syringomyelia, and we parted in dolorous confusion. And now my house officer and I can talk confidently of *meralgia paraesthetica.* A simple neurologic condition it is, harmless, incurable, but leading to no serious affair that will paralyze or kill a human being. The catch is to recognize it, and therefore to be able to put the patient's mind at rest.

Turning to the patient, I explain that because of her fat, her erect posture, and whatever else she has been doing, including canning fruit this fall, the two branches of the lateral cutaneous nerve of the thigh have been nipped by the fascia lata as she stands erect and sublime, mistress of her house. The tiny twigs of nerves do not like this, and the skin on the outer surface of the thigh begins to burn in a specified area. She can diet and cut down her weight, or can allow the process to go on to a final area of anesthesia which becomes part of her soma and is so accepted and dismissed from her mind. An alternative is to cut these nerve twigs and so hurry up the process and bring it to its expected conclusion. The disease can be unilateral or on both sides. In most cases, however, the patient, knowing what is going on and the final cost, is happy and satisfied to do just nothing.

5

Good morning! On my way here, I had to pass Saint Patrick's Cathedral. It is a building of Gothic inspiration, but dull and of no great interest. Alongside is a square, red brick building with a mansard roof. The bricks are so red that they shine out, intense, brazenly, as if afire on this dull and damp autumn day. Here lived Jonathan Swift throughout the years he lacked the preferment he sought. God send us pity for this tortured man who is now dead and at peace for over two hundred years. His relationship with Stella will evermore be as mysterious as the disease process that gave him roaring in the ears and vertigo. All we can say is that he, like kingdomed Achilles in confusion, raged and battered down himself.

At dinner one night an eclipse of the moon was heralded. Common people thronged around and shouted. Swift sent out word by his footman that by order of the Dean the eclipse had been postponed. The crowd melted.

I have a man here who complains of dizziness. This strikes him where and when he least expects it. The world revolves around him; he is nauseated and vomits, and he falls down prostrate. His life is spent in dread of such an occurrence, and he can not depend on his coming or his going.

For ten years he has been annoyed by a sound in his right ear. It is high-pitched and is compared to that of a water mill. Hearing in the same ear has been failing, so that he now uses the telephone receiver altogether on his left side. Two years

17

before he had his first attack of vertigo. This was terrific! At his place of business he was struck as if by lightning, and fell on his face amongst his papers and vomited all over them. He was carried home and put to bed, where he lay for twenty-four hours with his eyes tightly shut. He did not dare to move trunk or limb. Each time he opened his eyes the room swam around him, and he vomited anew and retched thereafter incessantly.

He recovered from this attack by being quiet and motionless, for a week, and was free from any trouble for three months. He regarded this as a single episode never to be repeated. At that time the iron had not entered his soul.

Remorselessly, however, the attacks of vertigo, nausea and vomiting recurred and kept occurring. These attacks of ringing in his ears, nausea and dizziness come more frequently, but as a recompense are less severe and of shorter duration. The noise in his ear is greater before an attack of vertigo, and the deafness is more marked.

And now we see this fifty-year-old man at peace with the world, except in so far as he has no guarantee that he may not be felled prone in his pleasures or in his devotions; he enjoys both and wishes to continue them. He has deficient hearing in one ear and a constant noise in it. Results of the neurologic examination, including tests for nystagmus and corneal reflexes, are negative. Caloric stimulation of his labyrinths with ice water syringed into his ear shows reactions relatively less on the right side.

The psychologic side is paramount here. Displacement in space is a grievous affliction. Few patients tolerate it gladly. Deafness can be adjusted to, tinnitus can be ignored, but to be suddenly distorted, avulsed and misplaced in the old, well-known, solid, happy earthy medium is something that produces a nervous shock, invites a neurosis. This disease, called *"Ménière's syndrome,"* does not leave all at once. If only these patients were taught from the beginning that their trouble is disagreeable but not serious, something would be gained. Unfortunately, they fear the worst, and concepts of tumor of the brain fill their minds. An attack of vertigo is more demoralizing than a headache. Pain is in one's being, but vertigo is a translation to another sphere.

And what shall we do with this man? I shall certainly give him words of comfort and assurance. A barbiturate or bromide is indicated for taking over a three months' course. He will be instructed that as the eighth nerve dies, the vertigo ceases. But what if he has a wife and five starving children? Also, what if he has an occupation that depends on hazardous work involving balance and co-ordination? To this there is the answer: we can destroy the eighth nerve by approach through the mastoid process or intracranially through the posterior fossa of the skull. In practical medicine it is seldom that this choice must be made. Ménière's syndrome runs its course over months or years, and once the eighth nerve is finally dead, causes no more trouble. Hughlings Jackson said we can not expect positive results from negative influences, and he is indeed right.

6

I COULD HAVE gone sideways from this next patient. He had so many interesting traits and would develop a theme of fascinating conversation leading away from his physical complaints. Ruthlessly, I kept him on his mark and there we stayed and will now stay.

He has a progressive paralysis of the right ulnar nerve. There is limitation of motion at the right elbow, and the nerve is swollen, thickened, indurated and lying in a groove one half as large as it needs. As a boy he had fractured his elbow; it was treated well and to this he has paid little heed over the years. At forty-five years of age he noticed increasing numbness of the little and ring fingers on the ulnar side of the arm with the broken elbow. There was a shrinkage of the muscles between the thumb and index finger, and the hand became more and more like a claw. Surprisingly, he could use the hand for almost everything; he could write, shuffle cards and tie his shoes. It was only at the urging of his family that he sought advice; they were worried over the appearance of the atrophy of his adductor thumb muscle, and those of the interossei. His hand is of the claw variety. There is anesthesia for all forms of sensibility over the ulnar border of his hand; this includes the little and one half of the ring finger. Pinning him down, I learn that his difficulties are trouble in picking his nose, in abstracting letters from their envelopes, and in snapping his fingers. There is some difficulty in buttoning his collar and the buttons of his shirt.

This is a case of *tardy ulnar palsy*. The original injury to the elbow joint has led to a progressive diminution of the groove wherein the ulnar nerve gets the protection it needs. Every movement from then on injures the nerve in its unhappy position, and it responds, accordingly, by progressive degeneration. Part of the damage to the nerve is caused by the uneven pulley action and part is the exposure to trauma. The only way to meet this situation is to transplant the nerve to a safer position. This can be done surgically. The nerve is brought forward and in front of the epicondyle, where it enjoys a secure and happy new home.

One hour of life, crowded to the full with glorious action, and filled with noble risks, is worth whole years of those mean observances of paltry decorum.
—Sir Walter Scott: *Count Robert of Paris.*

7

Good morning! It is cold and there is a flurry of snow. The ducks in the ponds in Saint Stephen's Green have sought shelter. The Shelbourne Hotel, flanked by its light-bearing and kirtled goddesses, carries on frigidly as it did when captured and re-captured during the troubled times of 1916-1923. The Liffey River smells as it always did—and it smells bad!

This man aged thirty-three has consented (after the payment of some largesse) to be shown to this class. I am grateful to him that he does so. I have known him some years, and I appreciate his integrity, but what I can do for him medically is in sad default. He is a little runt. Look at him, I beg you, for the first impression in such a case counts in the long run. When resting he has a tremor in his right hand and foot. It is slow and regular, but if allowed its pace it rises to a greater and stronger to-and-fro movement unless he changes his posture and sits on the hand or puts the foot in limbo; otherwise it goes on indefinitely, harder and harder and harder. There is no tremor of his head. The muscles of expression of his face are frozen in a mask, but mark you, and as a contrast, intelligence and responsiveness shine glowing from his eyes; like a dog he dumbly demands and craves friendly recognition. His shoulders are bowed, but he sits on the edge of the chair as if poised like a bird for flight. His speech is monotonous and flat, and he repeats his verbiage, but there is no defect in the intellect.

He is now rising to walk. Many false starts are made, with

21

appropriate curses, but finally he propels himself into an erect position.

And what a slow, wooden gait! His arms do not swing; he is stooped over, and his body moves as does a glue-dipped puppet. Movements such as we perform unconsciously and automatically simply do not occur. The fixed facial mask of expression is again shown, and the lack of bodily movements that are characteristic of one individual as compared to the next. One recognizes the loved one's step before arrival. In this disease all is leveled to a sterile similarity. On being asked to wriggle his fingers he starts out bravely, but then the movement is engulfed in the ceaseless tremor, and it just quits and is merged in the same useless shaking. Tying his shoes and buttoning his clothes are slowly and painfully done. What handwriting he has left is characteristic of the head and front of his affliction. It starts boldly enough in large type, but as it progresses it gradually shrinks to a tiny size which, mixed with the tremor, is characteristic. I have friends suffering from *Parkinson's disease* who write me, and the status of their disease is ever currently visible. It is the epitome of the disease, in that the handwriting shows a progress from brave hopes to an eventual narrowing, shrinking sense of abysmal frustration. The curses on attempting to get up from a sitting position are expressed as incense directed in a reverse direction to the gloomy underworld. On sitting down these patients go so far and drop the rest of the way.

And now the drama! This patient was a professional pugilist. I have shown him as one instance of *Parkinson's disease,* but he illustrates also one of the most dramatic features of that malady. He fought as a bantamweight, and was well on his way to becoming a champion in his field, but a Parkinson syndrome developed and although he could still fight, he was not well enough to count on in a final victory. He is, in retrospect, either a sufferer from the chronic phase of epidemic encephalitis, or a person with the degenerative type of disease that is forever with us and which was so well described by Dr. James Parkinson. The prognosis and treatment are the same for both.

I have ready a gramophone recording of a fist fight and also a floodlight centering on a white wall near where he is sitting.

When I give the signal, this patient will box an imaginary adversary in the form of his own shadow to the noisy clanging background of the roar of the ring. He will return to a crowded hour in his past life when he was a budding champion and not as he is now, a "has-been."

The sound recorder is started; the floodlight is on. *Now* look at this poor little erstwhile muscle-locked man. He is jabbing and furiously attacking in increasing measure his own shadow. Note that in spite of his disease all foot, arm and trunk component movements are in one crashing riot of co-ordinate activity. In his excitement his pupils are dilated, his face sweats, his nostrils spread, and he is hilariously back in the ring wherein his life career was so gloriously set and so pitifully lost.

The record stops, the light is off, and now our small friend is back in his chair, immobile, stiff, and to all intents and purposes as he was before. It is small comfort to say to a sufferer from Parkinson's disease that "if there were a fire in this building you would be the first one out." There is no such thing as a perpetual fire, except in Hell.

In clinical practice in the field of neurology, Parkinson's disease is something to be reckoned with. The old term, "paralysis agitans," should never be used. Its inexactitude lies in the fact that such patients are never paralyzed and not always do they shake. These middle-aged persons who have the disease, whether due to encephalitis or degenerative changes, are not a happy lot. They are moreover shrewd, understanding and acutely observant. Their problem cannot be passed by in a happy and universal formula. They realize only too well that they are becoming slower, more clumsy and less efficient in bodily movements. If they are right-handed, and the disease begins on the right side, so much the worse is it, as shown in their handwriting.

I think it is best for these patients to face up to the issue. They seldom want to do so; they crave a cure, and palliative treatment, while accepted, is misunderstood. Hyoscine hydrobromide is the time-honored drug, and now we have Artane (Lederle). Both relax the rigidity and diminish the tremor. Neither cures the progress of the disease, and it goes its inevitable way. These "most potent, grave and reverend seigneurs" can not comprehend as sufferers of Parkinson's disease such limitations in our therapeutic skill. As a result, our letter files are filled with savage indignation. Better tell a patient with Parkinson's disease that there is *no cure* but only palliation, lest he send you letter after letter, by air mail, registered and receipt-demanded, as to what to do next.

It is, therefore, a far better thing to talk long, wisely and kindly to these poor patients, outlining their infirmity and their future. Emphasis should be placed on their retention of intellect and the need of carrying on as they have been doing and for as long as they can. They should go on with their flags flying and their guns firing in a useful existence as long as they are able. Resignation is a fatal step for them. While few can galvanize into intense activity, as our patient above did, most of them can less dramatically fulfill a gainful career for an indefinite period.

James Parkinson of London lived between 1755 and 1824. He was a harmless, unobtrusive man, and why his more than scanty description of a very few patients gave him credit to fame is a mystery. Of such little things are our bids for fame. Would that you and I could have them made to that order.

Parkinson lived in an era of therapeutic nihilism. This humble London practitioner spent his life hunting fossils; at one stage the Law got him under its scrutiny. He had committed a woman to an asylum for the insane, and rightly so. An inquiry was held and he was found to be free from blame. Generally speaking, he left so little trace in medical history, and yet he lives amongst the immortals; it is strange. As Alice in Wonderland asks, "And why?" the answer echoes, "Why not?"

8

AND NOW, who is touching my gown? She is a poor unfortunate woman who can not control her face. She was not scheduled for discussion today, but I must and will show her. Overaction of facial muscles may be worse than fixity. Again, spasm may be more distressing than paralysis. And, of course, I have shown you pain in the face. She can not stop these spasms' occurring. As a differential diagnosis, jacksonian convulsions come to one's thought. The woman is, however, fifty-six years of age and has had her facial spasms ten years. During that time other structures inevitably would have become involved if she had had jacksonian convulsions. Moreover, cortical irritation is more slow and usually has an order of march to parts other than the face.

It is so simple a formula in these patients. We can cut her seventh nerve and cure her disease: you swap a facial paralysis for a facial spasm. One and all, and they are usually ladies, refuse. Recently there has been an operation to release from captivity the seventh cranial nerve in its tortuous canal. Ear specialists, operating through the mastoid bone, accomplish a relief of *facial hemispasm* by decompressing the nerve. How nearly permanent it is still remains *sub judice*.

Here is a woman who started out with a twitching of her eyelid on the right side. And now, like an atomic chain reaction, the contraction starts in the orbicularis muscles and brusquely passes over into the levators of the mouth and to all other facial muscles, including the platysma. Contractions are short, sharp and forcible, and keep coming as long as this patient is on parade. They are less marked when she is alone. These contractions can not be simulated; only a powerful electric galvanic shock applied to the facial nerve can produce such a phenomenon. It is therefore not of psychic origin, and by such means can not be produced. This is a case of facial hemispasm, one of the many rampages the seventh nerve may indulge in. These flashes continue indefinitely and are very embarrassing to the patient. Those who have unroofed the facial nerve in the fallopian canal claim that there is a thickening in the nerve and evidence of chronic irritation; hence, the operation of neurolysis. Other surgeons have deliberately cut the facial nerve and have done a spinal accessory facial anastomosis, in the hope of shunting impulses. It has not been successful.

NOVEMBER

Falstaff: . . . *that, Master Brook, there was the rankest compound of villanous smell that ever offended nostril!*
—SHAKESPEARE: *The Merry Wives of Windsor.*

1

Good morning! I passed down the Quays of Anna Liffey, our river, before coming here. The stream smelled as usual to high heaven. It is only one of the smells in this fair city of Dublin, wherein it is boasted that a blind man can find his way by smell alone. Coming out of Guinness Brewery there was a cavalcade of carts loaded with barrels of that black bitter beverage on which the Irish live, talk and romance, as they drink. The horses with their broad glossy rumps went clop-clopping on the cobblestones. Huge, well-disciplined, friendly beasts, they smelled of fresh, clean oats. Over all there was a canopy of the cloying, sweetish odor of malt fermentation. How can one hate a city where every corner has an individual personality, and to each is given a personal odor?

Here we have a man aged twenty-eight. Three years ago, and suddenly, he experienced an unpleasant odor which he can not describe, since it is apparently out of this world. It was only a short whiff, but following this he had a partial loss of consciousness. He felt as in a dream, and that he saw and heard things he had experienced before, and by now recognized them. But, mark, he can never remember just what he has seen, thought and heard, although when in the attack he feels that he certainly can. His behavior was not unusual, only he ceased whatever activity he was engaged in. He could not reply to questions, and he looked confused, but he feels that if he were being robbed of his pocketbook at that time he would know it and resist manfully. The attack lasted a scant few minutes, and then he was himself again.

These attacks of an olfactory aura and a subsequent dreamlike state have recurred at irregular intervals, averaging about four to five times a week. Recently they have been occurring daily. Added to these peculiar phenomena there has been a progression of more grave complaints in the evolution of the disease.

Two years before, the olfactory hallucinations were associated with sound and visual effects. In these more recent attacks he hears the loud sound of a clanging bell. At the same time, there appears to the extreme left side of his field of vision gorgeously colored fortification spectra. These immediately start moving from left to right, and within a few seconds they end up in the midline. The sounds of a bell and the unearthly odor then disappear with the visual aura. He becomes thereafter dazed, stupid and confused, but only for a few minutes, and then he feels normal. Recovery, as before, is prompt and without residue. He is by profession a draftsman, and he has sketched in colors these visual effects, which I show you now; they are, to say the least, artistically done.

During the last six months conditions have been those of a breaking-down process. His memory is failing, and his vision is becoming poor. He is not alert as he was, and just one month ago the climax came, when, following his triple-formed sensory aurae he had a general convulsion. Headaches are plaguing him early in the morning, waking him up and making him vomit explosively. Let us examine him.

He is vague in his replies to questions, his emotional tone is blunted, and most irritatingly, he yawns at every interrogation. He rubs his nose persistently, and it seems as if he does not want to be bothered. From his family we learn that before this mental slump, and as of three weeks ago, he was possessed by a tremendous anxiety, fear, restlessness and hostility; he was difficult to manage at home, and now his attitude is that of a complacent child.

The pulse rate is sixty beats per minute by average, but ominously, at times it drops to thirty and lower. There is, therefore, pressure on the cardiac centers in the medulla oblongata, and sudden exitus is something to be aware of and be prepared for.

Examination of his eye grounds shows a gross swelling of the nerve head, with hemorrhages and exudation. We were fortunate enough yesterday to catch him in a lucid interval, and the study of the perimetric fields of his vision showed left quadrantic hemianopsia in the lower quadrants. Evidently something in the right temporal region of his brain is pushing upward. Roentgenologic studies of his skull and brain show a dense but scattered granular calcification in the area of the right temporal lobe. The electro-encephalogram showed delta waves localized where the calcification appears. The visual-field charts, the roentgenograms, and the electro-encephalographic tracings are there for your examination, now or later. The one thing to think on is the excellent co-operation of our staff in gathering signs and symptoms. Diagnosis and localization are now possible of what is certainly a *tumor involving the right temporal lobe of the brain,* with all the rich symptomatology of such a lesion; one can pinpoint the area involved.

In the history and subsequent findings you can see the march of events. Possibly I am more impressed by the history, and one can visualize the remorseless progress of this tumor from the uncinate gyrus wherein the sense of smell is served, to the superior temporal convolution of sound value, and then backward to where the posterior temporal structures meet the occipital lobe, and formed visual hallucinations appear in the clinical picture. The later mental changes, headaches, vomiting and apathy indicate general pressure. This pressure irritates his gasserian ganglion, hence the scrubbing of his nose with his forefinger. So few neophytes in medicine know how to, or try to learn how to, take a careful history. This brings shame on them in later life.

The question arises as to what we can do for this sufferer. My surgical collegues can answer that better than I can. The roentgenologic findings indicate a slow-growing calcified tumor of the right temporal lobe of the brain. They suggest that it is an oligodendroglioma, a benign tumor and one not likely to recur if extirpated *in toto.* He already has hemianopsia, and this is something to which one can become adjusted.

Brain surgery as of today is more than radical. Exponents of that art have to be bloody, bold and resolute. There is no place for tinkering decompressions that end up with a patient whose brain sticks out far beyond the skull, and in whom the protruded mass is larger than the brain itself. Should the tumor be intra-cerebral, this patient should have a resection of part or all of his right temporal lobe, with the tumor cleanly removed in the center. It is some consolation that the right temporal lobe is the one involved: the left is not so amenable to surgery because of the speechlessness which operation would be certain to cause in a right-handed man.

NOTE: Two weeks later. This patient whom you saw previously has done splendidly after surgical intervention. The tumor was entirely removed, although it was a glioma and in the brain. He has a slight left-sided weakness which I think will clear up. The hemianopsia remains, but the papilledema is subsiding in both optic nerves. Whatever convulsive attacks he has after surgery can be controlled by drugs. Above all, his mind has cleared, his headaches are gone, and he will live on, we hope, to a useful existence.

2

LET US GO upstairs to the female wards. I would warn you that generations of students have fallen and broken their bones on this *Scala Santa* of stone steps.

This woman, aged forty-six, is not a resident hospital patient, but comes in to give her complaints. She is the hard-working wife of a carpenter and has four children, aged twelve to twenty years. Her troubles are always at night, and are such that she goes to bed in normal condition and wakes up preternaturally early, with numb and tingling hands. It takes an hour or more before normal feeling returns. In the meantime, she shakes and pounds her numb and aching digits so that she can use them to dress, and adjust her garments. Her greatest difficulty is to put pins in her carroty hair, now streaked with gray. These attacks of numb hands come on almost every night, but worse still, they awaken her, usually after midnight. She admits that her favorite posture in sleep is to lie on her back with her hands above her head. The psychoanalysts would call this a "posture of surrender." Nevertheless, and in token payment, she suffers for her nocturnal passiveness in the morning, and greatly so. Better would she be sleeping on her abdomen, free from all this temptation!

She is a tiny, small-boned woman barely five feet in height and weighs less than one hundred pounds. Inquiry leads to the fact that for four years she has had no domestic help. Naturally hardworking, she has done all that is necessary in the home, and that is plenty. There is no question here of a neurosis; she is a stable, well-adapted woman.

This problem is not uncommon. In England, during the time the nation was fighting with its back to the wall, women had to work long hours and do hard physical duties to which they were not accustomed. There was an epidemic of these nocturnal numb sensations in the hands in middle-aged women. They are due to this unaccustomed hard work, to the muscular flabbiness of the menopausic age, an unusually sound sleep from exhaustion, and to the narrow outlet of the thoracic cage in women. The cure is in more rest, and physical therapy to build up the muscles to a better tone.

The syndrome of numb hands on awakening occurs largely in middle-aged women; rarely does it occur in men. It is classified in general by the unsatisfactory clinical term, *"acroparesthesia."* Less succinctly but more descriptively, it is called the "hyperabduction syndrome of the shoulder girdle." I do not intend to give you the impression that posture is the prime factor involved here. Many patients continuously change their posture during sleep. Again, even if a device is used to keep the hands by their sides, these nocturnal acroparesthesias may still continue to plague them. Actually, we know so little about its clinical origin and treatment that we are ashamed.

We caught the tread of dancing feet,
We loitered down the moonlit street,
We stopped beneath the harlot's house.

Inside, above the din and fray,
We heard the loud musicians play
The Treues Liebes Herz *of Strauss.*

. . . .

Then, turning to my love, I said,
"The dead are dancing with the dead,
The dust is whirling with the dust."
                    —OSCAR WILDE: *The Harlot's House.*

3

Good morning! A barrel organ was playing just now outside the Ormond Hotel on the quays. Its strident notes were clashing with the medley of sounds on either side of the river, but they could be heard well above the rumble of the current traffic. A few seconds later the tune came to an end with a harsh clang, indicating a change-over to another measure, and forthwith it took place.

This was a bright and merry number, with a lilt that transfigured even the gloomy cabmen waiting frigidly across the street, slapping their chests to get warmth. Moreover, the skeletal horses looked up and shook their empty nose bags. I stopped, watched and listened.

Suddenly a torrent of dirty, ragged, shoeless little gamins debouched from a dim alley that led to the noisome slums behind the hotel. After a few seconds of open-mouthed, stilly wonder, they started to dance in perfect time, with abandon, and with no self-consciousness, the movements becoming more and more tu-

34

multuous as they danced, singing at the top of their reedy voices. It was a typical Dublin street scene, where all the children sing on the way to school, the old ladies talk to themselves, and the men preserve a dignified and safe silence.

Again came the harsh clang of changing theme. A melancholy, nose-fed patriotic dirge smashed out. Like scared mice, the children disappeared into their jungle fastness. I moved on.

And now to our clinical problem. This is a man of thirty-seven, admitted to this hospital because his relatives and wife say that he is daft and nervous. He appears to be both. These conditions have been coming on for over five years. His disorder of nerves antedated his mental break by three years, but this latter is now paramount, and constitutes a serious problem. For this reason, let us take it into consideration first.

There is no need, as you have observed, to use delicate mental tests to find out what is lacking. He is not in favor in this hospital. Last night he fell out of bed and thereafter wandered naked and unashamed into a midnight tea party given by the Sister in charge. Today he ate an egg as it was served, shell and all, and withal wet his bed. He is combative and quarrelsome over trivialities, and definitely mad and bad and not the best person to know. He does not know time as regards days, months and years, and he is very vague as to where he is at present. In dressing he gets confused as to what he is to put on and where on his body it fits.

You have heard me ask him whether he has any mind at all, or is he mad and insane.

His answer was, "What time is dinner?"

He has, as it were, no insight into his condition! He asked the nurse for a urinal, but before she could bring it he had taken one of his shoes and filled it with a golden, yeasty fluid; also the floor has suffered. He is now going to the open window; we shall watch him closely. All he does is to throw the urine-filled shoe into the garden. I think you will agree that he has a crumbling and progressive decay of the brain. According to his family, this is getting worse.

And now to the other complaint of nervousness, which was his earliest trouble and came on three years before the mental breakdown that is now so very obvious. In its earliest stage this nervousness was only what could be called "the fidgets." Restless movements of arms and legs, so that they were never still, and later, facial grimaces, appeared. At that time this man was smart, intelligent, and in a highly competitive business where he did well and made money. His mind was good, as was his judgment, and what we see now in these later stages of a remorseless disease represents the end stage of complete physical and mental collapse.

The movements are quick and rapidly changing. As we watch his hands and fingers jerking and twitching, out of the tail of our eye we can see his toes do the same diabolic dance. His diaphragm also is involved, as his frequent grunting shows. His trunk muscles take part in the dance, and the movements are irregular and purposeless. His face has a riot of expressional and expressionless movements. His speech is hardly intelligible. He can not write.

Words fail to classify such movement disorders, but roughly, this man's affliction lies midway between a myoclonic disorder wherein single muscles and groups of muscles unassociated physiologically fire off in sudden and flashlike contractions and the purposive co-ordinated movements of psychologic tics. Poor man, he has not enough psychologic processes left to indulge in tics! His trouble is *chronic chorea,* a word from the Greek, *choreia,* a dance.

There is here a negative aspect in his dementia and a positive component in his universal muscular discord of movements. The latter is probably also a negative factor. The movements must be a form of release mechanism, as a result of destruction of cortical control.

Let us get him walking. Herein is the essential drama of this case. He walks in a stilting, grotesque and dandified fashion. His arms, legs, trunk, head and neck fly in all directions. This gait has been described as that of the dancing master. We had one such *maestro* here in the earlier years of this century, and I have seen him myself. Professor Maginnis walked something like this, but his movements were purposive and controlled. He carried on his terpsichorean interest on the street, in a slow and solemn measure.

It was what he thought was the correct gait; to walk was to dance; to dance was to be elegant. He *was* elegant.

This man has **Huntington's chorea.** The dual factors of mental failure and choreic movements are present and you have seen them.

There is a corroborative avenue still to explore. The disease is hereditary, and its pathway through the ages has certain standards. This patient comes from a family that came from Germany and settled in the southwest of Ireland during the eighteenth century. As far as his family history goes, there is just one generation after another that has died in mental hospitals, helpless physically from the chorea and socially extinct from the subsequent dementia. Strange is it, however, that if one member of the family fails to show the disease, his branch remains intact, now and forever.

Nature, ever trying to root out this foul blight, has the disease appear earlier in each succeeding generation. As the disease begins to appear before the marriageable age in each offspring, so does it kill off the carrier before he begets successive human catastrophes. Women are equally affected in proportion to men.

Because of the inherent ugliness of nature of these families, they were hanged as witches in Massachusetts in the Colonial days. That should have stopped the breed, yet the disease persisted. There are few mental hospitals in the United States of America and Europe that have not examples. It crops up in even the best of social circles, and it behooves you to know it and to look for it with eyes of suspicion. People lie more in relating their family history than they do about their income tax.

4

THERE IS upstairs in the women's ward a patient I would have you see who has what is an example of a completely different type of movement disorder than that which you have just observed. . . . We are now with her. She is rather an engaging, good-looking girl, aged twenty years. She is a student of architecture in the University. Her trouble dates from the age of thirteen. At first it was a matter of waking up in the morning, and finding that her hands would not behave themselves and would fly in all directions. In the beginning she would come down to breakfast, but she had so many accidents during the meal that she now stays in bed. Actually, in the last few months, before going to her work, she has been fed by members of the family.

Her complaint is simple, in that everything she touches in these early hours of arising flies from her hands, and if such objects are breakable, they are dashed on the floor. This is because of sudden lightninglike spasms of her arms and hands, completely beyond her control. The movements are so sudden and violent that she can not anticipate them; hence the breaking of crockery and the spilling of food.

Sometimes these jerky movements are severe—at other times less so. The ominous feature is that after a morning spent in bed with the jerkings getting more and more violent, she usually ends up by late forenoon with a severe general convulsion. Once this has occurred, the jerkings cease. If the movements are mild and she can carry herself over that period, she can then get up by noon and go about her business.

For this reason, and in the earlier stages of her trouble, I was asked to appeal to the University to have it arranged that she attend lectures in the afternoon. However, the disease has progressed, and with her morning jerkings and midday convulsions, her University career is coming to an end. More recently the sudden flashlike movements have appeared in her lower extremities, and frequently when out walking she will have her legs taken out from under her and will fall heavily.

The third element of this sinister triad has appeared during the last six months. She originally had at least high-average grades in her studies, but now they are rapidly falling off, and mental deterioration is beginning to appear. Myoclonic jerkings, followed by convulsive seizures, and in the end, dementia, are the sum total of *myoclonic epilepsy or Unverricht's disease.*

This girl is lying quietly in bed, but there is a continuous play of galvanic shocklike movements in both upper extremities. They involve muscles, solitary or in groups, and even portions of a muscle. The movements are quite different from those of the patient we saw earlier, in that they are more rapid and completely outside all voluntary movement pattern. I give her a glass of water to drink; part of it is successfully swallowed, and then the glass and its contents are sent flying to smash against the wall. In chorea the object would be dropped or fumbled, but in this latter malady a propulsive movement occurs with respect to anything held in the hands.

The electro-encephalogram shows a very marked dysrhythmia, indicating a profound disturbance of cerebral action currents. This condition is one of the epilepsies and is of the worst type. The prognosis is one of dementia and ultimate helplessness, and treatment is without avail. It is of an earlier age incidence than Huntington's chorea, and the hereditary influence is not so marked.

Today you have seen two patients: one has a chorea of hereditary character and progressive dementia; the other has a myoclonic disorder which afflicts younger people, and which has the same lugubrious ending. These two conditions are similar living manifestations of the matchless drawings of Holbein's Dance of Death.

I, that am curtailed of this fair proportion,
Cheated of feature by dissembling Nature,
Deformed, unfinished, sent before my time
Into this breathing world, scarce half made up,
And that so lamely and unfashionable
That dogs bark at me, as I halt by them.
    —SHAKESPEARE: *King Richard the Third.*

5

Good morning! The wind is onshore, and from the sea has come
a predatory, greedy horde of sea gulls. They are mad for the kill
in the garbage pails left out for collection in the early morning on
our doorsteps. Big, strong, hungry chaps, with beady, calculating
eyes, they miss nothing. As I passed along they were furiously
fighting amongst themselves with high-pitched raucous cries like
those made by an infant dying of hydrocephalus. Later, there will
arrive the simple folk gleaning for their own ragpile or hogpen.
Their business is so genteel, quiet and polite that they deserve
infinite credit for preserving the neighborhood peace.

Of such a one as these is our patient this morning. He has been
scrubbed to the limit of his epidermis and ceases to smell, *Deo
gratias!* Withal, he is known to his fellow professional garbage
prospectors in affectionate terms as "Twisty Tim." His deformities
are physical and not mental, and he is a most fair and honest soul.
As long as he can remember, his body has been twisted out of
shape, so that one shoulder is higher than the other, with one hip
projecting out of line; hence his sobriquet. To him can be applied
the old nursery rhyme of the crooked man, the crooked stile and
the crooked sixpence.

The Germans have a word for this. It is called *Missbildung*, and
it indicates that in the formation of the individual the hand of the

40

potter slipped badly. It is strange that such things do not occur more often. There is indeed a divinity that shapes our ends, rough-hew them how we will!

Twisty is now twenty-seven years of age, but he has adjusted to his congenital difficulties, hoping that they will not increase as time goes along. For an indefinite period he has found that he can cut, burn or damage his arms and hands painlessly, particularly the right. He smokes cigarettes incessantly, or rather, as he can afford them. There are many scars on the fingers of his right hand, from burns that he felt not in their coming, and they were grudgingly slow in healing. For two years he has dragged increasingly his left leg, and now his right is similarly affected. What capped the climax was that three weeks ago his right shoulder apparently disintegrated. It suddenly became enormously but painlessly swollen, and power deserted the muscles around it. He had noticed some clumsiness of his hands before this and that the smaller muscles were shrunken and twitched, but he had a surprisingly efficient use of his arms and hands in searching out that which his old competitors, the sea gulls, had missed.

At this stage, I must say that the patient's history is unreliable and his physical examination even more so. He has grown up with his infirmity, has adjusted to it, and to separate his psyche from his disease is more than a serious problem. Moreover, this is the one disease of the nervous system wherein the patient *must* be entirely undressed and examined in the nude.

The man is intelligent, he is smart and wants to help us, but years of patient adjustment to a very slow-growing disability have exhausted their force, and they are now almost coming to an end. I hope not entirely.

This problem will take up all our morning; there will be no time for anything else. If you can understand and appreciate it, you have conquered one half of neurology, and so your time will have been well spent. Let us look at him first from afar. He is mis-shapen and crooked, and walks dragging both his legs. His hands have scars of burns, and as I see today, there is one fresh, unhealed one. They are mostly between his right index and middle fingers, where he holds his cigarette. (In a woman, they are on the radial margin of the forearm, where on reaching into a hot oven, she burns herself there unconsciously.) His right hand looks and feels like a piece of warm beefsteak that the cook has rejected. It is warm, sweating, swollen and red, the so-called "juicy hand" of *syringomyelia*. The combination of trophic, sympathetic and sensory changes in one or both hands is diagnostic in the extreme.

There is more, however. The thumb muscles and the interossei are wasted, and a frank fasciculation plays over both upper extremities and chest muscles like trout jumping in a pool on a sullen day in May. Tendon reflexes are lost in both upper extremities, but are exaggerated in the lower. Babinski's sign appears on both sides when the sole of the foot is stimulated.

And now let us get our cameras closer up for a nearer view. The man has a definite scoliosis of his spine, and fasciculations appear universally in his upper extremities and chest. We saw those before, but they seem now more widespread as he becomes chilled, and there are many in his tongue muscles, with one half, the left side, atrophic, and looking like a shrunken bag of worms. He has nystagmus on lateral and vertical gaze. His gait is spastic, more marked on the left.

It is only on testing his deep and superficial sensibility that the full flavor of his disease problem is to be appreciated. Herein, nevertheless, we are dealing with an unconscious trickster who is outwitting everybody, including himself. Except in a few areas, touch stimulation is rapidly and efficiently responded to. Pain and thermal sensibility require a more meticulous investigation.

My staff and I have repeatedly examined this patient's responses to pain and thermal sensation. We have pooled our findings. As a result, it comes out that there is bilateral loss of pain and thermal sensation or a severe depression of the same from the first and second cervical dermatomes to the level of the sixth dorsal segments of sensory innervation. This conclusive finding was not made easily.

We found the man had an uncanny ability to differentiate the point from the head of a pin by tactile discrimination, as it were. Moreover, cold stimuli, being lower proportionally than thermal, had a sting and an unpleasant sensation so different from the neutral sensation of the warm applicator. Thus, this man who we knew had no manifest sensation of pain or certain degrees of temperature on parts of his body fooled us all of the time.

My house officer became interested and tried to cut the Gordian knot. He tested this patient's sensibility to thermal stimuli with an actual cautery as compared with a large chunk of ice. Neither was allowed to touch the skin. Heat was recognized each time by the patient, but only in terms of the smell of burning hair. The ice caused spasms of his legs and was so recognized.

At an early age we learn that the highest point in neurology is testing sensation, and that the Mount Everest of all our laborious climbing comes along in syringomyelia. Tabes dorsalis runs a close second. Involvement of the decussation of pain and thermal sensation in the brain stem and spinal cord produces the jacket distribution of dissociated anesthesia; later, when the longer pathways of pain and thermal sensibility are involved, the clinical picture is not so clear.

And now to the joint involvement of the right shoulder. The roentgenologic studies have shown that the opposing parts of the head of the humerus and the scapular glenoid fossa have been destroyed. There are no signs of repair. It was suggested that this arthropathy was due to an osteogenic sarcoma, but its painless character and the ability to pull the joint into all sorts of grotesque positions fixed it as a neurogenic arthropathy or Charcot's joint, as was consistent with the diagnosis of syringomyelia.

There is some increased heat in the swollen joint, and a telescopic passive to-and-fro movement is possible. It does not hurt the patient but sets *our* teeth on edge.

And what is the explanation of this weird disease? The terms "hyperplasia" and "neoplasia" must be understood; there is little between them to fight over! At an early age in the development of the embryo and in the medullary-cervical region of the neuraxis, a pencil of restless ependymal cells appears. These cells multiply rapidly. The common site of these changes is in the base of one of the posterior horns of the cord, and not around the central canal. They multiply beyond their blood supply and thus die and leave a cavity. A hollow tube in Greek is a *syrinx;* hence, a syringa bush, or in medical parlance, a syringe. The sway toward neo-plasia can be understood, in that so many patients with syringo-myelia also have intramedullary tumors. The border line between simple multiplication of existing cells and formation of new cells is an indefinite one.

The pathways of pain and thermal sensation decussate in the center of the spinal cord. It is thus that early in the disease the sensations to temperature and pain are lost. The area of gliosis in the upper cervical cord may push its invasion upward into the medulla. Homologous disturbances of the bulbar mechanisms will thus appear. To atrophy of the muscles of the upper extremity there is added atrophy of the tongue and the face on the same side, with corresponding paralysis and fasciculation. To anesthesia of the neck and shoulder girdle there is added the same dissociated anesthesia of the face, gums and tongue.

Diagnosis here depends on a certain suspicion on the basis of the history and examination of an alert, fully undressed patient. There can be only one differential diagnosis, and that is leprosy. The skin manifestations of this latter disease, the patient's geo-graphic residence, and the peripheral rather than central nature of the signs are of themselves decisive.

For treatment, there is so little to offer. Surgery can not make up for a destruction already accomplished. Roentgen therapy to the cervical part of the cord and medulla may be used to keep the hyperplasia or the neoplasia in check. If only there were not so much wishful thinking in vogue, this would be the treatment of choice.

As to the future of our twisted, gnarled, deformed and smelly friend, there will be nothing that will happen tomorrow, next week, or even a year from now. He will continue to adjust; even a Charcot joint may become quiescent, and he can continue to ex-tract commercially valuable fragments from the city filth and suc-cessfully combat the savage birds from the sea. The rapidity of decay of his spinal cord is on the lap of the gods. I have seen a man of over seventy years who had obvious syringomyelia and who, going back in his history, distinctly remembers having sus-tained a painless fracture of his arm in adolescence. Again, our friend may go downhill fast and become helpless in too short a time. Such things are unpredictable, but it is my earnest and fervent hope that this brave and likeable "snapper-up of unconsidered trifles" will be still fishing in the garbage pails of my successor in Fitzwilliam Square after I have gone to where there are no eldritch, cacophonous screams of ravenous sea gulls to wake me from my eternal sleep.

When asked what he would take to let a man give him a blow on the head, he said, "A helmet."

—DIOGENES LAERTIUS.

6

Good morning! We have here in this bed a man whose head has been shaved and anointed. He is therefore an urgent candidate for surgery of the brain. I am fidgeting and fussing lest it be postponed too long, even in terms of fractions of the hour. He was admitted to hospital yesterday afternoon and seemed to be in fair condition, in that he cursed me roundly in terms I had never even heard of. I made what examination I could, keeping a weather eye out for a sudden blow in the face. This morning he is in coma, his blood pressure is rising, his pulse is falling steadily, and his respirations are becoming slow. It would be better for him to have his head opened as soon as possible. It will be, if I have my say in this matter.

He was so confused when I saw him yesterday that for his history I had to depend on one of his cohorts, who was, *Deo gratias,* unusually intelligent and helpful. As you see on his chart, this patient's name is given as "Bartholomew Gorman," and his occupation as police officer. Actually, he is known as "Flash Gorman" of the Garda Detective Division, a man with a high record for duty. The term "Flash," I understand, is used because he can pull out his revolver in a flash, just a fraction of a second before his opponent can do so. He has been brave and resourceful beyond belief, and he strikes a balance between the love and admiration of his friends and the hatred and fear of his enemies, sordid criminals and political assassins in the underworld of violence, threatening and attacking established law and order.

Three months ago he was in a raid on a slum district to capture

46

a man known to be dangerous. It seemed an easy affair, and he did not have to draw his gun, but out of the shadows a henchman of his captive suddenly appeared and broke a full beer bottle over Gorman's head. He was momentarily dazed, but was able to grapple with the new menace, and both men were captured and brought to the police station. There were no lacerations or abrasions of Gorman's scalp. He treated the affair lightly and without comment.

For some weeks thereafter he went about his business, seemingly normal, but then he began to complain of headaches in an ever-increasing refrain. About a month ago his friend noticed that Gorman had become slack in his duties, untidy in appearance, and that he often fell asleep over his work in the office. In the words of his friend, "There was a change had come over him." His memory became poor, and his previous alertness on which his rapid promotion had been based seemed to be on the wane. On occasions the sergeant had been obliged to admonish him for dereliction of duty.

A few days before his admission here, things took a change for the worse. He stayed at home altogether, complaining of headache and clutching his scalp; he abused not only his wife but all and sundry who chose to come and call. It was thought that he had a mental breakdown, and preliminary steps were made for commitment to a lunatic asylum.

I was contacted only yesterday by his *fides amicus*, and in view of such a history I had him brought here without delay. Believe me, he was no pleasant patient in this quiet and tranquil ward. I have sufficient knowledge of invective and abuse to admit freely that here I had a Master of Arts to my simple Bachelor's degree. For hours on end without much repetition he called all of us unprintable names, fought with nurses, and spread his bodily excretions lavishly and without thought. I have stayed with him all night to witness what I had expected and what inevitably appeared: a gradual change during the night from overactivity, confusion and delirium to stupor and later on to coma. When he was admitted his pulse was found to be normal, as were his respirations. During the night his pulse varied from fifty to eighty beats per minute, and the respirations from ten to twenty per minute. At times, in the early hours of the morning, his breathing took on a Cheyne-Stokes character.

Strange as it may seem, during the night his stupor relaxed, and while for part of the time he cursed and fought, for even a few minutes at intervals he seemed to be rational, and his pulse and respirations were corresponding in character. Later, the curtain shut down again, and he would become comatose and almost stop breathing. I am blaming myself now that his head was not opened just then. The struggle between life and death takes no account of a physician's amenities, and death comes regardless of time, place and circumstance. If one fails to stop this advent by ordinary care, skill and determination, there is not the slightest tissue of an alibi left. One has simply neglected the call of duty and will forever be blamed, and rightly so, but self-blame and recrimination will always be the worst.

I see now, however, the carrier to take the patient to the operating theater, and we will go along and watch the drama evolve itself to the end of recovery—or otherwise.

My surgical colleague has kindly consented to let us sit on the visitors' racks in the gallery. Already there has been made an incision in the scalp in the parietal area. Now a burr hole is being made in the skull, and the dura presents itself: tense, nonpulsating, and of a deep blue. I am thankful that we are not too late. The dura mater has been nicked, and to my great relief and joy, a huge liquid blood clot wells up! By suction it is completely evacuated. The hole in the skull is enlarged and the solidified portions of the clot are taken out.

This procedure was done entirely with the patient under the influence of local anesthesia. To my intense delight and wonder, this semicorpse has begun to show signs of life. He has started to curse again, in no uncertain measure, and what words he used yesterday are now being amplified and can never be recorded. Will you listen to them and rejoice in such a masterpiece of abusive diction?

But this is not enough for a complete cure: our surgeon has turned this cursing, blaspheming dog's body around, and he is putting a hole into the other side of the skull, in the same area. Again a liquid blood clot is found, but it is less extensive than the first; now it has also been evacuated. The cursing dies down, and now peradventure the patient is asking timidly and weakly for a drink of water. He has changed from coma to stupor, from stupor to belligerency and blasphemy, and from this latter now to normal mentality—all in the space of a few minutes. A surgical procedure has in a short space of time completely changed an impossible personality, and moreover rescued its owner from death. How many such patients have I lost by masterly inactivity and the lack of a suspicious mind!

Now that we are back in the medical ward, I can talk more freely. We shall see this patient in a few days from now, after he is free from the pains of surgery, when I am sure you will find him a very likable and sincere fellow, well on the way to a complete physical and mental cure and a return to his normal social and economic functions. "Flash" Gorman will be himself again, and there will be no aftermath of illness and suffering.

You have followed today in a most dramatic fashion, which I admit was forced on me, a case of *chronic subdural hematoma.* I am most elated and satisfied that I was but one small part in this drama that concluded with a happy curtain call. How many have I, on the other hand, let go down the drain for want, as I have said, of a suspicious mind? So many similar ones have died, unwept, unhonored and unsung. In any case of rapid and yet fluctuating signs of increase in intracranial pressure, even without a history of injury, and even without focal signs of brain damage, let there be made a hole in the skull as quickly as one feels it is indicated. The primitive Indians in America did it with flint knives; in their own time with their own methods, they may have been wiser than we.

Cynically, I have stated that whenever one thinks of a *chronic subdural hematoma,* it is not there. I had one patient who was riding on the mudguards of an automobile which, when it turned a sharp corner, shot him on his right side onto a pile of stones. His acromion process was broken, as was his clavicle, and his head was cut over the parietal area. He became increasingly stuporous and left hemiplegia developed. His head was opened, and a rapidly growing glioma was found right in the fronto-parietal area of the brain. He evidently had fallen off the automobile because his left arm had become weak, letting him fall when the corner was being rounded. By contrast, I have stumbled on these chronic blood clots more by luck than by judgment, as we have seen today. There is supposed to be a small hemorrhage at the time of the original injury which, by some process of physical osmosis, increases to take form as a semisolid blood clot, with a markedly fluctuating course of clinical signs. While the physician is waiting to make up his mind, however, the patient may suddenly die, with Cheyne-Stokes respirations and a pulse beat that slows to zero. Too late, too late, is the knell that strikes finally on our mentality that is only just more fluctuating than the course of the disease we would like to circumvent. There is no excuse for this, as we learn after several disagreeable experiences. This problem is so different from the more acute middle meningeal extradural hemorrhage of a few hours' duration. Here all our wits are sharpened by the background of recent acute injury. In chronic subdural hematoma there may be no history of injury, in that it has been so slight that the patient has forgotten it, but three to six months later a syndrome such as we have seen this morning appears, spreads itself, and surely keeps us all on our toes as to its proper evaluation and treatment. In such cases a suspicious mind is worth untold gold.

7

AFTER OUR urgency and anxiety earlier this morning, it will be a relief to settle down to a problem that is chronic and one not involving too great a stake as to life or even as to the ability to earn a living. Yet, no problem is too small in diseases of the nervous system.

This woman, about forty-five years of age, is a hard-working housewife who cans many fruits and vegetables in the autumn months. Last October she complained greatly of a numbness and a burning pain in the ball of her right thumb and in the pads of the last phalanges of her index finger, and less so, in the middle finger. She found it difficult to pick up pins, threads and the like, and to button her clothes with her right hand. The work of canning fruits and vegetables made this condition much worse, and by November she found a shrinkage of the muscles in the edge of her thumb, confined largely to the meaty mass near the palm of her hand. This alarmed her greatly, and her local physician suggested that she might have creeping paralysis. This of course made her feel no better. Further, she thinks that there is a similar burning numbness appearing in her left thumb and index finger, but there is as yet no atrophy of the thenar eminence.

Examination shows a discrete atrophy of the muscles of the right thenar eminence, taking in only those muscles nearest the radius. There is no anesthesia of the ball of the thumb or of the tips of the index and middle fingers. She insists, however, after stimulation there by pinprick, cotton wool and hot and cold bottles, that "it is not right." She is clumsy in sorting small objects on a tray. There is little to be found in the left hand. General examination of the nervous system shows nothing abnormal. All there is to be seen is that there has occurred a loss of a carved-out-looking chunk of her right thenar eminence at its outer part. There may be also some color changes in the area of the skin supplied by this twig of the median nerve.

This is a case of *median thenar neuritis.* It is associated with long-continued pressure bilaterally or unilaterally of radial fibers of the median nerve as it goes through a carpal tunnel under the transverse carpal ligament. Persistent hard work causes thickening of this ligament and continued damage to these tiny nerve fibers. The ultimate result is to produce a numbness and pain in the median-supplied areas of the thumb, index and middle fingers. This causes awkwardness in picking up fine objects as well as suffering from concomitant pain and burning. The weakness and atrophy of the thenar eminence are less disabling.

The treatment is to slit the carpal ligament with the aid of local anesthesia, unilaterally or bilaterally, followed by a career of lady-like rest with both hands in the lap. If the condition is too far advanced, results are not so good. As usual, too late.

8

Good morning! I go out very seldom at night. Occasionally, when forced to do so by my friends, I find that the night life of the city is given up mostly to eating, drinking and long, loud argumentative conversations. Dancing is only a screen for these arts, and to attend the theater or moving-picture houses is but a preamble to many hours thereafter of the use of the jaws, tongue, and vocal cords. I have here a poor man who is bereft of these civilized activities, for in pursuing them, he has such horrible pain and agony that he would willingly stay at home, be silent, starve, or die of thirst.

He remembers the day, hour and minute when, four months ago, he took before retiring a cold bottle of beer, which, by the way, he never finished. After the first few swallows, an ungodly pain struck him in his throat, in the region of the right tonsil, and extended like lightning to his ear on that side, going deep into that structure in the region of the drum. He tried again to drink his beer, but the same flashing pain occurred, with a hacking cough superadded. His wife, who was with him, asked him what was wrong, and as he tried to explain, one paroxysm after another hit him, rendering all conversation impossible. His family physician was sent for; he gave him an injection of morphine, and our patient went to bed to suffer an uneasy night's sleep.

Next morning at breakfast, the first mouthful he tried to swallow, just as it reached the back of his throat, produced the same severe pain. From that time on he has been living in a state of semistarvation. He could force down a few mouthfuls of food or a few swallows of liquid in order to appease only partially his hunger and thirst, but a dread of all deglutition and its accessory muscular movements developed. A specialist in ear, nose and throat diseases examined him and could find no cause for his pain. He did one thing, however: he cocainized thoroughly the area of his right tonsil, and sent the patient out to get a meal and such fluids as went with it. He was then able to eat a hearty collation at a restaurant nearby and to drink all he wanted. After an hour or two, the anesthesia wore off, and he was as bad as he ever was. This procedure of anesthetization of his fauces was continued, and he was thereby enabled to eat and drink enough to keep body and soul together, but by default he lost twenty pounds.

After a month of this palliative but unsatisfactory arrangement the pains ceased as mysteriously as they came. He had a remission that continued until a week ago, and he gained back some of the weight he had lost. The pain then returned in an even more unbridled form, and he comes here today to get, if possible, permanent relief.

As you see him this morning, he is sitting silent and immobile, with his mouth open and his head bent forward. There is a continual flow of saliva dripping on the floor between his feet. He can not talk, and his face wears an expression of extreme misery. He dare not swallow his saliva, and so lets it run. He has not eaten or drunk for three days and looks it. There are two things that I must do for the purpose of diagnosis. I have to reproduce his pain, and conversely, I want to stop it quickly and effectively, even if only temporarily. Not only the diagnosis will then be assured, but also treatment of a permanent nature.

I have here on a table two applicator sticks with a pledget of cotton wool on each. One is in a container of saline solution; the other is in a strong cocaine solution. At the side, there is on another table a pleasant and well-balanced meal, prepared in the hospital kitchen, all smoking hot and appetizing.

I ask him to open his mouth, and quickly, before any saliva can reach it, I simply touch his right tonsil. He jumps violently and jerks away from me; his face is contorted with anguish, and he acts as if a sudden violent pain had struck him. There is a sharp cough. He indicates his pain by putting his right forefinger over his neck in the region where the tonsil lies underneath, and points to its extension in the direction of his exterior auditory meatus. Successive minor paroxysms occur and he resumes his previous attitude, silent and fearful, with his head forward, and the un-swallowed saliva again trickling from his mouth. I ask him to take a drink of water, and he refuses point-blank, with a silent, cautious shake of his head.

The second applicator, soaked in cocaine, is then introduced. Again, a terrific spasm of pain, but willy-nilly I scrub his tonsil vigorously, so that it is fully anesthetized, taking at least three minutes in the process, and introducing fresh solution as quickly as I can get it into the mucous membrane of his fauces. What a metamorphosis then occurs in his bodily and mental attitudes! He is now a changed man. His head comes up, he swallows all collected saliva, and then as if seeing it for the first time, he reaches for the tray of food.

You will note that he seats himself closer to his coming meal and looks it over. There is no semblance of hurry. He knows that he has sufficient respite so that he can at least enjoy it, and not gulp it down like a starving dog. The first item he reaches for is a large glass of orange juice, which he swallows with great relish. The rest follows in easy stages until the tray is cleared of all it contains. He knows, however, that he is a man still living on borrowed time.

He now talks freely about his trouble and gives the history I have already related. We ask him if he would submit to an operation that would cure him permanently, and he is all for it. He has had enough misery, pain and suffering; moreover, his very existence is at a hazard from starvation and dehydration. You may be sure that he will be taken care of as soon as possible, and that the result will be eminently successful.

This case is one of **glossopharyngeal neuralgia.** The cause of this condition is just as obscure as that of trigeminal neuralgia. Of the two, the one just presented is the more severe, and the more threatening to life itself. There is no question here of the injection of alcohol into the glossopharyngeal nerve, since this nerve can not be reached successfully, and section of the peripheral portion in the neck is not practicable, since as soon as the nerve regenerates, the pain recurs. The only permanent cure is to open the skull and cut the glossopharyngeal nerve intracranially, and proximal to its ganglion. Under usual conditions, the risk of surgery is not so great, and complications are few. Numbness over the corresponding tonsil and pharynx is not greatly complained of, and even a palatal and vocal cord palsy, occasioned by taking part of the vagus nerve, are conditions that can be adjusted to later on. We can promise this man a way out of something that makes life impossible, and which is not necessary to be endured any more than the time required to arrange for his much-needed surgical intervention. At that, we can cocainize his tonsil if there is a need for fluid, nourishment, rest and sleep before surgery.

9

WE SHALL GO to a ward now that is being cleaned and that therefore has been vacated. It will be silent there. I am going to show you something that will appeal not only to your vision, but also to your sense of hearing. Let us be quiet on entering, and remain quiet.

Behind this screen, and hidden from your view, there is a patient whose main complaint is a clicking noise in his throat and ears. Not only can he himself hear it, but others can, even at a distance. Let you be the judge of this latter observation. As you stand here around this screen and silent, you can, I hope, hear a rapidly produced noise as if a watch were ticking, but not at the same speed. I can see by your expressions that you hear it. Will those amongst you who have watches with second hands on them —as yet not pawned during term—kindly time this ticking noise, and tell me how rapid this steady beat happens to be? There is a blackboard and chalk. After sufficient time has elapsed, please write down your estimation of the speed per minute of this ticking sound.

You have done so, and now I shall strike an average. . . . I find that I have a most intelligent and observing class here today, whose calculations singularly coincide. The rapidity of the clicking noise works out to one hundred twenty beats per minute. This figure is one agreed to by all competent observers of this strange phenomenon. The screen will now be taken away.

This man sitting here is sixty-eight years of age and he looks it. He has evidence of peripheral and central arteriosclerosis. During these last few years he has had a number of minor vascular thrombotic lesions in the central nervous system, but as yet not one of them has unduly incapacitated him. Two months ago, and suddenly, he had an accession of difficulty in swallowing and imbalance on awakening in the morning. He also had some trouble in articulating. As happened after his other minor central nervous system vascular accidents, he recovered in a few weeks. From the beginning, however, he noticed this clicking sound heard in his ears, but seemingly coming from his throat. As you get nearer to him, this sound of course becomes louder, and it is a sore affliction to the patient. When he opens his mouth, you will be able to hear it still better.

Examining him from where you are, you will notice that his larynx, or as shown on the surface, the Adam's apple, is synchronously moving up and down, and the muscles below his chin are taking a large part in this. When you look at his palate and pharynx, you will see that the same up-and-down movement is occurring. The tongue is still. With a laryngoscope, you could see that the ostia of his eustachian tubes are opening and closing, and it is here that the noise you hear is being produced. It is just as if you opened and shut your compressed lips at one hundred twenty beats to the minute, and produced some such sound. No wonder that this snapping of the orifices of his eustachian tubes irritates and bothers him with its ever-present noisy clicking.

This man has a clinical phenomenon that is rare but easily recognizable. It is called by various names. *"Palatal nystagmus"* is one, and *"palatopharyngolaryngeal myoclonus,"* another. The anatomic lesion is in the medulla, in a triangle comprised of the superior olive, the restiform body and the dentate nucleus.

This disease has as pathologic causes thrombotic lesions of the medulla, epidemic encephalitis, severe craniocerebral injury, caisson disease; and in one instance which I saw, it was associated with a paramedullary ependymoma in a child. Once started, it persists indefinitely, and there is no remedy. It is one of those *rara et curiosa* syndromes of disease of the central nervous system.

In the instance at hand, the condition obviously is due to arteriosclerosis of the brain, and is a result of one of many thrombotic insults, this being the most recent one of our patient. You may never see such a condition again, but it will give you food for thought, and a realization of the fact that diseases of the nervous system have always something new to flog your jaded sensory perceptions, and while preserving you from intellectual boredom, they will keep up an enthusiasm lasting throughout your professional career.

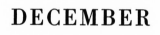

DECEMBER

> *. . . Funglus grave and the great tribune's barrow all
> darnels occumule, sittang sambre on his sett, drammen
> and drommen, usking queasy quizzers of his ruful con-
> tinence, his childlinen scarf to encourage his obsequies
> where he'd check their debths in that mormon's thames,
> be questing and handsetl, hop, step and a deepend, with
> his berths in their toiling moil, his swallower open from
> swolf to fore and the snipes of the gutter pecking his crocs,
> hungerstriking all alone and holding doomsdag over
> hunselv, dreeing his weird, with his dander up, and his
> fringe combed over his eygs. . . .*
>
> —JAMES JOYCE: *Finnegan's Wake.*

1

Good morning! I saw a fallen horse in the street on my way here.
Poor dumb beast, he lay on his side, his limp, tired, overworked
body steaming in the cold air, with an immense crowd around
him shouting advice from every angle. Some of the onlookers
were actually fighting each other to be allowed to get him up
before he was shot and carried to the knacker's yard to be made
into glue, dog meat and leather. I mused on the fact that a fallen
epileptic has no such following. It is only the good Samaritan
who remains to rob the stricken man of his watch and scantily
filled purse. Should one of you neophytes arrive on such a scene
later on, do pass on like the Jew in the parable, for by that time
the victim may possibly be conscious, and you may be accused of
the theft.

We are not so stupid today as to think that every case of epilepsy is devoid of cause. In every case there *is* a cause, if only we
can find it. With modern methods of investigation, air encephalograms, arteriograms, and electro-encephalograms, more and more

of the so-called primary and idiopathic epilepsies are being explained and treated scientifically. There is still a large number we cannot explain; hence the "cryptogenic" and "symptomatic" members of the epilepsies. The first term means simply that we do not know the cause but hope to. More recently, therefore, epilepsy is being classified on the basis of clinical, anatomic, biologic and pathologic studies. A step in the right direction as to the problem of why and how, is that the epileptic discharge is now made manifest, and where in this colorless jelly of a brain it originates. At present, however, the cryptogenic group of unknown origin or cause dominates the field of all the epilepsies, but that group is shrinking year by year. Let us begin on some problems wherein no clue as to etiology is available of this sacred disease of our ancestors and of our present generation less holily inclined.

This patient is a sad and sorry object of humanity, literally dragged in here by members of the Civic Guards. About four o'clock yesterday afternoon he was picked up from the gutter, limp and unconscious, covered with mud and blood, and his clothes were soaked with urine. At first it was thought that he was drunk, and the Guards were all for carting him away to the Bridewell, but some members of the quickly gathering crowd identified him as one having frequent fits, and accordingly he was brought here.

This morning he shows a gash on his right forehead extending into his right eyebrow. Both eyes are blackened, and he has sundry assorted bruises from thrashing his limbs on the ground. He is dull, sullen and unfriendly, but quite conscious and oriented as to place, time and circumstances. He has no memory of falling or of being brought here. His first realization as to where he was came to him last evening near midnight. Actually, he ought to recognize the place, for he has been brought here many times before. Each time we have examined him carefully, using every modern method, the last time being no longer than a month ago.

When he gives his life history it is short, to the point, but infinitely tragic. As he talks one notes the expressionless, smoothed-out facies, the low, toneless voice, and the complete absence of emotional reaction. There is nothing dramatic about his recitation; it is merely that of a sordid, depressing series of experiences such as he had yesterday and their effect on his life up to the present. Like Ishmael, his hand is raised against every man, and every man's hand is against him. He is dwelling in the presence of all his brethren, for no one else can support him.

He is twenty-six years of age. At the age of ten, he found himself afflicted with short periods of confusion or actual unconsciousness lasting just a few seconds but coming repeatedly every few hours for several days. In these attacks he ceased what he was doing, stared vacantly, became pale and blinked his eyes rapidly. In those days he did not fall, but it was obvious that he was more or less mentally absent. Some weeks would elapse between these crops of absences, and between them he was actually normal. These short attacks came closer and closer together, and when he was about twelve years of age his first convulsion appeared. This followed an unusual number of frequent minor attacks, a little more severe than heretofore. From then on his life was changed from a happy childhood to one of frustration, despair and degradation. He was now an "epileptic"!

In this new and more severe phase he suddenly lost consciousness and fell heavily and without warning, usually striking the right frontal region. On one occasion he fell on a red-hot stove, burning himself severely. On the ground his body was rigid, his breath suppressed, and he became deeply cyanosed. A few seconds later clonic jerkings appeared in all the muscles of his body, his eyes rolled upward, hands were clenched and legs extended. He breathed again, but respirations were loud and stertorous. Bloody foam came to his lips from the biting of his tongue by his clashing jaws. A few minutes of this, and after a few more extra-hard jerks, he would lie limp and still breathing heavily. Just toward the end of the attack his urine would escape and occasionally he would defecate involuntarily.

After half an hour or so of coma he usually roused to a confused state, was restless and complained bitterly of a severe headache and then went to sleep for some hours. When he awoke he felt wretched and miserable, sore in all his muscles and profoundly depressed.

These attacks have recurred again and again, usually being preceded by a crop of minor seizures. Each time he prays devoutly in all anguish that this may be the last one, only to be plunged once more into the abyss of frustration and acute misery. The attacks occur at any place and at any time, regardless of what he is doing. The only factor he knows of that precipitates them is overindulgence in alcoholic beverages. Year by year he is getting slowly worse; he has more frequent and severe attacks, and his range of activities has perforce been gradually diminished.

He is becoming more forgetful and apathetic, and often after an attack he is irritable and impulsive and will strike out at those around him who are concerned only with his welfare. He can not hold any gainful occupation for long but just drifts aimlessly around. He lives in his married brother's home, a sore burden financially and an evil influence on the younger children in the home who see him in his convulsions and are horrified by them, and who fear his surly, mean, bitter and hostile reaction to their innocent childish behavior.

All medication has been unavailing in controlling these attacks, although every modern drug has been used judiciously. During the previous occasions he has been here under our care we have sought earnestly to find the cause of his affliction. There was no familial history of his complaint. His birth was normal, and he had had only a few of the childhood diseases, none being severe or complicated. A few injuries in childhood were cited as possible causes, yet these were trivial. Roentgen studies of his skull, air encephalography and studies of his eye grounds showed nothing abnormal. Studies of his blood chemistry as to calcium and sugar content helped not at all. From a psychiatric standpoint he was neither worse nor better than one would expect as a result of his affliction and its effect on his personality. Repeated convulsions may have brought about mental deterioration, but that possibility has to be weighed against the psychic effect of being an outcast and a useless member of society, with, even worse, the intrinsic shame of public degradation. The only positive finding was in the electro-encephalogram, which showed that the smooth, normal wave impulses of the brain were in this patient in a state of diffuse dysrhythmia; there were no focal signs in the reading.

I am showing you this patient this morning as exemplifying *a severe malignant type of epilepsy,* or if you want a more pleasant term, a convulsive disorder. Happily this is not the most common type, but rather one of those cases you find in institutions—but mark this point, and that is that the patient you see is the one envisaged by the laity when the term "epilepsy" is used. This man will probably end in an institution, but there are, in extreme contrast, many, many others who because of a milder and more controllable type of disease are leading happy useful lives in their own environment, and who will continue to do so.

Will you note that our physical examination shows just nothing that can give us any clue as to the essential cause of the disease? Even the electro-encephalogram has a pattern that is found in 10 per cent of the general population who have never had, and never will have, fits. True, this patient's siblings and one or the other parent may show abnormal electro-encephalographic patterns, but the members of the family may not necessarily ever have epilepsy. Again, 20 per cent of known epileptics may have a normal electro-encephalographic pattern. The trail becomes even more tenuous, the ultimate cause of epilepsy even more obscure, except in that group of patients in whom there are obvious causes for convulsions, and they are by no means in the majority. I have shown you one extreme of this disease; let us see the other.

2

THIS PLEASANT, intelligent, friendly, co-operative girl, twenty-four years of age, presents herself with a problem ironically originating in the *benign* character of her trouble. I have been following her condition for some three years, and what to do now for her is difficult to say.

At the age of fifteen, she had her first minor attack. It was merely a transient confusional state in which she became pale; her eyes were described as being "glassy," and she was partly unaware of her surroundings. About a year later this attack recurred. It was repeated over a few days and then disappeared. At the onset she felt an odd sensation in her abdomen, a sensation which rose to her face, with cessation for a few seconds of all her activities. She began to recognize these short confusional states as something she had experienced before and she knew them intimately as they came.

At the age of twenty, she had her first major seizure, with the same autonomic aura as felt before, but this time she fell down and had a convulsion. Again there was a gap of some months when another convulsion appeared, this time in her sleep. It was noted by her family, who were aroused by her heavy breathing and her jerking movements in bed. The minor attacks had disappeared by this time, and they have never returned. Another seizure, the third, occurred six months later; it was then that I saw her for the first time and admitted her to this hospital.

Careful clinical studies, including an electro-encephalogram, showed nothing abnormal. She was given capsules of diphenyl hydantoinate sodium (dilantin sodium) and advised that one containing 1½ grains was to be taken three times a day before meals. She was also given tablets of phenobarbitone, of 1½ grains, to be taken at night before retiring. This was three years ago. Since starting to take medication she has had no trouble whatever and is today to all intents and purposes normal. She works regularly in a store and is entirely self-supporting and socially active. The electro-encephalographic pattern remains normal.

The problem now is, where do we go from here? The girl wants to forget her past experiences; she wants to get married, and she has a satisfactory suitor in view. She has taken her medication religiously, and from her own description and that of her intelligent family we have no reason to doubt that, having suffered from epilepsy in the past, she has none of its symptoms now. Is her medication merely covering up a hidden disease that will spring on her again with added force once she has stopped her medication? It often does so, and leads to discouragement and frustration.

I think, however, after her three years of freedom I will now gradually reduce her medication for the next year, and then, if all goes well, stop it altogether. She feels that as long as she takes it she is an abnormal person; let us see if she is. I have seen many, many records in the Mayo Clinic in which patients in their forties and fifties reported having had fits from the teen ages until the twenties or thirties when, without medication or for any known reason, the fits ceased spontaneously. I pray indeed that this will be the case here.

And so today you have seen two extremes of epilepsy. In the first case the disease is one I call a malignant type. It has worsened steadily and remorselessly since the first minor attack, and will continue to get worse. Despite all our more modern remedies, medication has failed, and the patient is a total loss to society and a misery to himself. The second patient has what one certainly would call a benign type of epilepsy, easily controlled by medication, and for all I know, she might have recovered without any treatment. The attacks of the first patient began when he was ten years old, and the course was more like that of those patients with structural brain damage, although we found no evidence of that. The second patient started having trouble in adolescence. While the earlier the attacks start in life, the worse the prognosis, and while attacks occurring for the first time in adolescence carry a more happy outlook, still no hard-and-fast rule can be made. There is no rule in epilepsy that cannot be broken; it is largely an unpredictable disease except for general experience and all the aids to diagnosis and prognosis we can get.

There is a third type of epilepsy and much the more common. In this type attacks come at *irregular* intervals, either as a minor form or a major one, or as both combined. Usually, a barrage of minor attacks antedates the major seizure, acting as a warning. There seems to be nothing to explain the periodicity except in females; with them attacks are more common during the menses, but again, no rule can be made, and too many times spaying of these women has been done without any effect whatever.

I saw professionally an attorney who had a large practice who had had five *major convulsions* in fifteen years, all in his sleep. Only his wife knew about them. He consulted me because his previous medical attendant had died. He asked me what he should do about them. I told him to kneel at his bedside each night and thank God that that was all he had to worry about up to date!

Some patients under medication do well, but so often the drug used loses its power and attacks start up again. Even without medication, attacks may cease for months or even years and then start again. At times epilepsy is one of the most frustrating diseases we have to cope with, but it has its bright moments, as in the second patient shown today.

It isn't really
Anywhere!
It's somewhere else
Instead!
—A. A. MILNE: Halfway Down.

3

Good morning! As I passed that famous tavern of Davy Byrnes in Anne Street this morning, I remembered a character here called Soapy Mouth Burke. He had a habit of chewing soap until a liberal froth was engendered. Then he would fall suddenly on the street corner nearest Davy's place of refreshment, convulse in a scientifically accurate fashion and surround himself with a crowd of helpful, sympathetic folk. Coming out of his fit he would gasp, "Surgeon MacCarthy told me many a time that if I had one of them fits in the street, I was to be brought directly to Mister Byrnes' public house and *made* take three glasses of raw brandy!"

Last week I dwelt on some convulsive disorders of adults and the difficulties of assessing their prognosis, except after long periods of observation. Today we are in the children's ward, a place I am very happy in unless it provides too many heartbreaking pictures of incurable disease.

This little moppet is six years old, a most engaging, pleasant, intelligent little girl. When she was four years old her trouble began, for no good reason. She began to have short attacks of mental confusion five to twenty seconds in duration. During these she blinked her eyelids rapidly; there was also some twitching of her eyebrows, but rarely of her hands and arms.

She continues playing, none the less. She has been seen careening down the circuitous driveway of her house on a bicycle while having one attack after another in a regular fusillade. She has climbed trees, and while hanging on to a limb many feet from the ground has been observed to be having many, many "blinking" attacks as if in imminent dread of losing her grip and falling to her death. In neither situation has she come to grief.

There is, therefore, during the attack some consciousness present that preserves her from evil, although she is not entirely conscious. She is having these attacks now, since the morning hours are the more likely time for their occurrence. If asked to count up to twenty, she starts to count, falters during the attack but picks up again after the few seconds are over and continues where she left off. She may have over a hundred of these attacks in a day. Occasionally, when they are very frequent, she is likely to stay confused.

At meals she will sit with the spoon poised, absently, for a second or two and then carry on eating. She never spills her glass of milk, but will hold it until the fleeting affair is over. The seizures start and end suddenly, but occur in what has been called "myriad of attacks."

The intelligence quotient, taken when the attacks are not too frequent, is above normal. The electro-encephalogram shows a pattern of a short and slow wave at rapid intervals, the so-called spike-and-dome pattern. This clinical pattern originally was called "*pyknolepsy*," and has now been regarded as "*the true petit mal.*" It is presumed to have a good prognosis in later life, with a disappearance of seizures in and around puberty. Unfortunately, however, one of my most cherished patients, suffering from this type of epilepsy, had her first major seizure at puberty and is now in an epileptic colony. The unpredictability of all convulsive disorders is notorious.

Let us move on. Here is another little girl, aged ten, who is likely to be showing her trouble right now. Yes, she is doing so. She has a momentary jerking of the arms and hands so that anything she is holding flies away from her. She is playing with a doll, but already, as we watch, it has been shot to one corner of her little enclosed crib. She recovers it immediately. I am placing a piece of chalk on her outstretched palm and telling her to hold it there. As you see, it is flung up and out to the farthest part of

the ward and onto the floor. These are called "myoclonic movements." They are unorganized and work as if a sudden galvanic
electric shock were sent into the muscles of the arms. She has
the attacks every morning, and her breakfast must be fed to her.
At noon she is allowed to get up when there is little likelihood
of shocks' appearing in her legs which might throw and hurt her.
She eats her lunch and supper without help. On the mornings
when these attacks are overfrequent and severe, she has had
minor convulsive attacks with pallor, staring and confusion. A
few times, again following a siege of myoclonic shocks, she has
had a major convulsion.

This type is called *"myoclonic epilepsy."* It is perhaps a shade
worse in prognosis than that for the first little patient who has
pyknoleptic attacks. In adults the myoclonus, the fits and a progressive metal deterioration have been described in a sad and bad
syndrome by Unverricht as "myoclonus epilepsy," a hereditary
and fatal disease. Personally, I feel that both myoclonus and myoclonic epilepsy as far as prognosis is concerned have a distinctly
bad odor.

Here is another child, a boy of five years. He has a bad history
of a long and difficult labor at birth. There were feeding problems
in the first and second year of life, but he rallied and had developed, as have the two preceding patients, normally, both physically and mentally, until he was three years of age, when he began
having falling attacks. Running around as a normal youngster he
would suddenly drop in his tracks, hit the floor and then arise
immediately and carry on normally. If he was unconscious it was
only momentarily, but his physical activities were obstructed in a
marked fashion. I will have him run around the ward. Within a
few minutes you have seen that he has fallen three times, but
that he gets up immediately, cheerfully and good-humoredly each
time, and darts off at another tangent.

He is in bed now, and playing with a brightly colored toy. He
has suddenly dropped it; he has become pale; his pupils are dilated; and he has fallen, his head forward and between his knees.
You saw that his arms were extended upward in the "salaam sahib"
movement just before he fell.

A few seconds later, and he is sitting up in his cot somewhat confused; then in a few seconds his color has returned and he seems to be normal again. These attacks occur every hour or less, and because of them he is kept as much as possible in bed. He resents this! He has no apparent memory of these attacks, but calls them "dizziness." He has not made much progress since the onset of the attacks, so far as his mental development is concerned; in some ways he has gone backward, his speech is less developed, and he is becoming a problem in the home with his brothers and sisters. The electro-encephalogram is a complex and variable recording.

This picture is called *"akinetic epilepsy."* It has a somewhat worse prognosis than do the other two epileptic clinical syndromes, and it may worsen as time goes on. Moreover, there is evidence of brain damage that is progressive and irreversible.

The condition of this last child we are to see is the nadir of all our hopes and prayers with respect to these epileptic children: it is the lowest of Dante's seventh hell. This child (shall I call it a vegetable; that is, less than an animal and more than a heap of clay?) was born five years ago, the first and only child, and apparently a healthy infant. It thrived and for the first year appeared to be normal, but how difficult it is for parents to assess normality in the first year of life, especially in a first child! However, at its twelve-month period a convulsive seizure wracked its tiny limbs, and a fever of more than 102° F. was recorded. Otherwise, there were no physical findings, but convulsions came thick and fast over a period of four days, with continued fever. The convulsions ceased under sedation.

Examination of the cerebrospinal fluid showed no evidence of meningitis. The child was listless after the fever subsided on the tenth day, and since then has made no progress mentally or physically, but has continued to have repeated minor and major convulsions. The minor attacks blend into the major ones, so that what is coming each time an attack starts is unpredictable. There are, moreover, twice as many minor attacks as general convulsions.

Some sort of convulsive manifestation can be expected many times each day, and only too many times. In the meantime, the child lies passive in its crib, has to be fed by bottle and cared for like a helpless idiot. There is no paralysis of its limbs, and urine and feces are discharged involuntarily, or rather unconsciously. The facial expression is dull, the eyes show no recognition of its parents, and after each convulsion the child sleeps inordinately.

Several times it has had respiratory infections with fever, and has been ill enough to have its life despaired of. At all times it has been difficult to feed. Mother Nature obviously has tried to balance the books, but some higher authority has kept this nightmare child alive. Why, we can never know. The parents as usual blame all the idiocy on the repeated convulsions. If only *they* could be controlled, the parents insist, the child would be well. It is impossible to explain that these are only part of the picture.

Our diagnostic ability based on a pathologic process appearing at this age is not so good because these children live long enough for early pathologic processes to become obliterated and covered by reactive changes that follow. Clinically, however, we regard this last patient's disease as falling into the vast and uncharted category of the *encephalitides* of childhood. There are also the children who start out bravely in life but due to heredofamilial blight, as in Tay-Sachs disease, pass, by amentia, convulsions and general physical failure, to death in childhood.

Last, there are the children who are born with brains only half-formed, who never develop normally, and who with convulsions and mental deficiency die at a tender age without the full explanation of their death being manifest at necropsy. The convolutions of the brain here are as few as the wrinkles of an English walnut, or, to change the metaphor, in these poor ones the egg is addled before it is hatched. Considering the delicacy of a child's brain, the wonder is that so many children are happy, normal, intelligent little elves and grow to maturity to become bank presidents or managers of a flea circus on Broadway.

I must confess that when illness is not too rampant here, these chubby, friendly little ones in their tiny white cots and clad in their gay little colored pinafores hold me happily and guiltily for most of a working morning. And yet the thought recurs that a child who is seriously ill is the greatest of all human disasters.

If it be the only one of a family, it may be the potential end of a dynasty, never to be replaced. If it be just one of a large family the anxiety is no less great, for that child is, as it were, the cornerstone on which the whole family is built and will remain so always, even though this favorite little one fails to recover and dies.

4

LET US DESCEND now from this cheerful, warm ward of children to the colder floor below, where there are the male adult patients.

This patient is a gray-haired farmer who has a small holding of land that would starve a paper-eating goat, and paper is now at a premium. He has fed, clothed and housed six children. As hostages to fortune, these children have needed incessant, laborious toil day after day both from himself and from his equally worn-looking wife. Although he is only fifty-eight years old, he looks as if he will never again see threescore years and ten. Up to six months before he came to hospital, he had been seemingly well, and complained only of increasing deafness, pains in his joints, and a tendency to dwell too much on bygone days. He had carried on the work of his tiny farm helped only by one near-adult son who had grudgingly stayed at home when the others had emigrated far afield to seek their fortunes.

The first appearance of his present complaint came in the middle of the night. His wife, who shares his bed, was roused by his noisy breathing and by his kicking and thrashing in a fit. She sent the son posthaste for the physician and the priest. By this time her husband had relaxed his rigidity and jerking and was lying limp, comatose, sweating and snoring. The priest came immediately and administered the last rites of the Church. The physician did not come.

According to the wife, it was May Eve, when fairies were abroad, intent on stealing small children and bewitching newly married brides. She excused the physician's neglect on this Walpurgis Night by saying that he had not the protection against evil spirits that His Reverence had. How could a physician have in his possession the proper triad of bell, book and candle with which to exorcise these evil spirits, even if he knew the proper ritual? Better let him remain at home in front of a fire with his friends, his punch bowl and a ladle. "Besides," she said, "it was a wet and stormy night, and the roads were dark and haunted."

The patient awoke just before dawn with a bad headache, but after taking a cup of tea slept again until the sun was well up on the horizon. Then, demanding his clothes, and seemingly as well as ever, he went to work grumbling that he was so late. He had no recollection whatever of the events of the preceding night. There was a great deal of work to do that morning, and he certainly did not believe in the trooping fairies, followers of the fallen Lucifer, in spite of all his wife had to say.

Since then there have been three nocturnal convulsions of much the same pattern. Additionally, he had one seizure in the daytime while digging potatoes. In this attack he had a warning in the form of dizziness, and of seeing bright lights in the right-hand side of his field of vision. On this occasion he tried to call his son, who was working alongside him, but was unable to do so and fell in a fit. This lasted only a few minutes, and he was carried into the house where he "slept it off" and awoke feeling as well as ever. This diurnal attack occurred between the nightly ones, and his last attack came on about a month before he came to the hospital, again occurring in his sleep.

The patient has been carefully examined here, and my gifted colleague, the house officer, has seen that for a man of his age his blood pressure, eye grounds and retinal vessels are not greatly changed. Roentgenologic studies of the skull disclose nothing and the chemical constituents of the blood are not altered. The electro-encephalogram, however, shows an abnormal focus in the left temporal lobe of the brain.

As to diagnosis at this stage, we know he has either a focal infarction in the left temporal lobe due to cerebral arteriosclerosis or a tumor in that area. A differential diagnosis between these two possibilities is as difficult as telling the sex of an infant before it is born. Even electro-encephalographic studies do not help. It is anyone's guess. However, and in order of probabilities, *cerebral vascular disease* is the more likely. Air studies of the brain are contraindicated at this age because of risk of further damage to a poorly endowed vascular tree; we can only wait and see what time will bring forth.

Direct surgical exploration of the brain in a patient of this age would be unwise, since even if a tumor is present it is on the dominant side and removal would likely be followed by hemiplegia and aphasia. Gliomatous tumors are more common after fifty years of age than benign removable meningiomas. Accordingly, we are going to advise anticonvulsive remedies, such as phenobarbitone, in doses of 1 grain three times a day, and re-examine him at intervals.

The French use the term, *"tardy epilepsy,"* for seizures coming for the first time in persons over fifty or sixty years of age. There may be no signs of general or focal damage to the brain. It is surprising, moreover, that for years the attacks may continue without any other signs of disease showing, and the patient pursues, for a time at least, a normal and useful life. Generally the course is mild, the seizures are infrequent and may come only at night.

It is possible that these patients with late-appearing epilepsy have always had a low threshold to fits, but whatever restraining influences there were present early in life had finally become worn out. Of course, in any given example, signs of physical and mental deterioration may appear at any time. The ultimate prognosis will have to be based on the presence or absence of physical signs of disease, both when the patient is first examined and later, on that which appears thereafter in periodic surveys of his or her general physical condition. Small doses of anticonvulsant drugs may control the seizures, but the dose must be kept low, since older persons tolerate these drugs poorly. At that, a few more years of a pleasant useful span of life may be enjoyed until the call comes and the number appears on that board which we are never allowed to see.

5

Good morning! My car refused to start this morning, so I hired a taxicab, in this cold and frozen Arctic bleakness. The driver was most conversational in the downtown traffic. He told me of an experience a middle-aged bachelor friend had had the morning before. He went out to get his milk on the doorstep. Flanking the well-battered pint can was a small baby wrapped up in an old grimy coal sack; blue with cold, it was yelling bloody murder. He took it and the milk in hastily to organize his defenses in such a problem. It was a newborn baby, and there it was, along with its food, arriving at about the same time. The milk was also half-frozen.

After we had missed a trio of bicycles by inches, I mentioned to the driver that this was probably a case of cryptogenesis.

"Begod," chuckled my Jehu, "I don't know what that is, but there will be a Holy War with his ould mother upstairs when they all get together."

"And what is that word?" he continued, inquisitive-like. "Is it anything to do with free love?"

I explained to him that a cryptogenic affair is one in which the origin of a physical phenomenon is uncertain, and its hereditary and familial concepts as yet little understood. The driver inhaled a long puff from his dirty yellow cigarette butt; then, thrusting his reddened, carbuncular face into mine, sighed in an odor of stale whisky, "You are right, sir, but there will be much more and then more for this poor man to explain upstairs, and he without legal grounds or otherwise to explain it." And so we turn to our first problem this morning.

This patient is an intelligent civil service worker of twenty-nine years. He has attacks which my house officer calls "peculiar," but then, *his* mind is virginal to such things. The attacks have existed for nearly five years now, are becoming more frequent and are disabling in his profession. By some of his friends he is regarded as being "mental," although between these short-lived seizures he is kind, friendly, considerate and well integrated. The attacks never alter in character, but sometimes do in severity.

Unlike the children of last week, he can not be expected to perform for your edification. The only thing I can find wrong physically is that his electro-encephalogram shows a complex and changing picture completely different from the short, rapid, high-voltage waves of grand mal on the one hand, and the stereotyped spike-and-dome waves of petit mal on the other. It is an example of brain recording suggesting a complex and variable disturbance.

Possibly, by administering a convulsant drug such as pentylene-tetrazol (metrazol), we may be able to initiate an attack. The difficulty here, however, is that given too small a dose, nothing happens; too large a one produces a major convulsion, which would be the end stage of his convulsive trouble and the least interesting to us. Let us at least try. The Chinese proverb still holds, that "one look is worth a thousand words." You have seen the patient's electro-encephalographic tracings. May I show you now a specimen of one of his numerous attacks?

He is willing to do all he can to help us, and the drug is being injected with every precaution. There is a short latent period, and now the devil's brew is working!

He is sitting up in bed. His pupils are widely dilated. His stare is blank, and his face is deathly pale. He is making chewing movements, and there are a few twitches in his face and arms. Look! He is out of bed and smacking his lips and frowning in disgust as if he were experiencing a foul odor or taste. His face now expresses horror and anguish. A few seconds by the bedside, and he is off, head low and eyes on the ground, searching and quartering each foot of the ward like a well-trained sensitive bird dog looking for game. And, just like such a dog, he has a thin stream of saliva pouring from one corner of his mouth. The game seemingly was at hand, but now is lost. Coming to the open door at the end of the ward, he darts through it in full chase into the cold and frozen yard in his night attire and with bare feet.

He is leaping over bushes, shrubs and fences as if they did not exist. My gifted junior colleague is on his trail, but a poor second, for the patient is long-legged and swift, the pursuer short and fat. He has now reached a stone wall and can not go any farther. At this stage one would expect a general convulsion, but it does not occur. He is standing quietly, leaning forward, his hands by his sides, his face composed.

Now the gifted one reaches him; he starts to lead him back to shelter and warmth, when suddenly the patient clenches his fist, draws back and hits my professional friend squarely in the jaw. Reinforcements arrive, and now the patient is back in the ward again, his color returning, his pupils back to normal, and he is recovering his senses. He is still somewhat confused; but automatically accepts a warm drink from the Sister. I check my watch: he is practically normal, physically and mentally, and it is just seven and one-half minutes from the time the injection was given. He will have no recollection of this attack, nor has he had of any of the preceding ones. These are called *"psychomotor seizures"*; of all the epilepsies they are the most complicated, variable, and yet the most informative of diseases of the brain. This attack was precisely that which he usually displays, but perhaps it was a little longer, due to its artificial induction.

With regard to this patient, the motor side is more marked than the other psychic component, but both are there. His expression of disgust and terror, his search for something not lost and not there, and his final belligerency show his mental processes to be still working, albeit on a lower plane. The pallor, the salivation, the automatic behavior, and the final blind, procursive chase into the open, are physical but intertwined with the psychic side of a primitive hunting beast. No wonder his friends think him daft and touched by the phases of the moon.

6

THIS LITTLE MAN with a waxed mustache and a humble air is a grocer's clerk. His trouble is much more complicated than that of our first patient, and yet more stimulating in its final analysis. He is thirty-four years of age and has had his unholy visitations for three years. Unlike the previous patient whose condition has not greatly changed in the process of years except in frequency, we see here an overt evolution, step by step, of an ever-spreading morbid process. I shall co-ordinate the story he has given me and develop it bit by bit.

In the beginning, the patient was not greatly disturbed. At times, weeks apart, he had certain attacks of dreaminess lasting but a minute or two. It was as if he were preoccupied and for a short interval detached from reality, but he was not entirely unconscious. A sudden wave would come over him in which he felt in a twilight state, as it were, in which it was hard to separate the real from the dream. The latter then was inchoate, and could not be analyzed. He was simply there and not there for a short period, but parceled up his tea and sugar in the shop automatically. All that was noticed was that he became silent. As time went on, however, there was added at the onset a strange whiff of smell that was not present on heaven or earth. It came suddenly, pungently, only to vanish immediately.

He kept on at his work, but in his spare time wondered at these things. Some months later, following the hallucination of smell and during the dream state, there was added a strange phantasy: he felt that he was somewhere he had been before, years ago. The scene at first was vague but gradually, like a jigsaw puzzle, it fell into shape. Places, houses and even a single room with well-remembered furniture came to him, and now voices were heard but dimly recognized. Usually, a single repeated phrase or a snatch of a song was heard. He even studied these memories as one looking on from outside a window, and frequently he could tell just what was coming, could anticipate the next act, the next scene, and the next line of the play. At the same time he heard the voices of his customers, only they were not convincing. At times the emotional affect was terrifying, but more often it was pleasurable. He seemed to look forward to his next experience.

By now his duties were more and more left undone, for during these brief few seconds, more often repeated, he was going deeper and deeper into a warping of contact with reality. In the shop he was regarded as becoming increasingly absent-minded and strange.

The psychic side became even more complex later. He would have his usual hallucination of smell, and sometimes of taste, and then a blinding flash of inward realization would strike him, as if all things were going to be explained, and if only he could wait long enough, all the wisdom of the world would be at his door. It was tremendously disturbing to this poor little grocer's clerk.

The attacks at the beginning were very short, a few seconds in duration, and he would return to his duties almost immediately. But later the absences became longer and a period of confusion followed, so that he began to mix onions with eggs and celery with sea kale. Once he was out of his attack, however, his memory of his trips into the *déjà vu* fantasies and of the flashes of intuition became blunted. In each attack he had felt that he could surely remember every detail, but in the gray light of reality these memories had faded.

A month ago he had his first convulsive seizure. He had had one of his usual attacks on a hard frustrating day of work. It was a severe one. He experienced the foul smell, then the vague character of his dream state; after that there was now, instead of mere confusion, total oblivion. His employer told him later that he had found him weighing a sack of potatoes, that he had stopped, looked as usual, blank, made a chewing movement of his mouth and jaws, and then had fallen precipitately in a general convulsion. After a half hour he had recovered and begged to be allowed to go home. He put on his hat and coat, took a streetcar, changed to another line as usual and paid his fare correctly each time. Arrived at home, he let himself in by his latchkey, undressed, laid out his clothes neatly and went to bed. Later, at about five in the evening, his wife found him sound asleep. In the morning he awoke, sore and tired, with the first of many severe headaches to come, and with no memory as to what had followed his usual psychomotor attack. He could not remember that he had had a convulsion or how he had arrived home as safely and expeditiously as he had.

From then on his downhill course has been progressive. He has had more seizures and increasingly severe headaches. He has been more dull mentally, and vomiting occurs with the headaches. There is a swelling of both optic nerve heads, and vision is failing, with left quadrantic hemianopsia. The left corner of his mouth droops and his left hand is weak. The electro-encephalogram shows random, irregular slow waves of the delta type in the right sylvian area. A diagnosis has been made of *"tumor of the right temporal lobe of the brain,* first in its anterior part involving the uncus and later spreading backwards." Surgical exploration in the hope of its removal has been advised and accepted.

Psychomotor attacks as shown in these two patients display a complex medley of symptoms and signs; as a whole, they show clinical signs suggesting organic lesions in the brain. These may be static or progressive. Scars of injuries or infections in the brain may produce symptoms for years; tumors may have a progressive course, as is seen in our second patient. Many times no cause can be found clinically or pathologically. Generally speaking, greater suspicion should be entertained of disease of the brain, static or progressive, in these patients than in the other epilepsies. The social repercussions are great, almost as bad as those accompanying frequent, recurrent, malignant major seizures.

Visual phenomena, simple or organized, aberrations of smell and taste, and more rarely, auditory hallucinations, appear. Automatisms of various kinds and states of furor may occur, disrupting social amenities. Autonomic disturbances, such as nausea, vomiting, borborygmi and automatic defecation, sweating, pallor and flushing, are not infrequent.

Psychic disturbances, such as fear, alarm, anger and belligerency, are more primitive emotional reactions. The more complex sense of things already seen and the dreamy, half-conscious states partly fill in the rest of the picture. It is a mixed bag and therefore an interesting one. Psychomotor epilepsy is not as yet clearly defined in all its boundaries, but it does shed some light on the functions of the temporal lobe of the brain, and to a lesser extent, on those of the frontal lobe.

My friend, the taxi driver, is now outside, smelling no doubt of fresh whisky as a result of his recent earnings. Can I trust him in the midday traffic? He is probably dwelling even more in gloomy thoughts on the fate of his friend faced with a cryptogenic offering of a blasted, nonwanted lovechild.

Next week we shall try to elucidate some more of the phases of epilepsy. By then the Sisters of Charity in their orphanage will have had their hands fuller by one more problem of hidden genesis in this wicked and godless metropolis. Shall we in turn be as successful in our search into the recognition, care and treatment of many of these problems of epilepsy of uncertain origin? Not so, I am afraid. We may have science of a sort, but lack greatly in charity, which is the greatest of all things.

7

Good morning! The shop windows are all brightly and colorfully decorated for the season, and Christmas presents for man, woman and child are inviting crowds of people to look at them. Many persons in the crowds are wistfully balancing the contents of their pocketbooks against the desire to give freely and generously. A fog dims some of the picture, creating an impressionistic effect, and a flicker of snow acts as a background, sharpening that which the fog has left uncovered.

The professional Father Christmas, with his plastic reindeer, has invaded the land. Poor fellow, he has had to stuff his midriff with a pillow to show an obesity where none exists, and to hide his lean and hungry flanks. A flowing white beard and stocking cap also hide what the ravages of a diet under normal have done to his face and skinny, pendulous neck tissues. Still, his eyes are bright and his voice cheery, since he knows he will not have to join the bread-and-bed line tonight at some grim "charitable" institution where piety prevails over kindliness.

At present he has his petty hour upon the stage, and for at least this one short period of the year he can give away gifts he does not possess, and wish all people some things he will never get, such as prosperity, happiness and the feeling of security for the coming year. At the same time, happily, he hides in a pleasurable anonymity.

The ward is well-nigh empty. Many patients have gone home

84

for Christmas, hoping to return after New Year's Day. At this season the Irish habitually postpone everything unimportant: even death comes into this category. They simply put it off during this period of the celebration of the birth of Our Lord. It would be impious to do otherwise. Ordinarily, they do not order their obsequies until after January the first, and therefore each year I can take during this time a week's vacation with a light heart and freedom from black, gnawing care.

Before I go away, I want this morning to round out the last three clinical lectures on the epilepsies, and I shall try to crystallize all we have seen and heard with a view to your future management of such problems. I want you to carry home something you can read, mark, learn and internally digest, along with mince pies, roast goose and plum pudding.

In essence, the problem is this: a patient of an age ranging from infancy to senility is brought to you because of recurring fits. These may be only transient losses of consciousness or downright convulsions. In the main, what the relatives demand from the start is the answer to the question of what is the cause of these fits and how can they be cured—a reasonable question, demanding a reasonable answer. Remember that a convulsion is something horrible to witness, and that, coming without reason, it strikes terror into the hearts of the onlookers, including those who are nearest and dearest to the patient.

Convulsions afflicting small children are accepted as something associated with a febrile childish disease. In the case of adolescents, a long skinny hobbledehoy may pass out at a long church session, from the effects of emotion, an empty stomach and standing for long intervals. An adult sensitive woman or man may fall down upon receiving bad news or from sudden, unexpected excessive pain and become unconscious. An elderly person may "black out" by virtue of impaired cerebral circulation. It is the more catastrophic, however, that a seemingly perfectly well individual in a public place may be normal at five minutes to ten and at the stroke of the hour, for no apparent reason, be lying on the ground, blue in the face, foaming at the mouth, and with all the body muscles jerking forcibly, a pitiable sight to all around and one of horror and anguish to those who love him, particularly if it is the first time such a seizure has occurred. More amazing still is the return to normal minutes or hours later, with no recollection on the part of the participant as to what has happened. Needless to say, our best knowledge, judgment and endeavor are required here.

There is always a first time in these attacks. A plausible reason is often given by the family, with the reservation that this is something which will never occur again. Lightning can never strike in the same place twice! When, however, fits recur, more severe and at closer intervals, there is certainly going to be asked, as mentioned before, the question as to cause, and inevitably the associated possibilities of cure. At this stage, or even anywhere along the line of an epileptic career, our best clinical efforts must be put forth always with an open mind as to the infinite possibilities prevailing. A cause should be assumed and extensive examination undertaken before the condition of the patient is put into the category of so-called "idiopathic," "essential," and "primary" epilepsy. A more honest term is *cryptogenic epilepsy,* indicating that we simply do not know the cause, but it should be applied only after every search has been made for a cause and none found.

In this modern age of facilities unknown to our predecessors, there is no place for a hurried, superficial examination in a consulting room or office. The stakes involved are too heavy and severe for that. It is even better for the patient to be admitted to a well-equipped hospital and there examined with every means in our power. There, at the least, the physician can observe him in the moments of a convulsion, instead of there being available only a garbled story given by a relative who was so terrified by the seizure that cold, unemotional and careful observation was out of the question. At the most, careful history-taking and a complete physical examination with a well-planned laboratory investigation can be done in a relatively short period and with a minimum of expense.

The approach to the problem should be that there *is* a cause for recurrent convulsive phenomena. Even after all causes apparently have been excluded, we grudgingly assume that this exclusion is only temporary, and that the final cause is unknown because of lack of evidence to date. Many times the cause of seizures is obvious, and with a minimal examination a program of attack on the problem can be launched. There must be, however, no guessing and no cheating ourselves with wishful thinking. There must be nothing like what the Indian proverb suggests, "Fools talk of a cat when a woman is brought to bed."

To pursue the gamut of things producing convulsions would take a longer discourse than I can give in a short clinical gab fest. Let us take the more common ones.

A history of injury to the head in childhood or adult life often is offered as a cause. In adults, however, such an injury must be reasonably severe. Convulsions are much more frequent when the dura mater has been torn or penetrated than in the so-called "closed" brain injuries in which both skull and dura are intact.

Chronic encephalitis in childhood, and less commonly in adult life, often is a factor, but here the history must be clear and definite.

Tumor of the brain, involving particularly the frontal and temporal lobes, or both together, must be excluded. Herein the history, examination of the eyes, roentgenologic studies of the skull, and the electro-encephalogram will be of help.

Metabolic disorders, such as hypoglycemia and hypocalcemia, are conditions that may slip our observations unless kept in mind. Studies of the blood constituents will help here, when these studies are done properly and by experts.

Toxic effects, as in eclampsia, uremia and alcoholic overindulgence, should be excluded by clinical examination and history. The so-called "whisky fits" occur while a patient is recovering from an orgy of drink, and not during the actual period of imbibing.

Cerebral vascular diseases, and the Cheyne-Stokes syndrome of heart block, appear in the older patients, but in these conditions there are many symptoms and signs other than simple convulsive disorders.

Syphilis *per se* never was regarded as being a frequent cause of fits; when it does cause them, it does so only in the early stages of general paresis. Serologic tests are always indicated hopefully, but seldom help in the final assessment of causes, now that syphilis is a dying disease and general paresis is becoming so rare.

8

I SEE that some of you are nodding, as in overpowering sleep, brought on no doubt by pre-Christmas celebrations. I have anticipated this, and we will move to another ward to see what I have laid out in films of air encephalograms, angiograms and some electro-encephalographic tracings. You may be examined severely on these in your final examinations, so you had better get at least a smattering of knowledge thereof.

We now come to the point wherein a given patient, after an extensive examination by all means in our power, exhibits just nothing to explain the convulsive malady that has afflicted him. Just as the relatives say, "There must be a cause," so cryptogenic epilepsy today is the convulsive manifestation of cerebral tumor tomorrow. Therefore, we must wait and observe this patient at regular intervals, always watching for a change in the clinical picture. What must be done in a therapeutic nature in the meantime?

The patient may live his whole life with convulsions of unknown origin, an "epileptic" to all around, and die either in status epilepticus or of old age. At postmortem examination nothing may be found to explain his fits. The brain grossly and microscopically may show just nothing. Spielmeyer described sclerosis of Ammon's horn in the region of the uncus of the temporal lobe. Pathologists are coming back to that in finding scars in that region.

In a motorcar accident the sufferer may have his head thrust violently into the windshield and the apex of the temporal lobe jammed against the anterior portion of the middle cranial fossa, without manifest signs of injury to the brain at the time. However, so many epileptics have no history of brain injury that this is begging the question, and the issue remains as to what to do for these patients who have epilepsy with no signs of organic disease, even after extensive clinical examination.

We have our anticonvulsive drugs. The earlier time-honored

bromides are still of use in certain cases. The barbiturates, such as phenobarbital and its side products, followed. The hydantoin group were next, and now there are a few of doubtful respectability because of the side effects they exert on the hematogenic system, particularly in that part of it which forms white blood cells. To date, the safe drugs are bromides, phenobarbital, and diphenylhydantoin sodium. More recent and less safe are trimethadione, methylphenyl hydantoin and phenurone (phenacemide). None of these *cure* epilepsy, but they may control it. There have been deaths from the last agents because of aplastic anemia, agranulocytosis, or in another term, leukopenia. In a cynical moment one might say an epileptic is better dead than alive, but none of us would want to be Pooh-Bah, the lord high executioner.

Chloroform was in use for a century, but because of a death of 1 in 10,000 it was abandoned for the less pleasant, suffocating and sickening ether. Accordingly, and in spite of the literature, I would advise using the least harmful drugs.

Trimethadione is supposed to be specific for psychomotor epilepsy and for petit mal. It is a dangerous drug. The side effects are photophobia, the appearance of everything around as being covered with white sugar, and a disappearance of white blood cells, with agranulocytic angina or aplastic anemia. Like chloroform, it is a helpful but powerful drug, and likewise has its serious demerits. Deaths have been recorded in association with its use. Psychomotor seizures and petit mal produce an electro-encephalogram that is different from that obtained in other forms of epilepsy, and the other safe drugs do not control these fits. Trimethadione does, but its dangerous nature necessitates excessive caution in its use. A single death is enough to make one abstain forever from prescribing it. Such also is the case with methylphenyl hydantoin and phenacemide.

The treatment of epilepsy is a most unsatisfactory problem, in spite of the enthusiasts who favor various drugs. All we hope for is control, and each drug loses its effect in time. No one drug *cures* the disease. Furthermore, the correspondence received from patients and relatives is depressing; every letter contains a request for "something new." The spontaneous cessation of the disease is like a miracle, as yet unexplained, but devoutly hoped for.

Too many patients turn to commercially exploited remedies. It is true that these contain phenobarbital and bromides, but they also contain remedies for constipation, and included in the package is a long and specific printed form of advice concerning diet, habits of living, the avoidance of stress and strain in everyday life and the overcoming of constipation. We physicians can do as much but rarely do; hence, the legally protected quack gets in and has no worry about dangerous drugs with serious side effects. Time however is moving on, and the drive to overcome epilepsy is ever increasing in vigor and determination. Let us, therefore, be not too despondent over progress to be made in the future but use judiciously whatever remedies we have confidence in, always on the watch for evil side effects. It is wise to be like the husband of Emma Bovary in Flaubert's novel, who never prescribed anything that could possibly hurt his patient and bring agony to the physician's soul.

The differential diagnosis of epilepsy, convulsions or seizures, whether they are of unknown origin or due to disease of the brain, is not difficult. If the patient is in a hospital and can be observed, there is no difficulty when whoever sees the fit is competent to describe it. Too often the observer is a nurse who runs for help at the first spasmodic contraction. It may be also a junior assistant, who is like the small boy at the zoo, who seeing a giraffe for the first time, said, "I don't believe it."

The history notes are peppered with details that were not present, and in the "name of a pipe" one asks what *did* the patient do?

"He had a peculiar fit of some sort!"

The staff should be instructed to see what there is to be seen, without comment, to stand right there and when it is over, to try to pen a picture equal to that of Gowers, whose writings I would have you all read as masterpieces of artistic writing and of scientific description.

Syncopal attacks are sometimes troublesome to separate from epilepsy, but it should be remembered that they usually occur in long lanky adolescents whose height is rapidly increasing, so that in parlance we may say that their head grows faster aloft than their heart. The attacks are not sudden, but with premonitory symptoms of hearing actual voices far away and with slowly dimming vision, the patient gradually fades out of the picture. He falls gently, and once on level ground or with head-between-knees he regains a consciousness which is abrupt and clear, not like a postepileptic confusion.

Hysterical attacks are just what they are: hysterical performances. They last a long time and are complex, with many emotional "sets." The cruciform attitude, the monologue of unhappy distress, the fully co-ordinated movements, such as hair-tearing, biting at those around, and tearing the bosom with the fingernails with the concentrated drama of frustrated existence that wears everyone else out before the sufferer falls asleep—all this is quite sufficient for a diagnosis.

Bromides, phenobarbital and diphenylhydantoin sodium can be given singly and in combination. It is a question of trial and error, finding the proper combination and efficient dose that may help in each case. Never should a patient be under the influence of drugs to the extent that he is stupid, drowsy and dull from overdosage, for there is an optimal dose that falls short of this. In the beginning of a regime of dosage the patient may seem to be drugged, but after a week this may pass. If it does not, the treatment is worse than the disease, and a reduction of dose should be insisted upon.

Use of the ketogenic diet regime, wherein children are stuffed with fat until ketosis is reached, with urinary findings corresponding, has waned considerably. One wonders if these children would have improved anyhow, without the lardaceous hegemony. At any rate, once they reached an appreciative and commanding age, they quit their diet and ate as they liked. Status epilepticus is the form of epilepsy that kills by exhaustion, following one severe attack after another; emergency treatment is the administration of sodium amytal intravenously or sodium phenobarbital intramuscularly until the convulsions are controlled. The regret is that another episode may follow later, and be uncontrollable by any means in our power.

As a warning, however, I must tell you that I attended one hysterical woman who had all that and more. I decided to give her a real convulsion, and with a very small dose of pentylenetetrazol I produced a violent epileptic fit. From that she went into status epilepticus and nearly died. Later, I found that although she was an epileptic, on coming out of her attacks she usually went into a hysterical and prolonged crisis. She proves the case that there is no such thing as hystero-epilepsy; it is either one or the other, but manifestations of hysteria may follow a major seizure in the confusion and depression that follow a fit.

The prognosis of epilepsy is just what one finds and observes over a period of time. If there is an underlying disease, that disease will be the outcome. If there is no evidence of progressive disease, one must follow the condition of the patient for two to three years to find out the essential trend of his malady. This will sooner or later establish itself, and can be interpreted in terms of malignant, benign or periodic forms. The response to such medication as we have is another factor. Generally speaking, a high degree of optimism should be embraced, for it is easy to give up hope and quit. The best physicians I have found who treat the disease are filled with the sense of relativity. To them a patient who is economically a total loss and a difficult member of the community is as far apart as worlds away from one who can support himself and his family, and still have epileptic fits. From that to the normal is only one step, and this gap is adjusted to gratefully and wholeheartedly by those suffering from the Sacred Disease.

May I now, since my time is over, wish you all a happy Christmas and a prosperous New Year? If you have a physician-father, tell him with my compliments that he knows nothing about modern medicine, and that all of us here know less!

JANUARY

Why should ye be stricken any more? Ye will revolt more and more: the whole head is sick, and the whole heart faint. From the sole of the foot even unto the head there is no soundness. . . .

—ISAIAH.

1

Good morning! I sincerely hope that you have had a happy Christmas season. You have, no doubt, received the appropriate gifts and have also given them to those who have rendered service to you. You have remembered your parents wisely and have not forgotten dear Aunt Tabitha, whose artificial dentures could not possibly have managed the box of hard-centered candies you gave her! Never mind, she has most probably passed them around to you, with your faultless chewing and a youthful craving for sugar. I hope indeed that you have not forgotten that fast-disappearing old servitor, the family maidservant, who helped rear you as infants and who has many times stood between you and parental wrath.

A word about these patients whom I show you here on Tuesday mornings. They have been selected mainly as to scientific media of expression. There is, as well, considerable thought given by me as to the effects of a gawking and curiosity-mongering crowd at their bedsides. They are actors with me in that show-of-shows, the teaching of the young. I usually discuss their part with them, assure them that they will be treated gently, without shame or indignity, and always I make a mental reservation that in so far as I am able, these poor people will not be frightened or hurt by anything that I may do or say. Let you do likewise! We are in the presence of sick and suffering human beings with an intelligence that may be greater than ours.

Before the holidays I had introduced to your notice a young lady not quite twenty-five years old. She was in this hospital for observation, and with a view to being helped during her periodic and severe headaches. At the time you saw her, she seemed to be in radiant health and good spirits. I explained that every laboratory test flung at her showed no signs of physical disease; even the results of an electro-encephalogram were normal. Roentgen studies of her skull, examination of her eyes and nasal accessory sinuses were carried out, and every chemical test of her blood that might have a bearing on her headaches was done; all showed nothing abnormal. About the only thing morbid that might have been observed was that she had a look of fear on her face; she seemed to be somewhat tired and worn, but I can assure you that there are days when she is our most eager helper in this ward and could pass a rigid life-insurance examination. And yet, the sands of time are running out for her with respect to obtaining employment which demands a regular and efficient attendance at duty.

The patient is the second eldest of a family of three brothers and two sisters, and her father and mother are still living. Her father by all accounts has had no serious diseases. The only flaw in an otherwise healthy family is that her mother had "sick" headaches until the menopause was over, in the sixth decade of life. In earlier life the mother's headaches were severe, and the patient often remembered her mother sitting quietly in a chair with a cloth dipped in cold water tied tight around her head. The patient has a younger sister who has mild headaches, but our patient and her mother show the maximal degree of a hereditary defect.

At the age of six, this girl had had intermittent vomiting attacks, and by the time she was ten years old, headaches were added. She remembers often returning early from school and shamefully vomiting in the omnibus that carried her home. At that time she missed many days from school, or at least, parts of days. After her return from school on these occasions, still vomiting, sick with headache, and listless, she would be put to bed by her mother, who doubtless understood a metabolic failure in her offspring, similar to her own, and who was accordingly sympathetic. These headaches were not so frequent or severe at that time, however, as they became later, when the patient was in high school and college. By dint of will and effort she finished these critical periods of her education without failure. Early enough in the formative years she had learned by experience what tended to bring on these paroxysms of headache and vomiting: a late sleep on Sunday, a missed breakfast and a period of excitement, such as a birthday party, the theater, or a football match, were paid heavily for in pain and misery. In fact, any laxity in a classic regime of regular habits of living brought a swift punishment, and although the regularity brought its own reward in general health, the payment in relief of pain was stingy. No matter what she did, her own efforts to prevent the attacks were never completely satisfactory.

There were not only the headache and vomiting that assailed her but also the general prostration, the coldness of her limbs, the sense of cessation of all gastrointestinal functions, the mental torpor conflicting with a hypersensitivity of all her five senses: all these contributed to her misery. During these recent years her problem has increased considerably. She passed her Civil Service examinations in college, and being a highly intelligent girl she holds today an important position in government service. There is, nevertheless, a series of disadvantages in such cloistered occupations, secure as they may seem. In every office given over to Civil Service there is a hierarchy of persons. As our Dean Swift said of such employes,

> *So, naturalists observe, a flea*
> *Hath smaller fleas that on him prey;*
> *And these have smaller still to bite 'em;*
> *And so proceed* ad infinitum.

Such has recently been the lot of our patient, and her economic history may become an exposition of a small hell inside the many government buildings subserving the State. It is not a good place for a sufferer from *migraine,* and particularly not for this patient here. In this regard one has to discuss the migraine type of personality, one which is so inextricably tied to these poor people.

Our patient is intelligent, sensitive, shy, ambitious, conscientious, perfectionistic and reliable, although she is prone to overdo in getting jobs done. If a migraine patient is a housewife she will literally never leave dirty dishes in the sink overnight. As with the epileptic personality, is this make-up a result or a cause of periodic convulsions, or of equally periodic blinding headaches? Does the chicken produce the egg or the egg the chicken? Let philosophers fight over this; they know scarcely more than we do, and at any rate we admit our ignorance.

The attacks of our patient come at irregular intervals, sometimes associated with the menses, sometimes not, and about equally so. There is usually, as has been mentioned, an increase in frequency and severity during periods of emotional tension. Hence the attacks were bad while she was finishing her college career and in the period of ambitious climbing to success in her earlier years of achievement. At the same time, they have continued to appear regardless of the background of circumstance, merely aggravated by certain events or conditions. Because of these we see her now at twenty-five years of age, struggling for mastery over the shears of Atropos and over the Greek gods of somber fate.

She is in a milieu of competitive, poorly paid and soulless activity, and there is not much chance now for her to go elsewhere for work of a different character. The head of her department is a petty official, yet he is a big flea on her horizon. She has escaped the little ones, but this big, wingless, bloodsucking parasite is biting her violently, without pity or a semblance of fair play, and apparently only for the reason that he hopes to enlarge his own ineffectual, constricted horizon by cruel and sadistic treatment of those in his power.

I am going to tell you what goes on during a severe attack of migraine, and then I shall show you the patient in an attack with all its accompanying drama. Naturally a severe type-case has been selected; you can, however, remembering the basic colors and outlines, sketch in your mental or physical notebook more lightly the less catastrophic forms. There are infinite variations in migraine, but all in all, they add up to a veritable headache for both patient *and* physician.

This patient whom we are following has abortive attacks, wherein she feels that one is coming on, but which never spills over the brim leading to the final explosion. She has milder attacks, also, during which she can work, but during the last six months all the attacks have been severe, prostrating and so frequent that her job is at stake.

Very often the day before an attack she feels, paradoxically, wonderfully well. At these times she covers areas of work impossible in ordinary periods, and moreover carries much of the work home with her to do at night, for she well knows that the next day may be productive of just nothing and a lost period of time. The day before an attack she acts almost hypomaniacal, laughing and giggling, the life and soul of the office, but underneath it all she knows that the following day will be the obverse of the medal.

On arising the next morning she is not so well and robust. There are a feeling of exhaustion, a dragging of her limbs and of her spirits, and she has a dull aching in her head in one or both temporal regions. She has little appetite for breakfast. Her face is pale and her hair seems to lack luster. Her eyes look as dead as those of a stewed fish. She goes to her work just the same and arrives there as usual, at 8:00 a.m. The dull grumbling in her head has by this time shifted to focus more on the left side, and her vision becomes misty, with, occasionally, colored spots in front of her which come and go. This visual disturbance lasts but a few minutes, but it is a definite prodrome to what comes after. Sometimes the attack aborts, the colored scotomas disappear, the head sensations clear, and the patient is normal again—until the next time! In less happy instances, the headache and other bodily complaints develop rapidly in intensity and furor. The dull, heavy headache becomes sharp, cutting, and above all, throbbing. It may be localized to any part of one half the head; it may be bilateral, and it may work in the cervico-occipital region. This latter is a *mean* type. The patient can not see well, can not bear the lights or sounds of her office, and she is rapidly becoming nauseated to the point of vomiting. She timidly asks leave to go home, and arrived there, often does not quite know how she got there.

She just reaches her apartment before vomiting. At first this was the tomatoes she ate the night before her attack, later the frugal breakfast of toast and coffee, and in the final heaves, gastric juice is erupted, followed by dark-green, bitter, foul-smelling and sickening bile, and her head pounds madly as if a devil had a nerve in her head under an anvil and was gleefully hammering it with a steel hammer. Behind this all is an obbligato of steady, sickening pain. Each stooping over the bowl to vomit increases this satanic symphony and the gush of bile.

We have already seen our patient in between her attacks, when she was seemingly well, efficient, and even sprightly. It was just her fear of further paroxysms and my desire to observe her in her further cataclysms of woe and discord that led me to urge her to stay on here. Another, and the most important, factor, was that here many remedies could be tried to relieve her before she went home and back to work. She was agreeable to that arrangement. Then I delicately introduced the subject, suggesting that I should like to show her to you students as an example of a patient with migraine in one of its periodic eruptions. She remarked, after this proposition was made, that she was so sick at these times that she cared neither for death nor for life, and that we could not hurt her more by outside influences than by what was already occurring within her bodily system. She was glad to think that by observing her we might help others in a similar affliction.

This migrainous patient is in the next ward, and her attack is well at its peak. I would ask you on entering to come in on tiptoe, without talk or noise, and above all, not to shake her bed. She is in one of those mysterious agonies of hypersensitiveness that are the pitiable afflictions of all sufferers of migraine.

She is in a corner bed, surrounded by screens to keep out light, and the window curtains are closely drawn. Sister has reduced all unnecessary sounds, smells and lights that may focus on a bed of suffering. The general appearance of the scene resembles that of the too-frequent setup of a dying person in a hospital ward, only here there is not the usual circle of agonized, pious, praying friends and relatives with their rosaries.

The screens have been removed, and the curtains have been raised. What a contrast now to what you saw of her before! She is lying curled up in bed, with her arms and hands around her head, which is buried in the pillow. Gently, I let you see her face. It is red and tear-stained, and her eyes are squeezed tightly shut. All previous make-up is a raddled mess, smeared around her lips and cheeks. Her hair is mussed, disorderly, and tumbled down over her neck and shoulders and into her eyes. Her hands are cold, and cutis anserinus is seen on both arms. Her facial contours appear to be swollen from weeping, with straining, gagging and retching. There is a vessel alongside her filled with *vomitus*, which is, at this hour of ten in the morning, beginning to be tinged with bile. She is vomiting once more. An ice bag which was on her head has been petulantly thrown aside. She stays very still and moves but little, except to vomit. There are no excitement, thrashing around, or dramatic hysterical gestures, such as the crucifixion attitude. She talks little, and her groans are manifested only as an aside. She seems to want to be left severely alone, to go through her own Garden of Gethsemane as quietly as possible until this trial ends.

I ask her a kindly question. Her only answer is, "Go away!" Let us begone to discuss this problem further in the ward from which we came. I purposely refrained from giving her any panacea this morning, even though we have found what will help her. You may be sure she will get it now, immediately on our leaving the ward. By tomorrow she will be herself again, although somewhat shaken and weak, glad to be free of pain but dreading the next attack.

You have heard this patient's life history; you have heard her own description of an attack and its usual evolution from the beginning to the end, and now you have seen her in the middle of an attack. I hope that you have perceived and appreciated its full significance and flavor. There is a total lack of drama—it is just a grim struggle against severe pain and a disturbance that racks every interstice of the body and every organ. The headache and vomiting are merely parts of the whole syndrome. As in epilepsy, we can not say here that such and such are cardinal features of the disease. The relatively normal status of the patient between attacks, and the serious prostrating character of the metabolic explosion, are features common to both diseases. Again, it is to be emphasized that epilepsy and migraine are cousins germane.

There is a life curve of migraine. It is severe during high-school and college years, reasonably bad but bearable during the third and fourth decades, and it grows severe again in the fifth, when it becomes atypical and plays all kinds of tricks. In the sixth decade, under favorable circumstances, it fades out imperceptibly and forever. Thus, patients with migraine seek help frequently in their second, and more often in the sixth, decades of life. It may blend in the fifth into syndromes of headache produced by hypertension and early cerebral arteriosclerosis, and it may unhappily persist to the end of life. Usually, sufferers from migraine have hypotension. Once the migraine disappears, however, hypertension may replace it, but not more commonly than in the usual run of patients; in fact, hypertension is probably less common in patients with migraine.

As to treatment, it must always be remembered that migraine is an inborn metabolic error acquired during the course of heredity. Worse still, it is a dominant inherited factor. In epilepsy the transmission of inherited disease is not so clear or definite. The headaches of migrainous patients are as much a part of them as the color of eyes and hair, and like these inherited physical traits, cannot be escaped throughout a lifetime. Therefore, there is no such thing as a "cure" to be spoken of with respect to this disease, but it can be mitigated.

You will find that migrainous persons often are philosophers. They accept their inherited burden and hopefully suffer the disease as an intrinsic part of their being. If the attacks appear but once in one or two months, or even less frequently, they are well satisfied, since this relative infrequency does not disrupt their path in life. But when attacks occur with such ever-increasing frequency that the patient either passes swiftly from one attack into the next, or can no longer depend on himself to be competent in the home, in society and in business, it is then that he comes at last, craving some relief from his intolerable burden.

Two forms of attack can be made on the problem of migraine: the first, through the general handling of the patient's life, and the second, by combating the actual attack in order to abort it or relieve it completely, so that the sufferer may go about his business and, above all, be relieved of his unendurable pain and suffering.

You have heard a description of a migrainous patient's personality. In some measure this pattern may be due to years of search for a proper regulating of habits so as to lessen the frequency of attacks. It is a good principle and a face-saving one for the physician to let a patient tell his or her life story. These persons have lived with their condition so long that they know from experience and intimately what errors they commit that cause disaster. They know more about *their* headaches than you can tell *them*. Therefore, leading questions, sermons and impatient homilies from you before they tell their entire story will just lose you one more patient. About their mode of living, they are the most solicitous, heedful, wary, prudent and painstakingly careful persons in the world, and the usual medical advice against irregularities in diet and living in their case is altogether fatuous.

Habitually, one ends the consultation by giving the patient the false comfort of such an assertion as, "Living as you do, you ought certainly to live to a ripe old age."

To this the riposte is as unfailing as it is immediate, and can only be expected: "Willingly granted, doctor, but I do not *want* to live a long time with these headaches; I would sooner be dead!"

Accordingly, let them give you the facts of their fight, and then you will be able to pick out what they have overlooked or thought to be nonessential. There is always some residue of sins, possibly more of commission than of omission, and one can skate gracefully, and perhaps efficaciously, along this patch of thin ice.

I was impressed by the relative freedom from migraine of soldiers during World Wars I and II. When in uniform and overseas, without great responsibility, leading a life that was close to that of an automaton, they were relatively free from that scourge. (Perhaps it was the general commanding officers who had had the headaches!) In face of imminent death on the field of war, what really matters and what is important? During a time past, now half-forgotten, they had served as white-collar clerks or executives in offices where petty irritations and a petty existence were more of a stress and strain than their regime in the theater of war.

Death they had seen in their comrades; it was not unexpected and was acquiesced in. A responsibility poorly borne, an unpaid loan, family troubles, and personal bickerings were each a major catastrophe in times of peace and much more devastating than being subject to a glorious ending of life and a cancellation of all current obligations.

In one of the short-short stories of O. Henry, *Let Me Feel Your Pulse*, a neurotic individual, presumably the author, found a cure. It was a plant that an old family doctor in blue jeans took him to find. For hours each day, in that wild, lonely part of the southern states, they climbed over hills, waded through marsh and streams to find it, with the result that the patient slept like a log each night. After a week or more of an arduous but thoroughly intense search, the doctor admitted failure and winked an eye. But there was no need to find that herb now; the cure was already found.

If attacks of migraine are coming closer and closer together, this status migrainus can be aborted by a return to an animal-like existence away from all modern civilization, with its thousands of incoming noxious stimuli. If at a certain period this is not feasible, a course of small doses of bromides for six weeks, as recommended by Charcot, or our more modern phenobarbital, may be of help. This, however, is only a blanket to suppress a fire that will continue to smolder, anyhow.

The drugs which can be used during an attack have increased in number in recent years, and are principally those of the ergotamine group. Many patients obtain relief with aspirin, or its combinations with acetophenetidin and caffeine. These patients (need I say?) you will not be likely to see. Morphine, and all synthetic analgesics leading to addiction, should be strictly forbidden. Happily, in most cases, patients with migraine are sensitive to them, and on taking them, vomit more than ever. The drug is excreted by the stomach, and the headache returns.

Ergotamine tartrate is a vasoconstrictor. It induces vomiting, and in too-frequent doses produces gangrene of the fingers. There are also painful and disagreeable withdrawal symptoms, when the patient because of pain or fear has been taking too much. It can be given, combined with caffeine, by mouth or in the form of a rectal suppository, under strict medical supervision. It is at times very helpful.

A milder preparation, such as dihydroergotamine (DHE45), given intramuscularly or intravenously in doses of 1 cc., often has a dramatic effect in severe, short-lasting headaches. The administration of this agent also must be strictly supervised by the physician in attendance. In attacks that are severe but infrequent, dihydroergotamine is valuable, or in those local severe head pains coming in clusters, usually at night, there need be no hesitation in using it. This type of migraine may occur in daily attacks for six weeks to three months and then disappear for a year or more, so that ergotism is less likely to occur. Inhalation of oxygen through a mask and from a cylinder has its place, but there are some practical difficulties in the administration of this in a patient's home, where his wife may light a cigarette during the process! Finally, there are those forms of migraine which nothing relieves, and then only prayer, sacrifice and trust in God remain. Actually, these things should have been mentioned first, and not as I have done, at the last.

2

THERE IS a man outside in the hall, waiting to see me; we will have him in. He is a most miserable object and looks like a dying duck in his own puddle, just barely surviving a thunderstorm. He clutches his shaven head in both hands and tells his story in a whining, lugubrious voice. He complains of a headache to end all headaches, or as he puts it, "I have the headache of the world." And yet it is *not* a true headache. It is a feeling of tightness, compression and squeezing, as if an iron band were around his head like a vise and were being tightened every hour. It is as if a heavy iron hat were on his head, the rim resting equally on the frontal, temporal and occipital regions of his cranium. As a side issue, there is at times a feeling as if an iron nail were being driven into the vertex; it is sharp and unpleasant but not a true pain. Not one of his head pains is so real as the joyous Katzenjammer he has had following an alcoholic debauch. He has had his share of those, he says, and has found cure in rest, purgation and abstention.

He finds no relief from ordinary analgesics, such as aspirin and acetophenetidin compounds. At one time his local physician gave him a hypodermic injection of morphine; it merely made him vomit, and there was no relief of pain. The sensation in his head is present first thing in the morning, lasts all day, and at night when he says his prayers, it is still there. Worry, anxiety and fatigue make it worse. He feels better when he is busily engaged. If he wakes up in the middle of the night it is still there, and yet he sleeps eight hours of the twenty-four. He never vomits with it. He is continuously searching his close-cropped scalp for signs of disease, but can find none. He is sure and certain that he has a tumor of the brain. He has had his skull examined under roentgen rays in every hospital in this city, and all films, including ours, have been reported as showing no signs of intracranial disease.

This man was a highly efficient grocery clerk in a well-known city business. His superiors recognized his energy, ability and worthiness, and from the first of the last quarter of last year he was promoted to local manager. According to his story, he has not had a well moment "in his physical constitution" since then. His head sensation has plagued him, and he is afraid for himself. He can not retire to his previous safe and happy position, nor, worst of all, can he see himself climbing higher in this hierarchy of tea, bread, vegetables, meats, and the like. He has been kicked upstairs to a place that terrifies him. He can not command those beneath him, nor can he consort on an equal footing with those in that celestial atmosphere into which he has been pushed. He is a fish out of water, a god without a Jehovah, a minister without portfolio. Therefore, he has headaches. Make no mistake; each one of *us* would suffer accordingly. And what is the solution?

This is a typical instance of **tension headache**, with an obvious mental cause for that tension. Good, commonsense advice can help a great deal here. It is imperative that this individual make a clean break from his present situation, without developing in the meantime a sense of inferiority and frustration over the whole thing.

Migraine and tension headaches are not so far separated. In any given individual they may coexist. A migraine phenomenon, by dint of frequent suffering and dread of more suffering on the part of the patient, may lead to tension headaches; on the other hand, a tension situation may bring out and aggravate previously existing migraine. It is for us to separate the two and treat each accordingly as it seems necessary for us to do, by friendly counsel and good advice. Drugs help least in tension headaches.

Headaches are strange things, and when dealing with them we swim in troubled waters. If they have persisted long enough and are severe, there is only one thing to be done. The patient should be thoroughly examined by every means in our power, with nothing taken for granted. Like epilepsy, an apparent migraine may have as its source a cerebral tumor, hypertension, vascular disease, cranial suppuration, renal insufficiency or even long-forgotten syphilis. The type of headache must be taken into consideration, and it must be emphasized that migraine and tension headaches have just as individual a character as have those pains in the head caused by gross intracranial disease. There is always, however, on the part of the physician some uneasiness that these headaches, supposedly benign and with no threat to life, may come back to roost like evil birds, dropping the filth of their *excrementa* on his head, bowed with shame and frustration because he had made a serious and vital mistake in overlooking a malignant disease process that is now past all cure.

Headaches are unpleasant things to deal with, in that after seeing three or four such sufferers in an afternoon, the physician himself is a candidate for pains in the head, especially so if he happens to have a familial and personal diathesis. At this stage of our discussion, I should like to advise you never, never to tell a patient with headaches that you suffer similarly, hoping so to give him the idea that because of personal experiences you have a more than sympathetic viewpoint with regard to his disease. The result is quite the opposite. The patient has no interest whatsoever in *your* suffering; you can have "the headache of the world," so far as he is concerned. Thereupon, from his point of view, you become a charlatan or a quack, no better than a bald-headed man trying to sell a hair-restorer. You have, in effect, become a man who claims to heal others of that which you can not help in your own case, and one who has blandly forgotten just that, a simple fact obvious alike to buyer and seller.

As I grow older, boyhood memories crowd in on me. There was the schoolmaster I had, the most brilliant teacher and the most stimulating, among the many droning misfits who had drifted somehow into the places they least fitted. He had a young, fresh face and long and prematurely gray hair. Every lesson he gave us in mathematics was inspirational. Every so often, however, late in the morning, his energy would appear to wane; he would drop his head on his desk, and with his arms around it, lie in silent agony.

Under ordinary circumstances, and at our age, the members of the class would have created a bedlam—a riot, a shambles of yelling, fighting, horseplay, and a blowing-off of suppressed energy from lack of control. Instead of this, the class prefect would immediately detail two scouts, one at each entrance to the classroom, so that if the headmaster were on a trip of inspection he could be seen from afar. Thereafter, quiet as mice, we would work at the preparation of our homework for the next day, until the moment when our master, whom we adored almost as a god, raised his throbbing head, and with eyes screwed almost shut, dismissed us, to go staggering out himself on his way to his home and his bed.

O dark, dark, dark, amid the blaze of noon,
Irrecoverably dark, total eclipse
Without all hope of day!
                    —MILTON: *Samson Agonistes.*

3

Good morning! I had to walk part of my way here and crossed
one of Dublin's bridges over the River Liffey, which as usual,
stank. A man was standing solidly and patiently against the curv-
ing wall of the bridge at the middle of its humpbacked curve. Between his feet he had a ragged cloth cap turned with its inside
upwards to receive alms. He had a cane resting against the wall,
and around his neck, hanging on a dirty string, was a blazoned
warrant of arms. It was framed, glass-covered against the weather,
and bore many pious sentiments. In the center, clearly to be seen
a long way off, there appeared the word, BLIND. Now, polite
blind persons wear dark glasses to cover up the appearance of
their eyes, but this man continuously held his uncovered eyes upturned to heaven so that the ghastly conjunctiva showed white like
a fish's belly—a dead fish at that! He held in one hand a battered
sheaf of yellow lead pencils, as if to show that he was an honest
licensed hawker of goods and not an impudent blind but sturdy
beggar who could support himself if he so desired.

According to my custom, I deposited a few coppers in the cap
and hastened on, pursued by a high-toned, singsong benediction
which I almost knew by heart, the usual Litany of the Blind as
said to their patrons, Saints Cyriacus and Lucy. As I neared the
end of the bridge, however, my hair began to prickle near the
nape of my neck, for like an old barrel organ changing its tune,
the blind man was now eulogizing me by name, by profession,
and by my personal habits as a friend of the poor. Blind people

are said to have a psychic gift; at any rate, through a surrounding darkness he apparently knew me and blessed me. I was reminded of Madame Bovary in Flaubert's novel. Poor Emma! The song of a blind man and all his lustful desires sent her to a terrible death by suicide with arsenic. . . . I may well increase my contribution next time, lest this man have it in his power to harm me. Perhaps, after all, he is a rogue who sees as well as you and I, and who needs a few weeks' correction in the Bridewell!

Our patient here is a woman thirty years of age who has come to me in a circuitous fashion. You will note that we are seeing her in the pleasant, softly decorated ward devoted to the god Hymen. She was sent here by her local physician because she has had no menstrual periods since she was twenty-five years old. The periods became more scanty and further apart, and finally ceased. She has remained unmarried. There were evident none of the usual causes of amenorrhea, natural or pathologic. My gynecologic colleague was ready to pass on her condition as a so-called primary amenorrhea and send her home under a regime of female hormones. Before leaving, the lady asked that her eyes be checked for change of lenses. She had no definite visual defect that she knew of, but her vision, particularly in the left eye, did not seem to her to be quite normal, although she could read normally and see across a street the clear outlines of faces and things. Her request was granted, and so started a serious train of thoughts and consequent advice as to equally serious action.

Our ophthalmologist was the evil genius here, disrupting all sense of self-satisfaction. He found the vision in both eyes fairly good for reading, but reduced slightly in the left eye. What held his attention, however, was that in that same eye, on examination of the fundus, there was a pearly white pallor of the optic nerve, not as yet an atrophy, but the stage of whiteness that leads to one. He tested her perimetric fields with various-sized objects, whereupon the tragedy of her problem began to become apparent. She has bitemporal hemianopsia, complete on the left side and partial on the right. Central macular vision is not greatly disturbed except on the left side. He asked for roentgen studies of the patient's head, and then things showed themselves to be really serious. The sella turcica is enlarged five times that of normal, the anterior and posterior clinoid processes are mere ghosts of themselves, and parts are missing. The little fossa which holds the pituitary gland, and which is usually just large enough to contain somewhat snugly the tip of one's little finger, now is large enough to admit freely the ball of a thumb. Further, this enlargement is to a great extent at the expense of the underlying sphenoidal air sinus. Something has definitely eroded the sella turcica, has expanded it, and has grown downward into the structures underneath it. Please observe the roentgen studies of the patient's head and compare these with similar films of a normal person of the same age and sex.

By a devious route, starting with the gynecologist and going on to the ophthalmologist and neurologist, we have reached a diagnosis. It is for the neurosurgeon to decide now what to do about a *tumor of the pituitary gland* that is threatening this patient's sight. I would have you note how insidiously this present problem has evolved. In the space of five years the tumor has been growing, and a hazard has crept up without the patient's or anyone else's realizing it. Nevertheless, it is fortunate that we know of it now and can deal with it. Without treatment, in a few months more or less, irreparable blindness would be inevitable, and there would then be no hope for her vision, no matter what was done. These tumors are like a snowball that, rolling down an incline, gains mass and momentum along the way until it becomes an avalanche; it will destroy vision and all vision means in life, plunging the victim into an abysmal existence without the ability to see, into a life pattern largely dependent on the help of others.

This patient has a suggestive bodily appearance which I would draw to your attention. Later, we can consider the results of her laboratory and other tests. Her hair is plentiful but dry and coarse. Her eyebrows are thinned out, and hair is lacking over her arms and legs. Her face is puffy; it is a yellowish white, with a mild malar flush. Her lips are somewhat thickened, and her voice is low and has a croak in it. There is a dull expression in her eyes, and her mental reactions are not so quick as one would expect for one of her class and education. I admit these changes are minimal. When looked for, however, they flash into sight. Her skin is dry; there is very little sweating in the palms of her hands. Axillary and pubic hair is almost absent. You have already heard of her amenorrhea of five years' duration, with no pelvic condition to explain it. She complains greatly of cold and asks for all the blankets Sister can spare in this winter weather.

As to laboratory tests, her blood pressure is 100 mm. of mercury, systolic, and 70 mm., diastolic. The basal metabolic rate is –20 per cent. The 17-ketosteroid estimation is 1 mg., and the corticosteroids are 0.5 cc. from a urinary output during twenty-four hours. There is a relative lymphocytosis.

All the above adds up to the fact that besides the threat to vision, this patient has an endocrine deficiency involving the complicated interlocking chain of the pituitary, thyroid and adrenal glands with the gonads. To know this is important, in view of possible surgical removal of this tumor. A certain amount of pituitary gland must be sacrificed at that time, and the influence of what Cushing called the "master gland" will be brought to a low ebb. In previous years mysterious deaths occurred on the operating table or shortly thereafter when this gland was attacked surgically. Now we have replacement therapy. Usually, cortisone is given in 200-mg. doses for three days before surgery, and a close watch for acute hormonal deficiency is instituted thereafter. The administration of cortisone can be continued for an indefinite period after surgery, so that these patients, after successful removal of a pituitary tumor, do not live out their lives as a primitive sluggish reptile, just existing and no more. The dose of cortisone can be regulated. Other endocrine extracts can be added as needed.

Generally speaking, surgical removal of these pituitary tumors is eminently satisfactory. Vision is improved, and the perimetric fields may return to normal. Hypopituitarism can be combated. In fine, the weightiest factor in regard to these patients is that they be seen early and treated early by surgical intervention. For patients who for one reason or another can not withstand surgery, roentgen therapy is often used. At times the response is good in selected cases.

So far, we have been discussing hypophyseal adenomas. There are, however, other tumors near the optic chiasm that may produce a similar effect. To proceed according to the ages at which such tumors appear, there are gliomas of the optic nerves and chiasm. These are bad, so far as restoration of sight and total removal are concerned. They occur in children, and happily they are rare. Normally, the stalk of the pituitary gland is formed by the meeting in the embryo of a pouch from the primitive pharynx and a down-growth of the floor of the ventricle. Sometimes, however, vestigial cell rests occur and may become tumors during the first, second and third decades of life. These tumors are above the sella turcica and may or may not erode it. They usually involve the optic chiasm, and a more complicated loss in the perimetric visual fields is a result. They nevertheless have the characteristics of a chiasmal lesion. If they extend upward, papilledema may appear, and involvement of the floor of the third ventricle may produce a complex clinical picture involving processes of growth, fat metabolism, water balance and sexual development.

To help in the diagnosis, there frequently are characteristic roentgenologic findings. Above the sella turcica scattered, minute, opaque granules appear in a cluster. These are in a cyst filled with a yellow fluid rich in cholesterol crystals. These tumors have many names—the common one, in deference to their embryonic origin, being "craniopharyngioma." Their removal is more difficult than that of primary hypophyseal tumors, but in this regard a tremendous advance has been made. Meningiomas, or tumors arising from the leptomeninges around the sella turcica, usually appear in the fourth, fifth and sixth decades of life. Endocrine changes are rare, and not only the chiasm here is involved but also the optic nerve itself. Again, as in craniopharyngiomas, there is in certain cases a highly suggestive picture in roentgenologic studies of the head. There may be seen a boss of overgrown dense bone in the region of the tuberculum sella. Aneurysms of the internal carotid artery are the most dreaded; these occur in middle age. Roentgenologic studies may show erosion of one side of the sella. During surgery, if such aneurysms are treated without gentleness, they may rupture and produce on the operating table death from intracranial hemorrhage. Surgeons have learned to look out for this disaster and to act accordingly.

By close co-operation among ophthalmologist, roentgenologist, surgeon and neurologist, some definite idea can be reached as to why a given patient is becoming blind; the endocrinologist helps to make the path to success the smoother. No one, however, can be absolutely sure as to what is squeezing out the life of the optic nerves and chiasm until the area is explored in the light of day by a surgeon who is quick to recognize what the trouble is, and who knows how to deal with it. It is a long and tedious surgical procedure fraught with risks all along the way, involving a burrowing into the very center of the cranial cavity with dangers to the right and left. Yet I recently saw a woman more than seventy years of age who had just had a tumor involving the optic chiasm removed *in toto*. She had left the hospital on the seventh day and had been sent home on the tenth, with her vision restored to normal and her perimetric fields almost so. Strangely enough, the tumor was a craniopharyngioma, the beginnings of which she must have had as far back as the time when she was still putting her dolls to bed for the night, after having her flaxen pigtails rewound and before saying her prayers.

Finally, the problem arises of the patient who is already blind, with only perception of light, or less. The report on the optic nerve heads is that they are atrophied. The disks are dead white, the lamina cribrosa is visible, and the vessels are reduced to mere threads. These optic nerves are dead, and they will not and can not return to life. You should verify this yourselves in other patients who have become permanently blind from the causes mentioned above.

What is the practical result of operating in such cases? There is no headache and no suffering. Endocrine dysfunctions can be taken care of medically as they are found to exist. Patients may live indefinitely, depending on the type of tumor involving the chiasmal area. To put a life to a hazard when nothing can be accomplished shows a want of judgment. To a blind person who has become adjusted to his loss, life may be sweet; rehabilitation centers are concerned with giving an incentive to live, and even a gainful occupation may be provided him by the state. Indeed, even failing that, a street beggar has his moments of bliss when there is a steady clink of coins falling into his cap! My friend of the humpbacked bridge seems to be in full pursuit of happiness. He is King of his Castle, and no one can depose him. He knows me now, and he knows that I know. We shall have more meetings, please God. There is nothing more flattering to one's self-esteem than to have a keen interest in a public institution, charitable or otherwise. I fear, however, that these copper coins will have to be replaced in the future by newly minted silver of the realm, for I do not doubt that, although to all appearances he is blind, he will be able to tell their current value by the tinkling sound they make as they drop into his greasy cap. I am afraid of this man, for I fear that he has within him the power of evil.

4

LEAVING the lavender-scented, rose-tinted abode of "female troubles," we arrive by degrees at our own grim ward devoted to stark male sufferers, neither tinted nor perfumed. There is a man waiting for me. He is a good friend of mine and I owe him many favors, not the least of which is his coming here today at my request to show you the infirmity which has pursued him nearly all his life. His hands shake at any movement he makes, but not when they are still. The shaking does not increase on movement; it is just there. It is present with his hands outstretched, even when he is trying to keep them still. Writing is his greatest task.

He is a meat cutter in a firm from which I buy all my meat for the family. He has an unerring instinct as to what I want, and he sees that I get it. No one else can select and cut a steak as he can. Usually I ask for his best, and he sniffs and feels over several half carcasses of beef until his choice is made and he is satisfied. He then unhooks the huge animal mass and staggers to a cutting table. Time and again have I watched him work. Once into action with saw and cleaver, he is the master of his task; it is a ritual. The shaking of his hands does not appear very noticeably in these crude but well-timed efforts. When he arrives at the stage of cutting, he reaches into the wooden scabbard dangling from his corpulent waist, and out come the knife and steel. His hands are as usual shaking, but the strokes on the steel ring out in quick succession, and a shaky thumb drawn across the edge of the knife satisfies him as to its sharpness. I watch the knife as it approaches the red and luscious flesh with its yellow fatty cortex. The blade is quivering, and I gasp involuntarily lest he cut himself severely. I need not worry, however, for it descends steadily and as swiftly as the intrinsic part of that "humane" instrument invented by our French physician, Joseph Ignace Guillotin. A few minor cuts more, and there is slapped on the scales a steak as wide around and as thick as the lid of an outdoor facility. I have measured these steaks with calipers, and have found that the size around their perimeter varied by not more than a few hundredths of an inch. I have never eaten finer steaks.

In public bars, he tells me, he has to hold his glass with both hands, but he adds that as the evening progresses one only is sufficient. It is at tea parties at which his wife presides that he is bad, and his cup beats a devil's tattoo on the saucer as he lifts it gingerly and restores it with contents half-consumed. As has been said, writing is his major difficulty. When alone, he can write quickly and yet legibly; when under observation, he writes a mere scribble, performed laboriously. He remembers this tremor's being present as far back as his grade-school years and chuckles even now when he tells that the master could not cane him on the hand, for it shook rapidly out of aim, and the master had to resort to caning him on the buttocks, which could be kept a steady target with his head between the master's knees and his rebel hands held out of the way.

He is now nearly fifty years of age, and this tremor, although it has remained confined to his hands, is definitely becoming worse; every other part of his body is steady and quiet. At work his main difficulty is wrapping up and tying with cord the meat he sells to a customer. He has obviated all clerical work by writing the price laboriously but legibly on the parcel with a large blue crayon. In a rush of work he bawls out to the cashier in her glass cage the amount owed and the name of the customer. There is as yet no reason for him to stop working because of his trouble.

I remember a world-famous surgeon who, at an abdominal operation, would hold his knife poised, shaking perceptibly, over the heaving, iodine-stained belly; then like a flash, lower it to make an incision as straight as an exclamation mark. Once he was into the abdomen, there was no fumbling. He dictated all his notes and signed his name with an indelible pencil. I know a plastic surgeon whose tremor is catching up with him with the years, but who does exquisite remodeling of faces hideously smashed or burned.

I have had our man bring a piece of paper on which he has written at home and alone a "Hail Mary." There are pen, ink and paper here now, on which he will write the same before you. After a long, ineffectual attempt he has completed this short prayer. I shall use the projector to throw both writings on the screen. That which he wrote when alone in his bedroom is legible; what he wrote under your Gorgon stare is not. Buttoning his clothes, tying his tie, and lacing his shoes also increase his tremor, but next time you are near his place of business, do go in and see him cut out a juicy steak—particularly for me!

There is more to come. My friend has a family, and by the laws of nature and heredity he is descended from one. His father had a tremor from an early age, but as a blacksmith he was able to pound an anvil until well on in years. His tremor became worse as he grew older, but he managed to work until he retired on the old-age pension at seventy. His mother was entirely free of tremor. As to the uncles and aunts, they emigrated early to America, and he lost track of them and of their offspring.

He had three brothers, older than himself. He recalls that two of them had shaky hands during the grade-school years. The third died at the age of ten from diphtheria. The remaining two brothers went also to America, where one was killed in an accident on the railroad. The other brother became prosperous enough to send home to Ireland at irregular intervals gifts of money to help his nephews and nieces. This man is now about fifty-five years of age and has a mysterious occupation which has something to do with horse racing. By luck, there is a letter available to show you, since the family received one from him last week.

Apparently the brother has a wife who writes his letters for him, for the characters are neat, legible and without a trace of tremor. At the end, however, there is a wind-up written by the brother, commending his nephews and nieces to God, and advising them with respect to their religious duties and daily conduct. I can not read it, and you likewise will not be able to do so. I throw it on the screen, and my friend can translate it for you, since he is accustomed to these messages of good cheer, wise counsel and pious exhortations. Moreover, they contain a generous sprinkling of largesse from an apocryphal source.

My good friend, the purveyor of excellent meat, has a family and an ever-loving wife. The latter does not concern us, except for the fact that she has deft and steady hands; I have seen her help her husband tie up packages during a Christmas rush period at his place of business. There are, however, five children. I have excluded the eldest and the youngest, and the other three with their mother are coming into the ward now. Notice how my friend's face lights up on seeing them. He has been a good father but is perplexed now, and I have tried to help him by counsel and advice, as well as through my friends.

John is twenty-five years old and has had a tremor of his hands since he was twelve; it has been gradually increasing. He works in a shop, in the position of a floorwalker. His firm found that he has marked native ability and promoted him rapidly. All he has to do with his hands is occasionally to initial a credit slip. Mary, here, is twenty-two years of age and is a schoolteacher. When she was fourteen, the nuns who taught her scolded her vigorously because her handwriting was not the Spencerian copperplate characters they demanded. Happily, her tremor is not marked, and she gets along by using the blackboard and wide, free handwriting. She can mark examination papers in private, and no comment has been made. James is twenty and is a plumber's apprentice. He can not remember when his hands were as steady as those of the other boys, but like his grandfather he took up a heavy, clumsy craft, and provided that he has not to go back too often for forgotten tools, he does well at it.

The two other sons are Matthew, aged twenty-eight, and Mark, who is eight. The former works in a bank and is entirely free of any tremor. He is the eldest, and having thus far escaped the family curse, he probably will remain free. The latter, Mark, the youngest of all, was apparently an "afterthought," since he was born almost twelve years after the last child. He is at present free from tremor, but it may yet develop. Time will tell.

We have tested the father and his three children for tremor as is done in the usual neurologic examination: the appearance of their outstretched fingers, the finger-to-nose test, and finger-to-finger—that you have seen. We shall work the projector once more and show you now the handwriting respectively of John, Mary and James. The writing of the last-named is by far the worst; the girl's trouble is slight, and that of John is midway between. Accordingly, there is no rule by age as to the severity of any given inherited defect. Sometimes a familial disease is more marked in the younger siblings, appears earlier and progresses faster than in the older ones, but that is by no means the rule.

From the imperfect and incomplete records we have had of this family, the inherited tremor, as far as we can tell, follows the Mendelian law of a dominancy of the disease factor such that out of four siblings, three show signs in varying degrees of being afflicted. For that reason, I think that the youngest son, Mark, has a fair chance of escaping, since three of the four siblings preceding him have been shown to have a tremor. Of course, he may be one of a possible succeeding four offspring who might have been conceived and born except that the age of the parents has now prohibited it. However, we can not be too rigid in this prognostication, for even, at times, the peas fooled Mendel.

Note the degree of involvement as shown in the handwriting of the offspring and in the tests I have used to demonstrate their individual tremors. Compare them with the father's handwriting and other evidence of lack of control of his fingers and hands. What degree of disability will these sons and daughter of his have when they reach his age? James may be worse than his father is now, and John may be just as bad. Mary probably will not be so badly afflicted. We are judging by the rate of progression.

A few more words before we close this lengthy session this morning. The condition I showed you is that of a *heredofamilial tremor.* It follows the Mendelian law, but family diseases are notoriously hard to collect in complete line of succession, and that which I showed you today, a two-generation vista of inheritance, is not always easy to produce for your edification. I might say that John had been selected for the priesthood and Mary intended for a nun. The Roman Catholic Church promptly rejected both on hearing the family history—a wise decision or not—yet there is no place for shaky hands in holy orders, where each member must be physically and mentally perfect. There is no medical treatment for the condition. A drug sufficiently powerful to stop a tremor will produce a state worse than a mere shakiness, and no drug can be taken indefinitely throughout one's lifetime.

Are tremors common, either acquired or hereditary ones? They are. There is a large class here today, but I shall not embarrass any one of you by a showing of hands. Besides, if any one of you has a tremor, it may be an acquired one from overnight carousing, and the only hereditary element might be that your granduncle was a "three-bottle" man, and one of *his* ancestors, a buck of the Regency.

Even though there should occur no increase in tempo somewhere along the course of the disease, still we cannot altogether satisfactorily answer the question of the prognoses, but the family should prepare for the worst and plan a program far ahead, and according as events progress. James, if he is industrious, may in years to come have a business of his own. He can then hire help in those divisions of the plumbing business where finer manipulations are required, and for tasks that are not based on brute force. John can continue as he is, rising to the position of a business executive, dictating all that has to be written to an efficient private secretary, who can learn even to sign his name better than he can write it. He should also learn to type, in order to anticipate conditions in which he may have to write his own correspondence and reports, possibly confidential. Mary is indeed the worst off. She is, however, still young and may elect marriage as a career, thereby avoiding the constant embarrassing supervision to which all teachers are subjected. But wedlock may be a long way off; so, in the meantime, I should advise her to learn typewriting, as her brother should, and to cultivate, by means of night classes, the finer arts of writing for publication, drawing, painting or etching, selection of textiles and design for women's clothes, and the like, for anything which gives her pleasure and helps her round out a satisfying and creative existence is all to the good. There is such a thing, I believe, as the organ-inferiority complex of Adler, wherein by reason of an infirmity we rise to accomplish greater things than we should if we were merely normal unambitious persons.

Note well that these children are already well on the way to a higher social scale than that of their parents and ancestors, including the mysterious American uncle! Even James can be included if he attains the stage of master plumber and owns his own business. At this point, my friend and his wife with their children are beaming with happiness and optimism. I have to thank them once again for coming and facing a curious and disconcerting audience. I have talked openly to you in front of them, and I see that the thought has struck home of overcoming a difficulty that has seemed to them insuperable. We can now let them go with, I trust, hope, faith, and charity in their hearts.

So sinks the day-star in the ocean bed,
And yet anon repairs his drooping head,
And tricks his beams, and with new-spangled ore
Flames in the forehead of the morning sky. . . .
—MILTON: *Lycidas.*

5

Good morning! It is cold this frosty day of midwinter. It is bitter-ly cold. I pushed my head out of my bedroom window on arising and saw a sheet of ice covering the street. Glittering, pointed, frozen daggers were hanging from the trees, threatening the heads and hearts of those who passed beneath. Farther off, a poor old cab horse was slipping and sprawling in terror, with all four feet splayed outwards, whilst his driver slashed him with a whip and yowled shouts of abuse and hopeful encouragement. The window was closed hurriedly and with a shiver.

There was no enthusiasm in me for this class this morning, but God is good, and the Devil not so bad a fellow, after all. As you see, I have succeeded in coming. Anyhow, my house was only a few degrees warmer than the frozen outdoors. I had one last thing to do before I left, however, if only to save a dynasty from extinction.

Some years ago a former student of mine sent me a little brass image from Alexandria. It is that of a deity in Royal Egypt of some three thousand years ago. Not more than six inches in height, it has the body of a man and the head of a baboon, one of the many forms of Thoth, the scrivener of the gods, who acts as secretary for the dead and guides them on their way. How old it is, no one can tell.

I took this little brass monkey-man, and wrapping him in many layers of wool, I put him with the family cat beside the fireplace.

This feline god of today, guardian of our *lares et penates,* is now also guarding this sacred manikin of ancient Egypt, and they are both certainly satisfied, since the temperature around the hearth is well above freezing point. Strangely enough, this old tabby was once called Cleopatra; she is now known as "Cleo," and she knows a lot more about things than we think she does!

This patient you are seeing this morning is suffering from that strange disease, **myasthenia gravis.** Please note her posture in bed. As an aside, I may say that every patient, whether nearly normal or seriously ill, takes up an individual position dictated by his or her personality, plus the disease suffered from. Advertisements for mattresses and bed covers exploit this fact.

This young lady is twenty-four years of age. She is sitting propped up in bed by pillows. Her right hand holds her falling jaw, and at the same time prevents her head from falling forward on her chest. She rests her elbow on her knee to act as a fulcrum. Her eyelids are drooping; the right covers the cornea, preventing all vision—the left nearly so. Ordinarily, with ptosis, the forehead wrinkles upward to overcome this drooping, but here the muscles of the frontales group are as smooth as glass. There is no marked squint, but the eye muscles do not work together. She complains of double vision. Pupillary reflexes and accommodation are normal in the two eyes.

She can not raise her hands to dress her hair, and when she elevates them almost ninety degrees, they tire rapidly and sag downward. As her chin and neck are released by these movements, the jaw drops open and the head falls down on the chest. Her tongue is weak; it can not push out her cheeks, and her palate and pharyngeal muscles work only feebly. It is because of this that her voice is weak, thick and nasal in tone. Unless she holds her head far back in swallowing—she can only do this lying down —the fluid is regurgitated through her nose.

As she is helped out of bed to walk, she has to hold her head up with one hand and with the other, pull up one eyelid in order to see. Her knees wobble under her as her quadriceps and iliopsoas muscles give way. Hurriedly, she has to be put back in bed lest she fall and injure herself.

We are giving her a piece of toast to bite on; as one would expect, she can not bite it, and because of her weak tongue and lips the morsel drops out of her mouth untouched. Now, soft pieces of bread soaked in warm milk are given her; again there is a failure in feeding her. The soft paste spreads itself over tongue, teeth and lips, only a fraction being swallowed, while most of it remains, this morsel of desperately needed food, caking up her whole buccal orifice. On checking her respirations, we find, ominously enough, that the thoracic cage has a poor excursion, the diaphragm descends but partially, and her cough is weaker than that of a kitten. It looks as if transfer to a mechanical respirator is only a matter of time. There is no atrophy of the muscles involved, no reflex changes, and no sensory loss; merely a weakness that is immediately intensified by fatigue.

I hope that you have taken fully into your mind the complete clinical picture of myasthenia gravis. It is a disease of muscles and its area of effect is situated in the neuromuscular junction. It is often most marked in the tongue, jaw, eye and neck muscles. It is less severe in the arms and lower extremities, but in each case the supporting muscles, such as the shoulder group and those of the pelvic girdle, are the most affected. Weakness in the intercostal muscles and diaphragm often ends the picture with tragic suddenness. The weakened muscles give way under the pull of gravity, and a drooping pattern is conspicuous. Certainly, the drooping of eyelids, face, jaw, head and arms is characteristic. These patients may be likened to a long-stemmed tulip raised in a hothouse, which, when brought into the home, within a few petty days wilts, its glorious head falling by degrees to the edge of the bowl. We know so little as to the cause of this disease. Pathologic changes found after death are few and are confined to mysterious infiltrations of lymphocytes between the fibers of voluntary muscles, and a persistence of the thymus gland that may undergo tumor formation.

The history of this patient is that four years ago she was attacked, more or less suddenly, by diplopia and difficulty in chewing and swallowing. One eyelid was noticeably drooped. Evidently, at that time, her condition was not a great cause for worry. She was sent to a leading neurologist who thought her problem was entirely psychologic and that she would recover. As if to prove this statement, all symptoms and signs cleared up within six weeks. Two years ago, weakness of her muscles again appéared within a short space of time. On this occasion her neck muscles and those of her shoulders were affected. She had trouble in holding up her head at the end of the day and had to sit in a high-backed chair to keep her head comfortable. She could do up her back hair in the morning without difficulty, but at evening time her arm muscles were so tired that she could not complete the arrangement of her hair for the night. In retrospect, she thinks that ever since her first attack, and even while she was apparently well, there was always present an undue fatigue with consequent muscular weakness after exertion; this was relieved by rest. Always during this first remission she was at her best in the morning. The second attack lasted about six weeks and cleared up spontaneously, leaving a slightly greater tendency toward fatigue than heretofore. At that time she gave up all her outdoor and indoor sports, but otherwise lived a normal life.

This last attack has been on her for two months. It has been severe from the start and has involved many more muscles, and particularly those essential to life. During her last remission, weakness of the muscles had yielded to rest, and there was no continuous palsy, but now her facial expression, her posture and her general appearance have altered and have remained thus continuously. Exercise merely intensifies it and brings into view the involvement of still other muscles. There is no question now that she is seriously ill, and all thought of a psychic-made disease pattern is an absurdity.

She entered the hospital early this morning, starved and dehydrated. There are signs of congestion of the bases of her lungs, and an oxygen tent is ready, but as yet she is not cyanosed. Further, a tracheotomy to clear out mucus in her bronchi has been arranged for, and it can be done at a moment's notice. This disease acts all too swiftly and is dangerous at this stage, so we must be equally swift if it is a case of saving life. While I have been talking to you academically, practical steps for resuscitation are in being. A mechanical respirator has been wheeled into the ward in case there may be need for it.

The patient is already receiving saline and glucose solution intravenously by the drip method and will continue to do so until her fluid balance is restored. Someone will ask why we do not pass a duodenal tube, since there is no obstruction, and give fluids and nourishment by this method. The answer to that is that such a tube would act as an irritant and produce more mucus to be got rid of, and the consequent gagging would further exhaust her muscles of respiration and deglutition; a vicious circle would thereby be engendered, leading possibly to sudden *exitus lethalis.* There is, however, a more efficient method of treatment whereby we may circumvent this complication, and I shall show it to you now, my gifted colleague being ready to demonstrate it. We shall see a modern miracle performed before our eyes. Watch it closely, for it will be dramatic enough to satisfy your love of strange and striking phenomena.

The patient is being given intravenously an ampule containing 1 mg. of neostigmine methylsulfate. In a few minutes, I hope, a change will occur in the whole situation at hand. While we are waiting, the theories as to the mechanism of myasthenia gravis can be outlined. The contractions of muscles are supposed to be affected by a chemical substance, acetylcholine, liberated at the motorial end plate and mediating between the nerve and muscle in producing the end result: the activation of muscle during a motor nerve impulse. Another substance, cholinesterase, destroys whatever acetylcholine remains after the contraction is effected. In myasthenia gravis there is an overabundance of cholinesterase, so that acetylcholine is removed before full contraction occurs. Subsequent attempts at contraction, with increasing fatigue, make the balance of available acetylcholine less and less, and complete loss of power ensues. Neostigmine is antagonistic to cholinesterase and renders available more and more acetylcholine. Recovery of muscle power should then occur. As we watch, this hoped-for happy result is certainly beginning to appear, for, look at the patient now!

You may remember the case of the man with the twisted lip

in the adventures of Sherlock Holmes. In this story the nimble detective with a bath sponge transformed a hideous, sullen-looking beggar into a young man with a prepossessing countenance. The same is occurring here and now. The eyelids have lifted, and with the ptosis almost gone, the face has regained expression, and the patient smiles engagingly on finding herself so much better. Her jaw is no longer pendulous, and she can clash her teeth together. Almost unconsciously she is moving her tongue to lick away the paste of bread on her lips and from her teeth, the erstwhile feeble tongue now searching into every crevice of her mouth. At last she is holding her head erect. Most gratifying of all, she can cough vigorously, and her respiratory excursion has returned to normal. See, she can raise her arms above her head and smooth her hair. She is talking normally to me and in a pleasant voice, expressing great happiness for this sudden relief.

Sister has a bowl of oatmeal porridge liberally sprinkled with sugar and covered with cream. She is about to feed the patient, when our young lady begs to take the bowl in her hands and feed herself. This she does with gusto, and rapidly shovels the strength-giving mixture into her mouth, swallowing it like one who has been starved, as indeed she has been. She tells me that the double vision is gone.

As the minutes tick by, she is becoming to all intents and purposes normal. As a last act, she is getting out of bed and taking a few steps unaided, although she is still weak from her illness. Even the expression of fear in her eyes, so far as her masked face could show it, is gone; she now feels confidence in us and a renewed hope for the future, which before she came here seemed to her to be black indeed.

Lest I build up in you too great an optimism, I have to spoil the apparently happy ending of this story by pointing out that the effect of this one injection is only temporary. Within a period of half an hour to three or four hours the effects of this agent will wear off, and she will be again as bad as she was before. However, now we can give a maintenance dose of this drug by mouth, and she can swallow it! In about half an hour from now she is to get two tablets, each containing 3 mg. of neostigmine bromide. Occasionally, atropine must be given, subcutaneously or by mouth, to offset the vomiting and diarrhea caused by the drug. This dose will be repeated every three hours for some days to come, and will be increased or decreased as the response to treatment indicates.

The hope is that we can keep her well and out of danger until a natural remission ensues. No one can tell whether this may come or how long it will last if it does come, for there are many variations in the response of patients to treatment. Some may stay well for years with or without the drug, which always must be kept as low in dosage as possible to maintain reasonable health and energy. Other patients do not do so well; the drug loses its effect, and in spite of all efforts, even the use of large doses, the patient fails to respond and is lost. As you know, I had the respirator ready and the tracheotomy arranged for, because I had no assurance that the response would be so good. Again, a patient may be in a remission, either taking no neostigmine or at least minimal doses, and seem to be doing well when, savagely and swiftly, an attack may strike, and within twelve to twenty-four hours *exitus* may occur. For that reason, the respirator will remain at hand, ready for immediate use. A physician who works with myasthenia gravis patiently must have a stout philosophy and suffer his losses bravely. Personally, I do not like this task, for I am a poor loser. One gets so attached to these patients, after taking care of them for years, that having them swept away in a few hours represents a bitter blow to one's self-esteem. It always seems as if one could have done better.

In a certain percentage of cases roentgenologic studies of the thorax (they must be technically perfect) show a thymic tumor, and many such tumors have been removed as a prospect of cure, but results to date are uncertain. Again, we may carry these patients along until nature produces a remission of indeterminable length. To date we do not speak of a "permanent cure."

In these demonstrations I try to show you instances of fully developed disease wherein there is no question as to diagnosis. If you are worth your salt you can, from now on, meeting early and fragmentary clinical syndromes, anticipate reasonably well their later and full development. This patient whom you have seen is now in her third attack. The first was so slight that it was passed by as a neurotic affair by a competent neurologist. All of us, given the picture as it was then, would have done the same. There is no history as to what the second attack was called; at any rate it was not recognized or treated as myasthenia gravis. Note the completely dissimilar appearance of the disease in those two episodes. So many patients with myasthenia gravis begin with ocular palsies and possibly a third nerve weakness on one side with ptosis and external strabismus, or *per contra*, a paralysis of the external rectus muscle.

If you take any textbook of neurology and look up causes of paralysis of the third or sixth nerve, the list will be very extensive, including among many other causes, myasthenia gravis. I have seen so many patients whose trouble started just that way, and an explanation for strabismus, diplopia and ptosis was not forthcoming. If one has a suspicious mind and tries out an injection of neostigmine, the ocular palsy will clear up almost immediately, as will facial weakness and speech difficulty, if they happen to be present. A diagnosis can then be made, obviating a long wait, over months or years, for other signs. Moreover, the patient's double vision can be relieved, and kept so by small doses of neostigmine by mouth.

One of our greatest difficulties in early diagnosis of myasthenia gravis occurs with neurasthenic individuals. I use this worn-out, old-fashioned term advisedly, and without apology to my psychiatric colleagues. There are persons who are chronically tired; they may have been born tired. In any event, they arise in the morning more fatigued and exhausted than when they went to bed. On reading, their accommodation muscles weaken and vision becomes blurred. They may call this "double vision" and lead one astray. Chewing hard objects and talking for long periods fatigue the muscles of mastication or articulation, and persons so afflicted may have to cease and rest for a while. Putting objects on a high shelf or combing their hair exhausts them, and they may have to call for assistance. Above all, their legs get weak, and they have to sit down after walking a paltry few yards.

These persons have myasthenia, but certainly not myasthenia gravis. There is at no time any actual weakness or any facial disfigurement, and their tongues wag joyously as ever, and far too long. A point to make is that they are also *mentally* tired, and after a conversation or concentration on a difficult subject, their brain processes become confused, and a rest is demanded before they can go on. At that, the physician himself gets a brain fatigue on listening to the long story of these worthy persons. An injection of neostigmine at the height of the alleged fatigue does just this—nothing. Curare, in one fifth of the pharmacologic dose by injection, does not bring out any muscular paralysis. The use of curare in such a dose is dangerous in true myasthenia gravis and the agent must be employed with extreme caution; most times it is unnecessary in the differential diagnosis but can be resorted to in a difficult case, with a syringe of neostigmine solution ready at hand in case the motor weakness gets out of control and danger signs appear.

Chronic bulbar palsy presents little difficulty in recognition, with the muscular atrophy of tongue and face, fasciculation, and the loss of the jaw jerk. Curiously enough, the muscles of mastication are seldom affected in this disease. The inability to chew and the drooping lower jaw are pathognomonic signs of myasthenia gravis.

The Landouzy-Déjèrine type of facioscapulohumeral dystrophy in adolescent patients may simulate myasthenia gravis, and worse still, certain muscular dystrophies may have an added myasthenic component. Repeated injections of neostigmine will separate in these cases the sheep from the goats. Muscular disease is as yet not entirely understood, but we are learning more and more from biopsy preparations. The electromyogram has not as yet come into the fulfillment of its promise in elucidating many of our problems of muscular disease, but there are great hopes that it will take its place along with the electrocardiogram and the electroencephalogram.

6

WE HAVE here an elderly male. He does not know when he was born, but since he anticipates his old age pension within three years, we shall put him down as being sixty-seven years old. His face in its upper right-hand part is badly scarred, and he complains of severe pain in this area of disfigurement. More specifically, the pain and scars occupy the forehead and beyond the hairline, the temple, the upper eyelid, and that part of the nose adjacent to the inner epicanthus. His cornea is so badly scarred that there is but little vision in his right eye. The scars are round, sunken and about the size of a split pea. The skin over them is acutely sensitive to touch, and yet is numb. He can not wear a hat or brush his hair because of this sensitivity, and despite this, stimuli by touch, pain, heat and cold are poorly perceived. We call this peculiar condition anesthesia dolorosa.

He describes the pain as a constant, burning, searing sensation—as if he were being scorched by a flame—accompanied by frequent shocklike pains in any part of the area involved, more severe in cold or windy weather or when the scarred area is touched. The corneal reflex is absent on the painful side. Mapping out the limits of pain and scarring, we find that the first or ophthalmic divisional area of the fifth nerve is affected; the second and third divisions have escaped. There is no motor involvement of the muscles of mastication. The patient had been in good health until this distressing malady hit him.

Six months ago his pains began suddenly, and after four days of suffering there appeared over the parts mentioned a papular rash which rapidly became vesicular. He had to receive opiates for his pain, since sleep and rest were denied to him because of it. The vesicles became infected, and he had a rise in temperature, so that, because of the red, inflamed appearance of his lesions, his physician diagnosed erysipelas and gave him penicillin, with local applications to the inflamed area, which included his eye. Because of the risk of sympathetic ophthalmia, it was thought that the eye would have to be removed. However, the inflammation died down in six weeks, and he was left with his pain, the

residual scarring and blindness in the right eye from corneal inflammation. It was hoped that his pain would then disappear,
but far from it; he undergoes almost as much suffering now as
when he was first acutely afflicted.

He describes the pain as being the same now as when it first
started, that is, a constant burning over the forehead and temple,
and deep in the eye. He also has sharp, lancinating pains coming
spontaneously, or when the forehead and contiguous parts of the
same nerve area are touched. The most severe pain is the constant burning one, but the sharp, sudden paroxysms make him
jump and groan aloud. He is in a pitiable state of misery and
has lost at least fifteen pounds. Sleep is still fitful. He has taken
analgesic agents such as aspirin and acetophenetidin, without
much effect.

This is a typical case of the residual effects of *herpes ophthal-*
micus or herpes resulting from inflammation of the ophthalmic
portion of the gasserian ganglion. It is more common in elderly
persons. Why only the ophthalmic portion of this ganglion usually
is involved is not well understood. The patient might have lost
his eye, but as it is, the eye is useless so far as sight is concerned.
Even if it were removed, pain would still persist in the socket.

The history and appearance of the disease now involve no
lengthy discussion regarding the differential diagnosis. The anatomic distribution of pain, the scars and the peculiar anesthesia
dolorosa speak for themselves. At onset, the condition may be
wrongly taken for erysipelas, and later for trigeminal neuralgia
involving the ophthalmic division of the fifth nerve, but the
clinical picture resembles neither. There is no great pain in
erysipelas and no sensory changes; in trigeminal neuralgia there is
no eruption or its aftermath of scarring, and there is not the constant pain, as there is in this condition. The paroxysmal pains
experienced when the zone involved is touched may bear a slight
resemblance to the pains of trigeminal neuralgia, but as mentioned
before, the latter are less unbearable than the constant, burning
agony experienced regardless of stimuli or motion.

Treatment here is a sad story of failure on our part to give relief. Opiates are certainly contraindicated because of rapid habit-

formation and addiction. A regius professor of Dublin University suffered from this malady until his death. When it became too intolerable, he would pick a time convenient to his colleague and medical advisor, and would walk quickly over to his office for an injection of morphine. It was strictly understood that the propriety and advisability of getting this relief were altogether the responsibility of whoever gave it. He could refuse or consent to administer the drug, and the sufferer would abide by his decision. Never was it self-administered. Further, the colleague who helped out was one equal in rank to the patient, and hence could not be browbeaten by command or influenced by undue sympathy. Minor analgesic agents are useless, and injection of the first division with alcohol, while it might relieve the pains produced by stimuli to the skin, fails because the underlying constant pain still remains.

Surgical exposure of the root of the trigeminal nerve and section of it have been tried and have failed; the constant, burning pain remains. The pain must arise at a higher level than the ganglion and its root. Possibly the descending root of the fifth cranial nerve in the medulla is involved at the time of the herpetic inflammatory process, and so-called central pain is evoked. In time the pain may lessen somewhat, but the sands of life are running out so fast that in the majority of cases the pain lasts until death comes from some other cause, and gives a merciful relief from human suffering. Many things occur in a medical history that are far worse than death, and the philosophy of old age includes a large chapter devoted to the virtues of resignation.

Do ye hear the children weeping, O my brothers,
Ere the sorrow comes with years? . . .
The child's sob in the silence curses deeper
Than the strong man in his wrath.
—ELIZABETH BARRETT BROWNING: *The Cry of the Children.*

7

Good morning! I left my car in a garage in Smithfield Haymarket to have various things done to it, and I walked the rest of the way to this hospital. There must be a grade school in the vicinity, and probably a convent school at that.

I ran into a group of little girls and boys, each carrying his satchel of books and lunch, wending in a common direction.

The little girls walked quickly and soberly along, and all the impact I made on their consciousness resulted in a few quick glances, a muffled remark or two, and then a cackle of high-pitched laughter from blushing faces suddenly withdrawn, to reach almost immediately an erstwhile sobriety and quietude of expression.

The little boys were different. They strode along, chests flung out, heads up, and singing loudly and merrily the more recent comic songs. A few caps were snatched off the heads of those in front and flung far afield with much scuffling. By and large, they were a merry crowd, with red button noses and eyes sparkling with the cold, and with primitive childish deviltry in full swing among them. As I drew abreast, a few boys separated themselves from the parent body and rushed at me with outstretched hands, demanding largesse. Always I carry a pocketful of copper coins for just such demands on the streets, and so I doled them out, as equally as was possible—enough coin of the realm to satisfy them.

The little boys scampered back to join their fellows and immediately a fight ensued. The larger boys, the bullies of the group, pounced on those whom I had just financed, and by sheer force endeavored to tear the coins away from them. Almost at once, the middle-sized boys, the rank and file, jumped on these overgrown bullies and overcame them, bearing them to the ground. Some just arrangement must have been made forthwith, for in the twinkling of an eye, peace was restored to the ranks. The boys again filed up in orderly procession and marched forward, singing joyously at the tops of their voices. . . . I should like to think that Dublin is the only European capital wherein little boys under ten years of age sing together noisily in the streets, and at the same time demonstrate an innate sense of justice.

I have noticed this morning also that these children seem to be well fed and nourished, and that their clothes, while cheap, keep out the cold. There was no child walking barefoot, a common enough sight twenty years ago, even in the stark, freezing winter cold.

I should wish that my friend, Dean Jonathan Swift of St. Patrick's Cathedral, had been with me this morning. His church and his house of the blazing red brick are just across the river from here. He would have noticed that these children, as compared with those of his time, are vastly improved as to their nourishment and well-being.

In one last explosion of savage indignation, the Dean wrote a small tract in 1729. The state of poverty, starvation and hopelessness in Ireland, his own country, led him to write a diatribe more ghastly than anyone can possibly conceive. He called it a "Modest Proposal"! The thesis was simply that since the Irish were prevented from being anything else than poverty-stricken, and still were blessed with many children, there was a corresponding remedy for this apparently insoluble problem. Let them take their younger offspring, he suggested, kill them carefully, spice them deliciously, cook them tenderly and then sell the product expensively, to be served at the tables of the high and mighty in both the capitals of London and Dublin. Naturally, no one took his proposal seriously, but as an example of biting satire and studied invective it caused some political commotion, and may have led to better social conditions.

Here is a small, unhappy-looking boy, aged eight years and three months. He is in bed and well covered up. It is not so cold but that I can have him wrapped in blankets and taken out of bed and into an armchair. This I shall do later. The clinical history is very interesting and was in some ways, earlier on, frankly misleading.

This child is the second eldest in a series of four children. His birth and earlier development were normal, and he seemed to be entirely well until two months ago. At that time, for no apparent reason, he started to vomit. The vomiting was sudden and forcible, and independent of his meals or of any activity. He would simply become pale, and without other warning, a flood of ingested food or gastric juice would gush from his mouth and nostrils. There were no other symptoms during those first three or more weeks, but he lost weight steadily and seemed also to have become weaker in a general way.

About a month before I saw him it was noticed that his gait had become staggering, and a while later that he had become clumsy and awkward in the use of his hands. He was now listless and apathetic, and more and more preferred to stay in bed. His local physician ascribed his trouble to what he called "cyclic vomiting" or "gastritis," and all other complaints and findings were put down to inanition. An intracranial tumor was not even thought of.

About two weeks before, things happened thick and fast. A squint developed, in which the left eye was drawn inward toward the root of the child's nose. His unsteadiness of gait was such that he needed considerable help in order to get around and he could not even sit alone without some support. His speech had become difficult to interpret, vision had become impaired and he complained of frequent, but momentary, attacks of blindness.

Headaches had appeared in the occipitocervical region and seemed to coexist with the vomiting. Now he would complain of a sudden, severe, early-morning headache, in both the back of his head and nape of his neck, and vomitus would shoot out until his stomach was emptied. After a few minutes, weak and exhausted, he would fall into an uneasy sleep.

Occasionally, hiccoughing would be present with the headaches and vomiting, and the nurse who looked after him mentioned that at these times his pulse at the wrist would go down to fifty beats per minute. He has been getting progressively worse up to date, and seriously so in this last week that has passed. Fluids have had to be given intravenously.

I am asking Sister and her nurses now to place this small boy patient, well wrapped in blankets, into an armchair. I must beg that this maneuver be carried out with the utmost gentleness, since sudden movement and jarring may evoke a fatal ending. As he sits in the chair, there is something so infinitely pathetic about him, and all these children who are suffering from this condition, that it tears at one's heartstrings to the point of breaking. They are usually intelligent, co-operative little ones, lovable to an infinite degree, and yet with a look of doom upon them, a doom which they seem to recognize by a subconscious intuition that is not present in children suffering from other diseases. They give the appearance of knowing their final possible fate and of simply waiting for it.

Never is there any difficulty in handling them, nor any signs of having been spoilt by their parents; they are grateful for the least attention and petty kindness, and somehow, compared with their brothers and sisters, they are the best child in the family. It is no wonder that the parents are indeed under a terrific emotional strain, and for that reason, difficult to be made to understand the tremendous responsibilities involved.

The small boy is in the chair now, but he can not sit up for any length of time, for his body lolls at various angles in the chair. His truncal muscles are in-co-ordinate. I ask him his name. It comes forth as "Al-ex-an-der Mat-thew Fitz-ger-ald" in a so-called "scanning" speech in which each syllable is sounded separately.

He has had a severe occipitocervical headache this morning, with projectile vomiting, and I do not want to start such a performance again. Besides, look at his chart made during these crises of headache and vomiting: his pulse rate drops to below sixty beats per minute, and his respirations become slow and irregular. All these suggest increased intracranial pressure which may at any time reach breaking point, and a sudden *exitus lethalis* ensue. The problem is entirely an urgent one, an emergency which must be dealt with swiftly.

Both his pupils are markedly dilated, but respond to the stimuli of light and accommodation. The fundus of the eye is easy to see. The optic nerve head is greatly swollen, up to a measurable three and four diopters of choked disk. The veins are engorged, and retinal hemorrhages are seen throughout. Just four of you students nearest the patient may look for this with the ophthalmoscope. If they are not proficient in this regard, will they please let someone else look, and not unduly prolong this examination?

The patient has, as mentioned before, paralysis of his left sixth nerve and internal strabismus due to paralysis of the external rectus muscle of that eye. This again is a sign of marked increase in intracranial pressure, wherein the sixth cranial nerve, by virtue of its long course in the base of the skull, and moreover, of its running between two large arteries, is bound to be squeezed somewhere along its path.

In the finger-to-nose test, each index finger fails to find the tip of his nose, and each is tremulous. Pronation and supination of both hands are imperfectly performed. For this phenomenon we have to invoke that horribly long word, "adiadochokinesia." Reaching for a glass of water, he overshoots or underreaches the glass, and is apt to spill its contents. He can not button his nightshirt because of this same in-co-ordination of fingers and hands, especially the upper buttons, where he can not see his fingers. There is a certain resistance to bending his head on his chest, and he holds his head stiffly and tilted toward the left side.

He has marked horizontal and vertical nystagmus in his eye movements. Experience teaches us that horizontal nystagmus may mean trouble in the inner ear, or at "end-organ" level, but the vertical component always means trouble deeper in, and involving the brain stem, that is, the medulla or pons varolii.

Sister, who acts as my stage property master, has produced a few old and cracked cups to pass around. Will you please percuss

these cups close to your ear, and using the middle finger? These
are not the fragile ceramics of the second Ming dynasty of China,
but a quick, sharp blow will bring out the typical sound of a
cracked cup struck suddenly. Do it, one at a time, and pass the
cup on to the other students. You can not hurt these cups; they
are ready for the rubbish pile.

Now we shall do the same to the patient. I want perfect silence.
Dividing the class into groups, I want just a few at a time to gather
close around, as I percuss this child's skull in the parietal and
frontal regions, just above the ear. The same sound is heard, and
moreover, there is a *feeling* of striking a rigid, globular body that
has actual cracks in it. I am asking four of our senior members to
try it. If done gently, it will not hurt the patient. This means that
before making any roentgen studies at all, we *know* that the child's
cranial sutures are widely separated. These should have been
firmly united at six years of age. . . . Here are the roentgenograms,
showing this spreading of the bones of the cranium. This again
means a severe increase in intracranial pressure in a child of this
age.

I have shown you, in the finger-to-nose test, that his upper limbs
are in-co-ordinate. In the heel-to-knee test, wherein his heel is
passed down the front of the opposite shin, there is also gross in-
co-ordination. You have heard his "scanning" speech. All this
means damage to the cerebellar hemispheres, bilateral and sym-
metrical.

Let us try his gait. You see that he walks with legs far apart,
lurching, and staggering equally to either side. His muscles are
atonic, and his knees seem ready to give under him; his head is
held stiff and tilted to one side, and now, with obvious great relief
to him, he is helped back into his chair.

One last thing, and that is the result of tickling the soles of his
feet. Both great toes go into extension, suggesting a bilateral
Babinski phenomenon, and therefore, the pyramidal tracts are also
involved.

And now, what is the interpretation of both history and the
findings? I want you to separate, in a sort of way, local damage to
the brain as compared with general disturbance inside the cra-

nium. His earlier history of vomiting, so misleading, was due to local compression and irritation of the vagus nucleus in the floor of the fourth ventricle. Later, signs of cerebellar destruction overshadowed this in his ataxia, in-co-ordination, scanning speech and adiadochokinesia. These signs suggested a midline cerebellar involvement, and being progressive, spoke for a *tumor of the vermis cerebelli, projecting into the fourth ventricle and compressing its floor.*

Evidence of blockage of the pathway of the cerebrospinal fluid, with increased intracranial pressure, is not far afield. It is characterized by paralysis of the sixth nerve, choked optic disks, cracked-pot note on tapping the skull, separation of the sutures as seen in the roentgenograms, vomiting (now from general pressure) and occipitocervical headaches. The stiff neck was produced by the jamming of the cerebellar tonsils into the foramen magnum, and the bilateral Babinski sign by general pressure, internal hydrocephalus and compression of the pyramidal tracts. To sum up, we have here a small child who has nystagmus, who staggers on walking, is clumsy in his hands and speech, and who shows signs of markedly increased intracranial pressure which is becoming rapidly worse.

The responsibility as to what should be done next to save this child's life is indeed a heavy one. First comes a review of our clinical diagnosis, and the certainty, or otherwise, on which it is based. The clinical picture is that of a rapidly growing tumor arising in, or compressing, the vermis cerebelli. There is associated intracranial hypertension and internal hydrocephalus. The lesion seems to be essentially a midline one.

Therefore, proceeding backward, what possibilities are there? The classic concept that a tumor of the frontal lobe may simulate a cerebellar one is well known, but is so rare as to be of little merit in our considerations. A tumor in the third ventricle may assault the optic nerves, and produce signs of involvement of its floor with obesity, polyuria, somnolence and fits of a diencephalic character. In this patient none of these signs are present. Tumors around the pineal gland compress the corpora quadrigemina of the midbrain, and paralyses of the third nerve occur, chiefly of origin in its connecting fibers in the brain stem. Paralysis of upward gaze and large fixed pupils are common; these, again, are lacking in this our patient here. Finally, the lesion is settled as being one invading the fourth ventricle of the brain, arising from its floor, or more likely bulging downward from its roof above the vermis cerebelli.

Inflammatory conditions such as chronic adhesive arachnoiditis of the posterior fossa and cisternal arachnoiditis come up for review. This pathologic condition may closely mimic cerebellar tumor. I see a gleam in one student's eye, and he suggests that we do a spinal puncture and examine the fluid for inflammatory signs, such as increased protein and an increase in its cellular constituents. This is a gallant question, and gallantly will I answer it. The rigidity of this child's neck suggests that part of the cerebellum (the tonsil) and medulla already have herniated through the foramen magnum. Simple spinal puncture would suck more of these vital structures downward. Within a short time after the puncture, the child's breathing would cease, and the pulse, getting slower and slower, would run finally to a thready end. The child would then be dead, dead, dead. And you, my friend, would be the executioner, never to forget it all your life, and never, never to do it again. In any case of increased intracranial pressure spinal puncture is contraindicated, unless in an operating room with a surgeon ready to tap the ventricles and decompress the zone of herniation. Usually, the surgeon prefers to tap the ventricles first and *not* do a spinal puncture.

A neurosurgeon is to see this child after this class is over. He probably will act as if this patient's trouble is one of emergency, which it is. Accordingly, as he sees fit, he may do a ventriculogram with roentgen studies to fix as clearly as possible the site of this malignant process, and anything else he may find. Actually, I think he will elect to explore the cerebellum and fourth ventricle directly, and assure wide decompression to relieve this tension inside the cranium that is threatening this little boy's life. What he finds, and what he can do with safety, will be the last answer to our problem.

As I remember, thirty years ago the mortality rate of surgical operations in this area was shocking. This is not the case today. Now, a generation later, results are vastly more satisfying. Having surveyed the field, the surgeon may do one of two things. He may attempt mass removal, amputating large areas of the cerebellum. (It is amazing how little incapacity results.) This is in the case of benign astrocytomas, with or without formation of cysts. The more malignant medulloblastomas he may remove as completely as he can, and he is not afraid of ependymomas arising from the floor of the fourth ventricle. They are benign, but certainly have their nests in and over the most vital portions of the brain. Many patients are given a course of roentgen therapy after surgery, corresponding in degree to the character of the tumor cells.

Occasionally, however, the surgeon may feel that he is licked, and after decompression and exploration he may close up the wound and resort to roentgen therapy without touching the tumor. The days of nibbling at and hen-scratching of tumors of the brain are ended. The dictum now is to get in, remove all one can with safety, taking serious risks, or do nothing and get out, leaving wide decompression and roentgen therapy to do what *they* can to alleviate and slow up the progress of the tumor.

NOTE: The child was operated on in the afternoon of the day I presented him to my class. His ventricles were tapped, and the pressure of the cerebrospinal fluid showed markedly increased intracranial pressure. Wide decompression was achieved, demonstrating the whole of the superior surface of the cerebellum. The cisterna magnum was opened and a large tumor was found, bulging into the fourth ventricle, arising from the vermis cerebelli, and not attached to the ventricular floor. The vermis and at least one half of each cerebellar lobe were removed *in toto* with the tumor. The gross specimen showed many cysts in the tumor, but no single large one. The diagnosis of the pathologist was that the tumor was an astrocytoma of low-grade cellular growth.

Convalescence was uneventful. The child was alive and active in a normal life five years later. At that time there was visible only slight ataxia of gait and of arm movements, such that his handwriting was poor and irregular, and he could not play games requiring speed and precision.

The final rapid course of his illness at the time we saw the child was assumed to be that the tumor had been growing silently until such time when, by its relatively large size, it suddenly caused occlusion of the fourth ventricle and aqueduct of Sylvius. The final notes bring out the point that no one can be sure about the character and size of intracranial lesions before exploration and direct visual assessment, with examination of those tumors by a skilled pathologist, are performed.

8

MAY I introduce this lady to the class? She has only one thing wrong with her, but it so exemplifies anatomic and physiologic principles, not to mention results of a certain type of injury, that it is an exquisite little jewel of a rare clinical observation. She is an expert golfer, or was, I should say, up to six days ago. She had been trying to improve her handicap on a particular day, so that when she found herself well ahead in her score she was determined to go one better.

There was a long and easy-looking drive ahead. She smote the ball with every ounce of such vigor as she had in her delicate frame. Three things happened simultaneously: (1) she missed the ball; (2) she broke the golf club near its head; (3) she felt a sudden and sharp pain around her right shoulder blade. She flounced off the golf course in rage, frustration and pain, vowing that she would never play again. That evening, the anger and sense of inferiority had already diminished, but the pain remained, and continued for three days. She fulfilled her oath, in that she has not played golf since.

The pain was gone by the fourth day, and that evening she and her husband were dressing for a dinner party. She was sitting in front of her mirror, doing her hair, and she noticed that to do the back curls higher up on the right side of her head was a very difficult project. Her husband came into her room at about that time and found her without her dress, and struggling with her hair arrangement. He made some facetious remark about her budding angel's wings. They both then discovered that the vertebral border of her right scapula was unduly prominent, and that when she put her hand out to straighten the mirror it was even more so. She then remembered how hard it had been to replace a heavy book on the top shelf of her library shelves the day before, and moreover, she had had to use her left hand to help her right to do so. I saw her the next day, and realizing the interest of this clinical material, I begged her to come this morning and let you see her shoulder blade, six days after her tragic Waterloo on the local golf course.

With the patient undressed to the waist, and draped in front, we can see all there is to see. With her arms resting on her lap, there is very little to notice, except that the right scapula is somewhat "winged." But now, with her arms abducted horizontally to ninety degrees, this "winging" disappears, and the vertebral border of the scapula is drawn nearer the midline than its opposite member. Now let her swing her abducted arms forward, with the palms of the hands facing each other. The "winging" becomes suddenly so marked that my whole hand can be placed between the scapula and the thoracic wall. I am having her push forward one of my hands with her right arm, as in shutting a door. Evident weakness is shown in this movement, and the scapula sticks out even more markedly. The inferior angle tends to swing slightly upward and inward, but the gross prominence of the vertebral edge of the scapula is the outstanding feature.

I am asking her to raise her arms above her head. She reaches the ninety degrees of abduction horizontally, and then tries to swing forward and upward with her right arm. She fails to reach any higher level. The deltoid and trapezius muscles have done their part, but a scapula poorly fixed to the thoracic wall is against any further degree of elevation.

In a good light, the digitations of the serratus magnus muscle in a spare person can be readily seen when he attempts to push against a heavy object. When this patient pushes a door shut against resistance, we can see them well on the left. On the right, there is not a flicker of these muscular fingers attached to the ribs, and the door remains open, even though weakly held against her.

The long thoracic nerve of Bell arises from the fifth, sixth and seventh cervical nerve roots close to where they emerge from the intervertebral foramina and before the brachial plexus is formed. The nerve pierces the medial scalenus muscle and enters the axilla, where it is the sole motor supply of the serratus magnus muscle. It has no sensory fibers. Each digitation of the serratus magnus is supplied by an individual nerve fiber from the long thoracic nerve. Hence, following injury, nerve grafting is unsuccessful, unless the parent trunk is found.

The functions of the serratus magnus muscle are chiefly those that keep the scapula plastered to the thoracic wall, and let the trapezius and deltoid muscles carry on freely with a scapula behaving itself and staying where it should. Sir Charles Bell also classified the serratus magnus as being one of those muscles accessory to forced respiration. Hence the word "respiratory" is often included in the term, "the long thoracic nerve of Bell." Length means vulnerability; therefore the long thoracic nerve is the more easily injured, as are the sixth intracranial nerve and the sciatic.

I think we have seen all that this gentle and kind lady has to show us in regard to her recent injury. Accordingly, now we can excuse her. I am to watch the course of this problem each week, until regeneration does or does not occur!

The long thoracic nerve is injured or damaged in a variety of ways, some obvious, others less so. Penetrating wounds in the supraclavicular fossa, direct blows over the shoulder and heavy burdens carried on the back and shoulder present no difficulties in their recognition as a cause. In amputation of the breast, the upper extremity may be very much overabducted to allow greater room for the surgeon to work. Muscles flaccid during general anesthesia may allow the arm to go so far as to tear the long thoracic nerve. Postoperative paralysis of the serratus magnus muscle is not an unusual complication after this kind of surgery, and it is very humiliating to the surgeon.

Below the clavicle, the nerve is well protected by the overlying scapula. I have seen, however, a seasick immigrant who found, a few days after arrival in New York, that he had paralysis of the serratus magnus muscle. During the seven days at sea, he had been so sick that he had slept day and night on a wooden and iron deck seat. He had lain on the same side constantly, with his arm under his head for a pillow. I had always assumed that his nerve was directly compressed by the seat, but now I can more readily assume that it was torn or stretched by hyperabduction of the arm. With respect to another patient, he and several other men were lifting a telephone pole, when the other men suddenly let go their hold. This heavy object, falling down, nearly tore the patient's arm out of his shoulder socket, and shortly thereafter paralysis of the serratus magnus muscle was noticed. The method of damage must be similar to what happened to the patient you have seen here this morning. By virtue of sudden wrenching of the shoulder joint, a tear occurs in the long, frail nerve.

Infections in the subscapular bursa may produce mononeuritis in the long thoracic nerve, or this nerve may, with other nerves, be affected by some acute infectious process around the shoulder joint. In these cases, the long thoracic nerve is the hardest hit, and while taking the longest time to recover, it carries a greater amount of permanent residual damage.

There is but little difficulty in the differential diagnosis. A preceding injury and a winged scapula, with inability to push forward the shoulder and arm, or to raise the arm above the head, are typical signs. Lesions of the spinal accessory nerve may cause winging of the shoulder blade. There is usually, however, concomitant weakness of the sternocleidomastoid muscle. The main weakness is shown in raising the shoulder to the corresponding ear, and when atrophy occurs, the smooth curve of the trapezius muscle is replaced by an angular outline. On the patient's shrugging the shoulders, the bulk of the trapezius between one's finger and thumb can be felt to be greatly diminished. Weakness and winging of the scapula in abduction are maximal on a horizontal plane in paralysis of the trapezius, and less on forward extension of the arms. The reverse occurs in paralysis of the serratus magnus. Anyhow, winging of the scapula is always greater in lesions of the long thoracic nerve.

Naturally, the first, second and last question my lady patient asked me yesterday was in regard to her future ability to play golf. The emotional effect of the prognosis of any disease depends on what the patient wants to do, be it ever so great or ever so small. I thought of plasterers, of painters, and of tic-tac men who signal the odds at a race meeting, with arms raised above the crowds. The power of elevation above the head of one or both arms is limited indefinitely in this nerve lesion.

I thought of a priest friend and patient of mine who could not elevate the Host without using one hand to grasp it and the other to seize that hand by the wrist, and then to raise the chalice by combined effort of both arms unequally paralyzed. There is often a compensatory horsetrading between muscles that usually do things and those that simply fix and hold. Some vestigial straplike muscles, such as the levator scapulae, may hypertrophy enormously and take over a partial share of the functions of the trapezius when the spinal accessory nerve has been cut accidentally or deliberately.

I told our patient in the end that she could play golf if it meant only the putting of the small white balls into holes just a little larger. As to the wild, free swing of her club, propelling the ball many feet or yards away down long avenues of green springy turf, time alone would tell. I said that a year was the least time in which one could envisage her permanent situation. With a scapula failing to act as a *point d'appui* for all the muscles attached to it, and shamelessly slithering all over the thoracic cage like a neophyte on roller skates, I could see no good golf in the immediate offing.

I recommended endless placing of books on shelves at a height above her chin, her eyes, or even above her head. During the winter and summer she should indulge in croquet, in swimming, and in fishing, of the kind that Izaak Walton lauded: for every ounce of fish, a ton of philosophy, and the smaller the fish, the more delicate its white flesh. She might even learn to bowl, shoot dice, and aye, pick up the money that she has won. Almost her greatest grief that I can see is that, on putting on a new dress, her husband will perforce have to help it over her shoulders, holding up meanwhile her right arm. But then, she will *have* a new dress, and as always, a solicitous husband. What more can a woman want? She has already a flock of adorable, affectionate children!

And what is golf? A selfish, irritating, exacting and frustrating game. The broken club, with its head lying in the hole she dug in that final fierce stroke, was symbolic of the act of an all-seeing Providence who has so ordered her nerve injury that it has removed her temporarily, if not permanently, from a situation as bad for her body as it was for her soul. There will be no more golf for this lady, and methinks it were better so. Perhaps subconsciously, knowing her limitations, she wants it so!

FEBRUARY

Now conscience wakes despair
That slumber'd,—wakes the bitter memory
Of what he was, what is, and what must be
Worse.
—JOHN MILTON: *Paradise Lost*, Book IV.

1

Good morning! What a foul winter day with its gusty squalls of wind and rain! As I came up the driveway I saw a line of patients waiting to see the physician of the Out-Patient Section. Each one clutched a red card and an empty medicine bottle, as if they were talismans to life eternal. Poor souls, what a feeble, shuffling line of prematurely aged, ill-fed, overworked, crippled, gnarled and discouraged creatures they seemed to be! My heart fell and a sense of frustration overpowered me. In private practice one sees chronic hopeless problems, but not to the same degree as in a City Hospital. Here, the end results of toil, starvation, vice and evil circumstance call for all your pity and commiseration. Let us for that reason then be nearer to God, and if mundanely possible, twice as charitable. With better social conditions this blight may pass from our land. I profoundly hope so.

In the following three clinical discussions we shall be dealing with a group of what are called "degenerative diseases of the nervous system." A stickler for clear and concise definition will ask, "What is 'degeneration of the nervous system'? How is it caused?" Referring to Webster, I find that degeneration is "A deterioration of a tissue in which its vitality is diminished." This is certainly no answer as to cause and effect. Hughlings Jackson, the philosopher-neurologist, wrote a learned discussion on the degeneration and regeneration of the nervous system. Like many

151

of his published works, this essay was comparable to "the peace of God that passeth all understanding." The term *degeneration* is a sop to the Cerberus who guards our ignorance. That ugly word indicates an irreversible process and is a negation to all progress in regard to treatment and cure.

Men become bald because their hair follicles die. In heredo-familial disease nerve cells and fibers simply disappear; yet it was only yesterday that the term "subacute combined degeneration of the spinal cord" was used. In its early stages this condition is now curable and not an irreversible phenomenon. Let us then keep an open mind on all matters dealing with "degeneration." There is, of course, the one real and inevitable process, and that is our journey along the path to the grave. It has to come sometime, since human flesh and blood have their limitations in time. In that regard I can not forget the lines written by that brave and resolute Elizabethan, Sir Walter Raleigh, in his *Bible* the night before he was executed:

> *Even such is Time, that takes in trust*
> *Our youth, our joys, our all we have,*
> *And pays us but with earth and dust;*
>
> . . . .
>
> *But from this earth, this grave, this dust,*
> *My God shall raise me up, I trust.*

I sincerely hope that, as in other diseases of the central nervous system, we may advance with respect to treatment and possible cure in what I am going to show you anon. Vitamin E gave a certain promise a few years ago, but the human hope of success died in its infancy. At this present date we must face the fact that we have so little in the line of help for these unfortunate, doomed sufferers. There is always that intolerable sense of frustration that I felt this morning on seeing the line of broken-down wrecks of humanity who will go home later with their medicine bottles filled with useless colored trash, hoping against hope. Not all of them are such fools, however; there are certainly realists of the first order amongst them. If there is any deception perpetrated, it is for the sake of their beloved family, who insist that they are getting better and better.

Our patient is a man whose given age is fifty-five, although he looks far older. His face is emaciated and expressionless, the face that has been called "the frozen mask of horror." Only his eyes seem to be alive, and they move around as if begging for help and succor. As a contrast to the lack of expression in the rest of his face, there is in these eyes a look of impending doom. His body is wretchedly thin, as if through chronic starvation; no doubt he *is* starved, since he can hardly swallow enough to keep him alive, and this failure of deglutition is becoming slowly but remorselessly more marked. His very life is being threatened, and this is no idle threat.

Generally speaking, his symptoms are few but serious. They consist of paralysis of muscles working his face, tongue and throat. He can not control his lips, so that saliva trickles out of his mouth, and he must carry a rag in his hand to sop it up. He can not close his eyes; when he tries to do so, the white of the conjunctiva shows up grimly. His speech is indistinct, and although what he says is intelligent, it sounds as if his mouth were full of mashed potatoes. There is no aphasia; what our ear can catch in terms of spoken words is to the point.

The most distressing and ominous complaint is that he can not swallow anything but soft food. If he tries to drink a glass of water, it first trickles through his nose; later it reaches the glottis and he strangles on it, coughing and spluttering. A pitifully small moiety reaches his stomach, where it is obviously needed, since his skin is as dry as old parchment. At night, as saliva pours into his windpipe, he starts to strangle, and racked with useless coughing, he awakens in terror of suffocation. All these symptoms have been present for six months or more, and he is failing in health because of chronic starvation, increasing weakness and loss of sleep.

Having heard his symptoms, we can now understand the horrible mask of a face he bears and read truly the expression in his eyes. His face, like his tongue and throat, is paralyzed. He can not blow out his cheeks, for the slightest tap of our fingers breaks the tension of the purselike muscles around his mouth. His tongue is a shrunken, useless organ, lying inept on the floor of his mouth; it seems like a bag of worms, for there is a constant fasciculation in its muscles. He can not push out his cheeks with it or lick his upper lip. The muscles around the mouth show the same fasciculations.

As to his throat, there is no movement of his palate on phonation, and on gagging, the curtains of the pharynx remain immobile. A tongue blade stimulating the oral part of the pharynx produces no reflex contraction. There is no pharyngeal reflex. The saliva which can not be swallowed and can not be retained by the weak mouth muscles pours out on the floor when his head is bent, or into the soaked rag he holds under his mouth. Tapping his lower jaw produces no response; the jaw jerk, usually not so active normally, is definitely absent in this disease.

In the simple classic functional nomenclature of our forefathers in medicine, our unfortunate patient has what was called "labioglossopharyngeal palsy." Anatomically expressed in terms of a specific anatomic lesion, it was later called *"chronic bulbar palsy,"* indicating that the damage is situated in the bulbar nuclei subserving facial movements, articulation and swallowing. The "medulla oblongata" and the "bulb" are synonymous anatomic terms.

As far as our present knowledge can tell us, death is inevitable here. Postmortem studies show simply a disappearance of nuclei in the medulla and "ghost cells" of those remaining. There is no evidence of inflammation or tissue reaction to noxious stimuli—no evidence of circulatory failure. Like the hair follicles of a man going bald, these vital cell structures, essential as far as life is concerned, simply disappear and give up the ghost. Up to date there is no treatment of any value, and speedy death is hoped for as a result of inhalation pneumonia rather than by a process of slow starvation, more dreadful still. Occasionally, these patients just die for no clear reason, as in the case of acute bulbar poliomyelitis, where the reticular formation of the medulla is attacked. The medulla oblongata and pons represent a crowded area of vital structures and do not suffer disease gladly. Chronic bulbar palsy is the first of our series of chronic motorial diseases of the brain and spinal cord that I am going to show you. Humanely speaking, one feels that it is the worst, and yet in one way not the worst, for the end of all suffering comes quickly.

2

THIS LAST PATIENT you saw had a destruction of the motor nuclei of the seventh, ninth, tenth and twelfth cranial nerves. The eleventh was but little involved, because a large part originates in the spinal cord but not in the bulb or medulla. From the fifth cranial nerves upward and their nuclei there was an escape. It seems that the disease of chronic bulbar palsy has a selective action on the lower motor nuclei of the brain stem. Chewing is therefore seldom affected, a point of differential diagnosis from myasthenia gravis. It is possible that the functions of swallowing are so vital that the patient dies before further upward progress of disease in the brain stem has time to occur.

Below the foramen magnum and in the spinal cord are the anterior horn cells, entirely analogous to the motor bulbar nuclei. The disease of destruction of motor cells may strike there in a similar chronic fashion and progress equally and remorselessly to death from respiratory paralysis or pneumonia. Clinically, the picture with respect to this second patient seems to be entirely dissimilar to the first, but in other instances and given enough time, each may merge into the other by degrees, one passing upward, the other downward. The former is the more common, since chronic bulbar palsy kills more quickly.

This man is sixty years of age. He has worked hard all his life and looks it. Five years ago he had noticed that the muscles in his hands were shrinking and that hollows were appearing between the carpal bones. In the fleshy portion of his thumb and ulnar side of his hand a similar progressive atrophy was taking place. He noticed fasciculations wherein the muscles would suddenly dimple and a few fibers twitch. At times this produced a jerking of his fingers. These processes of wasting and fasciculation were present equally in the two hands.

He is a mechanic by trade, and some months after the onset of his symptoms a clumsiness appeared in his hands, so that he could not manipulate a wrench or make finer movements at his bench. Occasionally, when the hands were used forcibly, the muscles would cramp. The atrophy and weakness gradually increased, and after two years he noticed that his forearms were also involved. There was no pain, numbness or sensory changes of any kind: this has been carefully inquired into. The fasciculations had now spread to involve hands, forearms, arms and shoulders. He was not altogether conscious of them, but in a mirror he could see these little dimpling, flashlike changes in the bellies of the larger muscles. His trouble has now reached such a stage that for the last year his hands and arms have been useless. He can no longer work, dress or feed himself, but as yet his speech and deglutition are unimpaired.

When he is undressed, the appearance of his upper extremities is by no means a pretty one. His arms hang uselessly dangling, and a pair of hands flapping idly by his sides are mere appendages of inaction. The muscles in his hands are shrunken so that they are flat like paddles. Normally, and even at rest, the hands have a curve of semicontraction. These hands here have been described as those of an ape, shapeless, and without those delightful contours that our artists delight in and find so difficult to paint. Sir Charles Bell, the Edinburgh surgeon, spent many hours drawing hands; next to faces, they were his chief hobby.

There is in our patient complete paralysis of the hands and forearms now, the muscles there are gone, and note, there are no fasciculations to be seen below the elbows. There is some slight use of the upper arms and shoulders, and in the latter, fasciculations are abundant. The neck movements and intercostal contractions are preserved. Further search for fasciculations shows them in every muscle of the body, and ominously enough, the patient's tongue, while still active, shows these rapid tiny contractions. They are also present, although to a lesser degree, in the muscles of the face. All sensory functions are present and active. The tendon reflexes of the upper extremities are gone; the lower tendon reflexes are active but not exaggerated. Babinski's sign of dorsi extension of the great toe is absent. Stimulation of the sole shows a normal plantar response. The autonomic or vegetative system seems to be unimpaired.

This, then, is an instance of *advanced progressive muscular atrophy.* The public calls it "creeping paralysis." Although this term covers a multitude of human ailments, it is correct here in its expression of what is going on and of what will continue to happen.

The differential diagnosis is not difficult, except, of course, in the early stages. Absence of all sensory changes, the reflex loss, the age of the patient and the symmetry of involvement are obvious signposts. Peripheral neuritis is excluded because of sensory changes being absent. Involvement of the small muscles of the hand in only one limb is unusual, but again, careful search for sensory changes, objective and subjective, must be instituted. The diagnosis of "progressive muscular atrophy" is too often made in progressive lesions of the ulnar nerve, due to damage to it by an arthritis or an old fracture of the elbow joint.

Chronic inflammatory processes affecting the muscles of the shoulder girdles with or without associated skin involvement are the most difficult problems in a differential diagnosis. Pain, occasional bursts of fever, elevation of the sedimentation rate, tender muscles, and the feel of both the muscles and skin help out considerably in the problem. In recent years electric myographic studies are helping more and more.

The prognosis and treatment remain as they were in the time of Charcot: bad for the former, and entirely wanting for the latter. Death usually occurs as a result of respiratory paralysis, or, as in the disease which ascends to involve the nuclei of deglutition and respiratory mechanisms in the medulla or bulb, it is a silent and quiet affair.

Which way shall I fly
Infinite wrath and infinite despair?
Which way I fly is hell; myself am hell;
And, in the lowest deep, a lower deep
Still threat'ning to devour me opens wide,
To which the hell I suffer seems a heaven.
—JOHN MILTON: *Paradise Lost,* Book IV.

3

Good morning! Again I am late. This time my path was crossed by a funeral cortege on its way to the cemetery of many of our heroes. The hearse was drawn by two draped black spavined nags, but on their heads were plumes of white, showing that it was a child who had failed to survive a promise of earthly endeavor and had died pure and without blemish. I wish we might all claim this privilege. Funerals are such a pleasure to the poorer classes here. In this procession of shiny black horse-drawn coaches the elders sat back and enjoyed themselves in an unaccustomed grandeur, and the children leaned out the windows, with sticky, dirty faces, sucking lollipops. And why not? Death should be to all parties concerned a happy event. It is at least final.

We were on a difficult trail these few lectures past, and those to come will be worse; therefore, now we must proceed carefully, as the Chinese proverb says, "softly, softly catchee monkey." Crossing the *pons asinorum* of all clinical neurology there is fear that by chance we may go reeling into the whirling, stinking river of confusion blended in equal parts with frustration.

You have already seen two patients with progressive destruction of the bulbar nuclei on the one hand, and on the other the quite analogous demise of the anterior horn cells of the spinal cord. From the anatomic standpoint these disease processes are simple

158

and easy to understand, and straight is the pathway of resultant clinical signs and symptoms. What I am showing today is something similar to what you have already seen, except that something now has been added. The additional factor still stays within the realm of the great voluntary motorial system of the brain and spinal cord. Need I remind you that there is such a thing as a pyramidal tract and its cells of origin in the motor cortex?

This patient is a woman aged fifty-seven. She complains that her legs are stiff, that they drag in walking, and that her ability to get from place to place is becoming increasingly slower and more arduous. Both lower limbs are equally affected. Her hands have become weak, so that she can not do her housework, particularly the small, rapid movements such as beating up eggs. She has trouble in wringing out her washing, and her hands are shrinking in the volume of their muscles. She has also noticed twitching in these muscles and those of her arms. She states that her speech has become indistinct, and it is getting hard for her to swallow food, especially dry morsels. Liquids strangle her if too suddenly imbibed. She has been wont to cry and laugh easily, although no great emotional factor has appeared. All this has been going on now for three years. As her symptoms have been given from the feet upward, so should proceed our course of examination.

Her gait is stiff, clumsy and slow. She pushes her feet along the ground, wearing out the toes of her shoes. When she is seated, the movements of her toes and feet are also slow and stiff; she can barely wriggle her toes. Feeling the passive pull of her leg musculature, there is a resistance to shaking her feet that can only be called "spastic." Correspondingly, with this increase in tone there is an explosive character to her tendon reflexes, and ankle clonus is present. Babinski's sign on plantar stimulation is also present; the great toe unequivocally rises upward forcibly. Corroborative reflexes indicating disease of the pyramidal tract are present and too numerous to mention. They are of value only as corroboration, or in the rare instances when the great toes have been amputated earlier on. It seems that every neurologist who makes a bid for fame now and in posterity describes a new sign

built around the foot of a spastic paraplegic person. Someone outlined these signs with a diagram of arrows pointing to parts of the
foot stimulated; on the opposite page was depicted a fat, par-
turient sow surrounded by a large brood, all sucking vigorously!
There are a few fasciculations to be seen in the spastic muscles,
particularly of the calf. The muscles are weak but not markedly
so; the disability is more from the spastic interference in function.
There is no atrophy of the leg muscles.

As we come to the arms we are reminded of our second patient
whom we saw at the last clinical lecture. The small muscles of
the hands are atrophied, the forearms less so; but both areas show
weakness and fasciculations galore. This patient's upper arms and
shoulders are nearly normal, but again, fasciculations are plentiful.
There is added, however, an element of spasticity. The wriggling
of her fingers, in so far as there is movement present, is slow and
stiff. The tendon reflexes are exaggerated, and Hoffmann's sign
is present. This is such that flicking the middle finger with the
hand partly closed produces a grasping response. We have here a
combination of upper and lower motor lesions, about equal in
caliber.

Her speech is indistinct; it is a grating, forced, labored enuncia-
tion quite different from the mush-in-mouth speech of a patient
who has chronic bulbar palsy. The jaw jerk is present and overactive. Most important of all is that if I stroke her lips or her hard
palate with a flat wooden blade, her lips pout like those of a baby
reaching for the nipple of a feeding bottle. These are primitive
sucking reflexes which indicate that the supranuclear pyramidal
pathways to the medullary nuclei have been damaged. The movements of her tongue are slow, but not so weak as they are spastic.
There are definite atrophy and fasciculation in that organ. The
pharyngeal and palatal muscles are slow and stiff in movement, as
when the patient is asked to phonate. The face is not greatly
affected. She can close her eyes readily and surely, but movements of her mouth are slow and insecure. She laughs and cries
without any antecedent emotion or cause. As it does in a patient
with chronic bulbar palsy, the saliva drools from her mouth.

And what are the anatomic factors involved here? As mentioned before, she has many of the signs and symptoms of our last two patients, but with something added. This addition is in the form of evidence of damage to the pyramidal tracts. These are the upper motor pathways ending in the nuclei of the medulla and in the cells of the anterior horns of the spinal cord. Somewhere from the Betz cells of the motor cortex of the brain to the medulla, and far down to the last anterior horn cell of the spinal cord, interruption of voluntary motor activity is increasingly making itself evident. The simple clinical pictures of our last two patients have been modified. This change should not be difficult for you to understand if you know your anatomy and physiology of the nervous system. If the principles of upper and lower motor lesions have been pounded into you, all should be well. In this our patient there is merely a combination of the two principles involved. Damage occurs simultaneously but in different degrees. Please think all this over now and hereafter.

The relative speed of the effects of damage to upper and motor neuronic structures counts heavily in the clinical picture in a given patient at a given time. Given a spastic condition of the upper limbs, the tendon reflexes will be exaggerated and tone increased. If the damage to anterior horn cell structures catches up with this, spasticity becomes flaccidity and reflexes become abolished. The reverse does not hold true, since once damage to the final pathway from anterior horn cell to muscle is complete, later damage to the pyramidal tracts has no influence whatever. Generally speaking, the clinical picture is a combination of two processes, confusing to the utmost to a neophyte, but not so hard to comprehend if the problem is thought out carefully and with anatomic understanding, step by step.

This patient is suffering from *amyotrophic lateral sclerosis.* The effects of damage to her upper and lower motor neuron pathways have fluctuated year by year and will continue to do so until the final resultant picture of damage to the two motorial systems in brain and spinal cord is such that existence is no longer possible.

The differential diagnosis is not difficult. The morbid process is so selective that if any sensory changes appear one must stop, look and listen. A tumor in the upper and middle medullary parenchyma might lead us astray, but pain in the neck and occiput with sensory findings in the skin, for pain, thermal and tactile changes, would change our viewpoint. Periodically, syphilis has been invoked as a cause, but this is academic, for antisyphilitic therapy has no effect and is not a deciding factor. In the main, however, this is a serious disease, common and widely spread amongst the population. It is familial and endemic on the island of Guam in the Pacific.

Such a diagnosis as amyotrophic lateral sclerosis means helplessness, despair and ultimate death. When the condition is early, therefore, let this diagnosis not be given without long observation, frequent consultation with senior and well-established colleagues, and above all, let there be that ever-present question given to ourselves, "Could this be something else?"

4

THIS PATIENT is the fourth member of our group of progressive and specific lesions to the spinal and bulbar mechanisms of voluntary muscular activity. As usual he is in the last decades of life, and his age is just sixty-three. His chief complaint is that there has been a gradual loss of articulate speech and difficulty in swallowing. Like our first patient of last week and of this one, he carries a handkerchief to mop up the continual flow of saliva, and it is becoming rapidly soaked.

Six months ago he found that he could not speak clearly to his staff and that the dictation of his correspondence was becoming increasingly difficult. This is serious for him, since he is a successful business man who all his life has sought to buy cheaply and sell dear, and so far he has accomplished this apparently simple process in which so many, particularly physicians, fail.

Added to his difficulties with speech, he had found it increasingly difficult to swallow, and he just about subsists on a diet of mashed potatoes, eggs, minced meat and jellies. He has many sons and daughters who would have him well, but nevertheless his trouble is slowly getting worse, and both he and the family are becoming desperate. An added and sad factor is that he is a man who for years has been celebrated for his gift of speech at any formal occasion or in a hot debate. Additionally, at the banquets where he had, like a dog, to speak for his dinner, he emulated that faithful dumb brute by eating all before him. Like Caesar, but yesterday his word might have stood against the world, and now there is none so poor to do him reverence.

I feel very sorry for this poor little man, deprived of the two things he has loved the most. It seems that in our later years we fail in that which we have used not wisely but too well. The heart of a physician is torn so many times by anxiety, worry and solicitude about his patients that it is the first organ to give way. Coronary sclerosis and thrombosis are professional diseases amongst physicians and they are increasing in recent years.

Since the presenting complaints in this patient are comprised of dysarthria and dysphagia, let us first examine his tongue and throat mechanisms. It is noteworthy that in the resting phase of these organs there is but little to see. The tongue is full and rounded; there is no atrophy and fasciculations are scant. The palate and pharynx look normal, and the facial muscles are not wasted. In action, however, the picture is different.

His speech is slow, rasping, labored, and each word is prolonged. It is dominant in lower tones and hardly intelligible. It is like the stiff gait of a spastic paraparetic patient moving with might and main but progressing ineffectually under heavy internal difficulties. He can protrude his tongue partly, but wiggling it to and fro is slow almost to the point of extinction. He can not push his cheeks out. Movement of the palate and larynx is slowly and only partially performed. Under laryngoscopic examination the vocal cords get together but slowly, and his hypopharynx is full of mucus. As a contrast, the jaw jerk is tremendously overactive, and sucking reflexes are present and easily demonstrable by stimulation of the palate or lips with a wooden tongue blade. He can chew well, but the movements are slow. The food thereafter is swallowed with difficulty and chokes him at times. Liquids do not go through his nose, but gag him in their downward course to the esophagus.

Further examination shows that the functions of all the other cranial nerves are normal. He has no trouble with his arms or legs, and generally speaking, the rest of his central nervous system is normal. The tendon reflexes are active and brusque, but as yet the plantar responses to stimulation of the sole of the foot are flexor. To sum up, this man has a disturbance in the functions of the muscles supplied by the nuclei of the bulb or medulla oblongata, but it is far different in clinical characteristics to that shown by our earlier patient whose condition we diagnosed as chronic bulbar palsy.

Our revered defunct ancestors in neurology were acquainted with such conditions which, to their virginal minds, were examples of "chronic bulbar palsy" but here there was not at all the same clinical picture. There was no atrophy of the tongue, fasciculations were few and far between, the speech was very different, and above all, the jaw jerk was not abolished but actually was exaggerated. And yet these poor patients could not articulate or swallow, and died the same way as did those with chronic bulbar palsy.

Our predecessors did not know their anatomy of the central system so well as you modern privileged students, and accordingly the horrible, confusing name of *"pseudobulbar palsy"* was coined! There was no falsity about the paralysis, but it was *not* of medullary origin. It was palsy, certainly, but not bulbar in origin, and so that name has persisted, one of the many to confuse medical students, and we would wish most heartily that it were never used.

This disease that you are seeing now was called, as I have said, for want of a better name, pseudobulbar palsy. There is no such thing as a "pseudoparalysis": the patient is paralyzed or he is not. The same clinical affliction is reached by the same disease, but a higher level is attacked than that in chronic bulbar palsy. Instead of the bulbar nuclei, the pyramidal tracts from the motor cortex are here affected; hence lack of atrophy, exaggerated jaw jerks, and the sucking reflexes directly analogous to Hoffmann's sign in the hand and Babinski's sign in the foot. The only difference in this disease as compared to those in the group we are following is that it may occur, nonspecifically, in the cerebral palsies of childhood, and in other bilateral diseases in the cerebral white matter in adults. This is a quite different problem.

Therefore, what is the matter with this man? What motor mechanism is involved? Already I can see a light on your usual sheeplike faces! The pathways involved in this slow but progressive degeneration lead from the motor cortex to the motor nuclei of the medulla. The nuclei themselves are in the beginning intact. The condition is entirely an upper motor neuron affair without atrophy of muscles, and with exaggerated tendon reflexes, sucking reflexes and spasticity. Fasciculations are minimal or absent. The speech is spastic and quite unlike that in chronic bulbar palsy. In amyotrophic lateral sclerosis we may get a mixed variety, and as with the patient, the woman I showed today, it depends on where the lesions are dominantly situated. Here, in this man, there is pure degeneration of the cells of origin and fibers of the cortical medullary pathways. The lesion is *not* in the motor nuclei of the medulla (or bulb).

The syndrome of pseudobulbar palsy (a curse on the name) may occur in other diseases of the brain than in the primary degenerations we have been discussing. It may be seen in children who have cerebral palsy or cortical atrophy; it may appear in encephalitis, in hypertensive encephalopathy and in demyelinating diseases of the brain. Usually, in these patients there are many other signs indicating a more widespread disease of the nervous system than is seen here in an isolated progressive degeneration of corticomedullary motor nuclear pathways.

I am showing this patient to round off the quartet of big names meaning *little*. You have seen chronic bulbar palsy, progressive muscular atrophy, amyotrophic lateral sclerosis, and finally, pseudobulbar palsy, all children of the same parental disease but given a misleading terminology. Next week I shall try to co-ordinate the whole line of thought on these individual problems, lest you leave here more confused than ever.

The final word comes, as it always should, what about our patient and Christian brother in the Lord? Some of his complaints and signs simulate those of the amyotrophic lateral sclerosis we saw earlier, but this first patient had so many other things wrong, and both bulbar and pseudobulbar damage were evident, probably more on the side of the bulbar manifestations, but yet a mixed picture. The prognosis in each is the same. I am afraid that future generations will have to solve this problem of decay. There is, however, an old French aphorism. It is on the bronze plaque commemorating Trudeau at Saranac, New York; in the Middle West it gleams through the stained-glass window of Balfour Hall in the Foundation House of the Mayo Foundation:

To cure sometimes, to relieve often, to comfort always.

5

Good morning! Coming here to meet you, I ran into the usual snarl of traffic where Grafton and Nassau Streets meet. A gigantic Civic Guard put up his hand, and everything stopped. I had time to think over dead men's names and of how hard it is to get rid of them. Minutes later I was released, and farther on my way here I passed Mary Street. The Duke of Grafton, Stadholder William of Nassau and Mary Stuart were three first cousins, but the first-named was illegitimate! The Hollander married his English first cousin, and each occupied a separate throne of England. The bastard Duke died in some petty fight in Ireland while serving under Churchill. What they all did for this country, and why their names should be commemorated in the corners of streets, is hard to say. But there has occurred recently a subtle revenge: under each name plate inscribed in English there is another plate, in a vivid nauseating green, carrying a laborious translation of the name into Gaelic script. What an unconscious insult, brought about by an unstudied anachronism! *We* are living in the twentieth century, the *first cousins* gamboled, fought and loved in the seventeenth, the *Gaelic script* goes back to time immemorial. Better to get rid of all these names over street corners and use only those of extinct animals and birds who became obliterated because of a too friendly, charitable, trusting and kind disposition. Let them be boldly inscribed in faultless Latin, e.g., *Didus ineptus,* representing the whole character of that noble bird, the dodo, a

167

large, heavy, flightless creature related to the pigeons, and larger than a turkey, last seen on the island of Mauritius. Such names will fittingly express this country in the past, now, and in the future, and for ever and ever, amen!

In medicine the same problem occurs, that is, the craving of workers in new fields to fix forever their names in history. Perhaps it is more true that it is their colleagues who do this embalming. It is cheaper than having a portrait painted or a statue carved out of stone. It is not strange that the names that survive must have a euphonious character to permit their survival. Jacksonian convulsions are clinical phenomena readily grasped by students. The very name is poetic, but who has heard of that very obscure disease known as the "nocturnal stertor of Buggins"? In my student days there was bandied around a syndrome called "duck's disease." To the innocent inquirer it was explained that this term meant a human anatomic deformity so crippling that the fundamental orifice of the sufferer was ever too near the ground. A murrain on all creators of eponyms!

Another and an even more serious source of confusion is that in which a research worker puts his own title on a disease he has claimed to discover, or at least on one whose many characteristics he has elaborated, satisfying himself as to the underlying anatomic and pathologic factors. He may even use a purely clinical term and not bother about cause and effect. If almost simultaneously his kind friends and colleagues working at his elbow and on the same problem use different terms, then everyone is confounded in his own confusion. It is just this confusion we have been struggling with the last two mornings. Once more I say that here is the *pons asinorum* of neurology, and on these problems I have had more questions put to me by students than on all the ramifications of neurologic dogma. Degeneration of the motor system of the brain and spinal cord is hard enough to understand without these dead hands twisting our modern brains into an inextricable tangle.

During the latter half of the nineteenth century there was an able and busy school of neurologic endeavor in Paris, headed by Charcot at the Salpêtrière. Duchenne of Boulogne, the big, bluff sailor-man, wandered through the hospitals without any definite appointment and was ably helped by Aran, who died so young. Vulpian was a scientific neurologist who started the crude microscopy of the day; his career paralleled that of Charcot, but his efforts led into too many different channels of research to help us here. Souques and later Déjèrine carried on where these worthies left off. It is these persons who are largely responsible for the terms: "chronic bulbar palsy," "progressive muscular atrophy," "amyotrophic lateral sclerosis" and "pseudobulbar palsy." They meant well; may their bones lie in rest and peace. It is possible that in the shadowy generations behind them there was an earlier phase of this nomenclature. No one can trace a name precisely to its origin, and this process of searching for original title deeds in neurologic nomenclature is of all things on earth the most sterile of occupations.

I fear these names are here to stay a while. Our reaction to the problem should be to remember that these nineteenth-century observers were each seeing different phases of the same disease, and calling the same disease by different names. They did not reckon on the fact that in any given patient all these four categories of disease may occur in varying degree, so that the patient may have at one time all of them. They did not appreciate that one may imperceptibly change into the other.

It is true that this may occur only from the simpler types into the more complicated: chronic bulbar palsy or progressive muscular atrophy may become later amyotrophic lateral sclerosis, and often does. The last-named disease is usually the stew into which all the above ingredients have been poured. What sets the pace of spread and into what final picture each one goes are unknown.

A patient may start out with progressive muscular atrophy or chronic bulbar palsy and end with death. In default of this, what he has may sooner or later go on to the more complex amyotrophic lateral sclerosis. In this latter disease, you may remember, he may start by having spastic paraplegia and subsequently go the whole gamut of degenerative diseases of the motorial system. Who is there to know what way these diseases will go?

Chronic bulbar palsy often is combined with pseudobulbar

palsy, and later the whole brunt of disease may descend into the spinal anatomy of the central nervous system, involving arms and legs equally. All this is not difficult to envisage if only one thinks of anatomy and pathology in the central nervous system. When a building crumbles into decay, it does not do so equally. Let us at least keep these archaic and false pigeonholes of our ancestors open and free from obstruction. As Horace said, when they crack wide open, the ruins will strike us fearless.

How often do these diseases begin as an atrophic flaccid weakness of the *lower* extremities with loss of reflexes? Very rarely is this the case. There seems to be a predilection for the motor cells of the medulla as well as the upper part of the spinal cord, and for the long supranuclear pathways of the spinal cord and brain.

There is a form of this motor disease occurring in earlier middle age, say in the fourth and fifth decades. It is extremely rapid in course, is patchy in distribution and has an onset of pain and cramps in the affected muscles. It has been called *"chronic anterior poliomyelitis"* without good pathologic evidence of an inflammatory process. Still, it exists clinically and must be reckoned with. It is the more deadly in that it strikes a patient at a comparatively young age and therefore at the height of his or her career, when there are as yet no signs of a wearing-out. The length of life following its onset is nonetheless much shorter than it is in the other forms of the disease. Even more caution, therefore, must be shown here as to the making of an accurate diagnosis and a prognosis postponed for sufficient time to enable us to be completely certain of that with which we are dealing.

In regard to these earlier-starting and more quickly moving downhill cases of disease of the motor system, the giving of a prognosis is an art in itself. The older type of patient has perchance already received his or her death sentence, perhaps not. In any case, it is so much easier to agree with the one who has already given the death sentence, since now the news has been broken. There is a class of patients or relatives, however, who adopt the attitude of "tell me the worst," and with their hands on your throat they force you into a corner to make you do so.

Harassed and annoyed, one is then apt to blurt out brutally and sadistically something that should not be said but merely hinted at, whereupon an inexpressibly depressing collapse ensues. A good practice in the giving of a prognosis is to beg for time, so that inevitably the patient and the family will come to realize more certainly than you can tell them what is now beginning to be apparent as to the final outcome and the stages by which it is reached. The modern public library and current moving pictures of the last stages of a given disease represent a channel of information to the laity, though morbid in the extreme. I might add that there is usually sufficient time for the patient to dispose of his mundane affairs.

Finally, it is possible that a cure may be found for these diseases, and posterity will laugh whimsically at these last few ponderous utterances. If the diagnosis is even suspected, appropriate treatment will then be immediately applied, and there will be no need to worry over death sentences and all that nonsense we talk of now. In my grave or out of it, I shall be the first one to join in that Olympian titter.

I have played with names throughout this discourse. Later I cursed them. It seems that if a man's name should be perpetuated, the reason for doing so should be frankly stated, and the name should occur only as a mere appendage to his chronicled work. Our Civic Guard who daily regulates traffic at the corner of Nassau and Grafton Streets knows nothing about these names and what they mean. As to the English laws of monarchic succession, he knows as much about them as a jackdaw knows about the Day of Pentecost. He is the better for it.

The problem of priority in medical nomenclature is the most sterile of all research. As that kind, quiet little doctor of the seventeenth century, Sir Thomas Browne, complained, "Man is a noble animal, splendid in ashes and pompous in the grave." Let your lives depend on what you do, day by day, and give no thought as to what is to be scratched on your tomb.

The epitaph on the headstone of William Stokes, of Dublin memory, is simply, "He fed fevers." It is all the more worthy, since up to his time countless typhus and typhoid patients died of dire starvation by the mere withholding of food by their physicians. There is a powder called Dover's powder that has been now almost forgotten. In fevers it was an excellent diaphoretic, antipyretic, and reliever of pain. How many of you know that the English Doctor Thomas Dover was a highly efficient buccaneer and that his fleet was the scourge of all Spanish and French vessels sailing the Spanish Main in the early seventeenth century?

If any of you here can discover a treatment for these diseases of which we have been recently talking, I will forget my rabid hatred for eponyms and let you go down to history as one who brought peace, happiness and life to patients otherwise doomed. I will even forgive you for what you do in your spare time.

MARCH

Surgeons . . .
Spend raptures upon perfect specimens
Of indurated veins, distorted joints,
Or beautiful new cases of curved spine.
—ELIZABETH BARRETT BROWNING: *Aurora Leigh.*

1

Good morning! This man here in bed is called Timothy McGrath, a name of quaint and pleasing combination. Of Greek and Gaelic origin, it indicates that he is the God-fearing son of a weaver. He is all that and more, and is now thirty-five years of age.

Young Tim, having watched large, painful and unsightly swellings develop about the gluteal bursae of his father as he sat toiling all day long at his loom, decided that a sedentary occupation of this kind was not for him. Having no desire to acquire a weaver's bottom himself, he ran away from home at an early age to become a seaman on a coastal steamer. The worst occupational diseases he could get in this profession would be too great a liking for strong drink, and a woman in every port where his steamer docked for the night. Such diseases have a pleasant side to them and do not involve a struggle with the Workmen's Compensation Act; they are strictly a personal problem.

We see here now my bucko having risen to the rank of a fighting bosun. He manages the tough crew admirably by the weapons God gave him: his fists, his feet, occasionally his teeth; if necessary, now and then, he makes use of a belaying pin to crack down on the skull of a disgruntled newly hired belligerent waif and stray of the sea. It is strange that his present complaint arises from no such glorious all-in fight, lacking any of the rules of the late Marquis of Queensbury. It came about in this way:

Three years before, and during a storm, he had to lift a heavy

175

drum of oil and bring it forward to soothe the turbulent seas. As he did so, he felt something snap in his lower backbone and just to the right of the lumbosacral joint. He fell helplessly to the deck and was carried to his quarters in the forecastle of the steamer. There he lay with severe pain in his back for four days, and he cared nothing about the raging storm. On the third day this back pain began to descend into the buttock, and from there went down the back of his thigh into his calf on the right side, along the course of the sciatic nerve.

The back and leg pains were excruciatingly severe, but on the tenth day after his trouble began, and when the weather became calmer, he was able to get out of his bunk and sit on a chair covered with cushions. The next day he crawled on deck and took charge of operations, still in pain, but able to carry on until the steamer reached port. The pain in the back and leg was intensified by coughing, sneezing and straining at stool, and he noticed that he had to keep himself bent forward, with his back kinked, so that there was also a bend of the body to the left.

From the ship he was sent into a hospital, and was put to bed on a hard mattress, with traction applied to both legs. Within three weeks all his pain cleared up, and he went home for a few days, after which he rejoined his ship, apparently well. Since then, and during the three years that have followed the initial attack, he has had four similar attacks, of varying severity, but this present one is the worst he has had.

He can not rightly say just what brings on an attack. It may be a sudden unguarded movement such as picking up a match he has dropped, or even turning in bed. He is not keen now to go into a fight with the crew, but even so, he has done it on occasion without evil consequences, whereas the next week he has been entirely crippled without obvious cause or reason, except that perhaps he moved his back in a way he should not have done. At the same time, he has realized that he has an infirmity in his back, and this is not good for him or for his employers. A man at sea under all sorts of conditions must be entirely fit to handle any emergency.

His present attack has been on for four weeks now. He made

a sudden, uncalculated movement and received, as he calls it, "a catch in the back." Severe pain appeared in the usual lumbosacral area on the right, with extension down the sciatic distribution in the leg. This time the pain has gone into the anterolateral aspect of his leg below the knee, and it is associated with a persistent tingling in the same area, felt also in the dorsum of the foot. There is some weakness in the muscles that dorsiflex his foot and toes. His favorite posture in bed is to lie on his left side, with the left leg extended, and right knee and thigh flexed. The pain is more severe on his attempting to get up out of bed; lifting objects is impossible, and he dare not cough or sneeze because of pain shooting down the right leg to the ankle.

It is better to examine him while he is out of bed, if it is humanely possible. He is willing. As he stands up, there is a marked spasm of his lumbar muscles pulling him to the left. Asked to bend forward, with knees unbent, he goes only a quarter of the way down, with much grunting and complaint of pain. Bending backward to the left is even more painful. The list of his body increases at this point. He walks with his back held stiffly, and he can not walk on his heel on the right side without the foot falling helplessly. He can walk on the toes of both feet without difficulty. Sitting on a chair, he can extend his left leg normally on the pelvis, but the right seizes at about thirty degrees, and if it is forced, great pain is produced. This is a positive Lasègue sign. Fist percussion of the lower lumbar vertebrae is painful, and his sciatic nerve is tender along its course behind the right thigh. Tendon reflexes of the right Achilles and external hamstrings are diminished. All other tendon reflexes are normal. Results of objective sensory tests of the lower extremities are normal, but he insists that subjectively there is not the same degree of sensitivity over the lateral aspect of the right leg and dorsum of the foot as there is on the left side.

We shall return him to bed. He now complains that this examination has greatly increased his pain, although I have been as gentle as I could possibly be. I ask him to cough hard; he does so, and the pain in his back and down the posterior portion of his thigh and leg is greatly increased; moreover, the tingling and numbness over the fifth lumbar and the first sacral dermatomes become much more evident. Careful palpation of the course of the sciatic nerve shows no tumor, and sensory perception over the glutei muscles and around the anus is normal.

Roentgenograms of the spinal column show no evidence of primary tumor in the lumbar part of the spinal column, and metastatic carcinoma has, as far as possible, been excluded. There is, however, significantly, a marked narrowing of the fifth lumbar and first sacral interspace, as if the intervertebral cartilage had been absorbed, and bone is resting on bone, without the friendly cushion in between. There are some signs of hypertrophic arthritis in the lumbar part of the spinal column.

What is the feeling you have about this patient, as to the cause of his trouble? Is it something that has descended on him that causes him pain, regardless of what he does, and that is damaging his spinal nerve roots, or is this a purely mechanical process whereby the onset of his trouble, its perpetuation and its aggravation depend on his bodily movements? I know you will vote for the latter. Rest and traction relieve his pain; movement exaggerates it, and his nights of rest are more tolerable than his frustrated attempts to do his work by day. Any increase in pressure of the cerebrospinal fluid caused by coughing, sneezing or intra-abdominal tension seems to push something more painfully against the spinal nerve roots. His first attack followed a sudden abnormal movement of the lower part of the back, and through several attacks the same factor operates, even though the particular movement causing trouble is obscure. He has a weak back on which he can not depend, for it is all too likely to give him trouble where it is least wanted, at sea, and away from medical aid. In sum, something slips out of place in his back and compresses one or more of his spinal nerve roots.

Between the vertebrae of the spinal column there is a cartilaginous disk, consisting of a hard rind called the "annulus fibrosus" and a soft mushy center called the "nucleus pulposus." Usually anchored in place by ligaments, such disks may be set free to herniate into the spinal canal and compress nerve roots. They may slip back into place again, with relief of symptoms. If they do not, and compression of the nerve roots continues, a surgical procedure can remove these derelict structures, and so relieve pain and suffering. The particular disk involved must first be found.

The disk between the fourth and fifth lumbar vertebrae and that between the fifth lumbar and the first sacral are the most common offenders; both may be herniated at the same time. What is the next procedure for this, our erstwhile fighting commander of men as tough as himself? He can not go on as he is; he can not even go home and help his father make imitation Aubusson carpets.

The procedure in these cases is to inject a medium opaque to roentgen rays into the spinal canal, after withdrawing sufficient cerebrospinal fluid. The patient is then put on a table that can be tipped up or down. Under a fluoroscope, the opaque medium can be seen to pass up and down the subarachnoid space of the spinal canal. If it blocks at a certain level, there is something protruding into this canal. Roentgenograms are made, and if the column of opaque medium shows an indentation at a certain level, our evidence is overwhelmingly in favor of a **protruded intervertebral disk** at that level. The protruded disk or disks can be removed surgically, and after some weeks or months of convalescence, the patient can resume his normal occupation. In some cases the orthopedic surgeon is called in, and if there is associated instability of the back, bony fusion with a graft taken from the tibia is done. Patients for this procedure are most carefully selected. There are no indications in this patient of ours for such an addition to his surgical requirements.

I have shown you a patient who has no other choice than to be operated on, since otherwise he may become an invalid and remain so all his life. Nevertheless, in other cases, removal of protruded intervertebral disks is not the whole answer. A patient who can afford to cease work at intervals and have physical therapy, with massage, heat and traction in bed, may weather more storms than this patient has, and may even never need to be operated on. Suffice it to say that our patient's state of affairs, economically speaking, is uncertain.

There was a time when this procedure for relief by surgery

was unknown. Patients got along somehow, if ingloriously. Reckless operation on patients who have few or no indications for surgery is something to be abhorred. The much operated-on back today is a scandal. Each operation worsens the original condition, and the end results are shocking. Such patients are truly the most pitiable, miserable wretches in existence. Repeated operations on nerve roots produce a chronic arachnoidal meningitis which engenders a pain that lasts as long as life lasts. Cutting nerve roots, cordotomy and finally lobotomy of the brain, leave even worse wrecks of humanity.

The first question that should be asked of every patient with a possible protrusion of a disk is whether the pain and loss of income from invalidism make him desire operation. Can he not get along with rest and physical therapy, a supporting lumbosacral belt, and a trust in God? If he is a common laborer—or like our patient, dependent on his muscles—with a starving wife and six hungry children to support; if he is a farmer, or the owner of a small business requiring constant heavy lifting, and can not survive economically without continual attendance on his work, then these are strong points for surgical intervention. If the patient is a "white-collar" operator, more dependent on brains than on brawn, that is another story. Physicians are not very quick to undergo surgery, except those thoracic or brain surgeons who have to stand many weary hours alongside the operating table.

From the standpoint of selection of suitable patients for surgery, women are bad risks, and correspondingly, among them failures to relieve are higher, and multiple operations the more common. Better give them months or years of conservative physical therapy before advising their going further. Women have a keener sense of discomfort and pain than men have. Their condition is the result of trauma, and further trauma may defeat our purpose.

The workman seeking compensation represents by far the worst of all results of removal of a protruded lumbar intervertebral disk. Such an adventure is best avoided, unless most rigid rules are applied as to the advisability of surgical interference. Compensation lawsuits may go on forever, and so do alleged pain and suffering. Furthermore, the surgeon who first operated is thereby discredited. Notwithstanding this jeremiad, there is still a group of patients, and a substantial one at that, who can be relieved of pain, returned to their previous occupations, and who will be very, very grateful.

We have forgotten Timotheus for the time being. I would ask you, as students of medicine, to use your powers of observation. Stripped to the waist, he is a very muscular person. His body is decorated with numerous tattoo marks. As usual, there is the ship he first sailed on, with crossed anchors, and its name in a scroll on his chest. On his right arm he has an almost undecipherable name, which has been nearly obliterated by the same art that put it there. I think the name is "Edith." It is faded, blotched and obviously of an old vintage. On his left arm, near the antecubital fossa, there blazons out in purple, blue and crimson colors a fresher declaration of his everlasting fidelity to womanhood. The name spells out as being "Anastasia." I look up his record here, and find that he is a happily married man with four children. His wife's name, as given, is the dearest, sweetest of all names, and the one nearest heaven—Mary. No! We shall move on to the next patient, and so save him his blushes.

2

THERE IS a divinity that shapes our ends, but the god who does it is so human in his imperfections that he seems to have more of humanity and less of divinity. The greatest mobility of the spinal column is in the cervical and lumbar region. The thoracic part of the spinal column supports a rigid cage guarding respiration, heart action, and the great vessels. It does not pay, in the human economy of life, that this bony support should at any time come adrift. Our God-fearing friend, whom we saw earlier this morning, had pain in the lower part of the lumbar sector of the spinal column and it extended down a special course in the back of his thigh and leg, into calf and foot. Our second patient, whom we are seeing now, has a pain in the lower cervical part of the spinal column and it extends down a particular area of the thorax, arm and forearm into the hand. There is a similar set of mechanics shared by these two patients, but with an extraordinarily different clinical picture, because so different are the parts of the body involved. They both indicate a laxity in development of the human body that may well take many thousands of years of evolution to catch up with.

This man is a gallant pilot who distinguished himself in the Battle of Britain in 1940. He has survived a series of air crashes with minor injuries resulting from short-lived effects of violent contact with Mother Earth. He remembers, at least on two occasions, that his neck was sore and stiff after one of these mishaps, but he recovered from all these previous injuries in a very short time.

Three weeks ago he was hurriedly called to substitute for another pilot who was ill, and he was a trifle late on starting for an observation flight over France. For that reason he jumped into the cockpit of his plane without the usual care to avoid hitting himself in so crowded a space. As a result, he struck the left side of his head against a projecting object. His head was correspondingly thrust backward by the blow, and to the right side. A small laceration of his scalp in the left temporal area began to bleed, but the hemorrhage ceased almost at once by digital compression and application of a first-aid bandage.

A few minutes later, across the English Channel and over French territory, he realized that his neck was hurting him severely, chiefly over the lower portion. From then on, minute by minute, the pain increased steadily and began to extend into the scapular area, clavicle, deltoid region and down the lateral aspect of his upper arm to the elbow. This pain and the enemy's natural annoyance at his visit made things rather hot for him. However, he finished his reconnaissance and flew home to his base, with ever-increasing pain in his neck, shoulder and upper arm. That night he had no sleep, and he has not had much more since then.

A few days later, the pain was as bad as it could be, and added to it was a numb, tingling, prickling sensation felt in the thumb and index finger of his left hand. At times, pain and tingling shot into these fingers like an electric shock, particularly on sudden movements, such as those jarring his neck. He could not feel small objects between his thumb and index and middle fingers, and had difficulty in buttoning his clothes and tying his shoes. Coughing and sneezing were avoided or stifled, since they caused sudden and violent jolts of pain in his neck, shoulder and down his arm.

During the last few days he has noticed some wasting of the left thenar eminence, with fasciculation in the muscles comprising it. In all his story he keeps coming back to the pain in his neck. It is at the site of the *vertebra prominens* and it extends into a few spines below. This is the center of his suffering, and he has to hold his neck stiffly in order to relieve such pains. He realizes that the pains in the chest, shoulder, arm, and forearm are entirely secondary in character, but they are none the less severe.

At night he has to sleep almost sitting up, because sleep is not possible in any other position, and he has plenty of pillows with a few last small ones at the nape of his neck and occiput, pushing his head forward. This, on the other hand, is not always successful. He has lately procured a high-backed chair with wings, and here he tries to sleep, sitting up, with a small foam-rubber pillow behind his head, secured to the back of the chair with adhesive tape.

As this man's history is short, concise and to the point, so his physical findings are equally definite. During the giving of his history, he holds his head and neck constantly rigid, and even when he turns toward me, his head, neck and trunk move as one mass, as if to avoid untoward and painful movements of the parts involved.

I have asked him to strip to the waist, and with his right hand to point out exactly where his pain is, even at the risk of tedious repetition. This is for emphasis of his clinical picture, and without apology to you who are listening.

He places his hand on the *vertebra prominens* and a few dorsal spines below it, as indicating the main origin of his pain. Thereafter his fingers follow the line of the spine of the scapula behind and the clavicle in front. He runs over the surface of the deltoid, and down the outer surface of the forearm to the external epicondyle of the humerus. There it stops. He next extends his left hand, and rubbing the index and middle fingers against the ball of the thumb, he shows where they are numb. Further, if he moves his neck unduly, the pain will extend down into the numb area.

There is a slight but definite atrophy of the thenar eminence, and there are fasciculations in the belly of its muscles. The left biceps tendon reflex is abolished, but the triceps and brachioradialis reflexes are brisk and active. The tendon reflexes on the right side are normal. Testing the ball of the left thumb and index finger with touch, pinprick, and thermal stimuli, we find a subjective difference to that in the right hand: although the stimuli are felt, they are not so keen. The movement of opposition of the thumb to the index finger is weaker than on the right side, but it still functions, if only partially.

Now comes the more important part of his examination, the passive movements of his neck. He cringes at this suggestion, and certainly we must be gentle and careful, lest we hurt him unduly and even cause damage. Pushing his head forward so that his chin rests on his chest produces no great pain. Turning his head so that he looks over his right shoulder is not greatly resisted, but turning the head toward the affected side is immediately resisted, and a sharp cry from him results. To force it now would increase this neck and shoulder pain, which, as you see, extends into his thumb and index finger, increasing the numbness already present. We do not force this maneuver, for it has already been productive of adequate, and at that, dramatic, results.

The next test is the most informative. Gently, his head is pulled backward. Before the least part of the journey of his head in that direction has been made, there is an even more bitter outcry of pain, and this maneuver dies almost before it is born. Again, his pain is suddenly and violently increased; it extends down the left shoulder and forearm and into the radial fingers in a sharp lancinating flash, with concomitant tingling and pins-and-needles sensation in the digits involved. He is very glad that we did not manhandle him. We, in turn, are glad, since we should not like to damage permanently the important functions of his left hand.

Pleasure and pain being opposite and equal, we try to see what will do the reverse of hurting him—that is, give him a sense of relief. He has a haggard and woebegone facies from so much suffering, and looks expectantly for me to hurt him again. I am placing both hands on his neck, so that I embrace both rami of his mandible. He is sitting up now, and I pull forcibly upward as if to stretch his neck, like pulling out the units of a telescope. I am using all my power. Look, a beatific smile is breaking on that pain-ridden countenance, and as the pull increases, he cries out, "That feels just wonderful!" As I let go, his pain promptly returns, but there is now given us a dramatic hint as to future treatment.

Roentgenograms of the cervical part of the spinal column show no gross lesions of the vertebrae, but two significant features appear: the natural curvature of the cervical part of the spinal column is obliterated, and there is a straight up-and-down alignment of each drum-shaped body. Further, there is a distinct narrowing of the space between the fifth and sixth vertebrae. The cartilaginous body between these vertebrae has been greatly diminished in width. It has been absorbed or has gone elsewhere. It has probably been extruded laterally, and to the left side, to compress the fifth motor and sensory nerve roots, causing all the symptoms of which this patient complains, as well as the physical signs. Note well that these signs and symptoms are in the area supplied by this root, and nowhere else.

I think that at this stage there is little more to be said as to diagnosis. As our clumsy-minded legal friends would say in their jargon, "*res ipsa loquitur.*" The thing speaks for itself. If you know your anatomy and physiology, you will know that only one such mechanical process could produce such a clear result, in a corresponding manner, and with such a sequence of events. There has occurred in this man *a lateral protrusion, herniation, or slipping of a cervical cartilaginous disk.* It is impinging on corresponding motor and sensory nerve roots; it is giving him great pain and progressive disability, and must be attended to as soon as possible.

What are we going to do to help this modern Icarus? He has

flown too near the sun god, and the wax of his wings has melted. He wants this to be remedied, so that later he can fly again faster and more deadly instruments of destruction. I think we can manage to do this for him. Our business is to cure him, and is not concerned with what he does thereafter. We should hate, however, to see all our skill and efforts annulled later on by circumstances that led to his failure to return from a dangerous mission. The science of healing takes no cognizance of unrelated principles of conduct.

You will remember how he experienced sudden and ineffable relief from my stretching his neck with my clumsy hands. This can be done efficiently and repeatedly by my colleagues in physical medicine. He can have a suitable padded halter put around his neck. From this a rope goes to a fixed point, and standing on a series of steps, he can gradually let himself down, so that his whole weight will dangle from this collar and his neck be stretched to its uttermost.

The cervical interspaces will be enlarged, and if ever this extruded piece of cartilage wants to return to its home, it will have the greatest temptation to return at this time and cease its assault on the nerve root. This stretching or traction can be repeated daily, so long as improvement occurs. Pain clears up, and numbness, with weakness of muscles, yields to this simple treatment. In every case, traction should be given a trial, but not too long in face of increasing numbness and weakness of the hand.

Unfortunately, in a large percentage of cases, it fails, and then surgical removal of this wandering piece of cartilage must be instituted without delay. There is much more urgency in these cases of protruded cervical disks than in their homologous cousins in the lumbar and lumbosacral areas. Resultant damage is more swift and more irreparable in the former.

I have shown you an instance of protrusion of a disk between the fifth and sixth cervical vertebrae. It is a classic one, and we can tell just where the disk is to be reached by surgical procedure. In a given case, a neurosurgeon can operate in just that site and reasonably expect to find something he can remove, and so produce a permanent cure. Sometimes it is not so easy. When the intervertebral disk between either the sixth or seventh spaces, or that between the seventh cervical and first thoracic, is protruded, the clinical picture is different. The pain is now down the inner aspect of the arm, and extends into the middle fingers, or into the ring and little fingers. Numbness may be felt instead of pain in these fingers. The triceps and brachioradialis reflexes are lost; the biceps, preserved. Now the question as to the site of surgical attack comes up. The cervical segment of the spinal column is small compared with the lumbar, but, considering the vital character of the spinal cord in the cervical area as compared with the cauda equina, the risks of surgical intervention are greater.

Some surgeons explore directly, according to signs and symptoms. This, I should think, they would do here. Where there is any doubt, a spinogram is done as a test, and according to the deformity of the column of opaque media, with roentgen studies, surgical exploration is planned to include that area. The results are, in the main, highly successful, and more so than in the case of a protruded lumbar disk. More amazing still is the fact that as the patient is coming out of anesthesia, he appreciates the resultant pains of surgery and expects them. At the same time, he cries out in joy that his previous pain is gone, that relief has been obtained, and from his half-conscious mental state, still fogged by the anesthesia, he is overwhelmingly aware that the operation has been successful. His present neck pain is a quite different one, and there is no trace now of the pain down his arm. He knows full well that something has been accomplished.

Perhaps I have indulged in a too great simplification of the problem of protruded intervertebral disk; anyhow, I have given you two classic cases. There is a large number of adumbrations, permutations, and complications in these cases. To take one example, the history of injury may be totally lacking. We speak of laterally protruded disks, of those in the midline, and multiple disks, and of those which recur. If you know the fundamentals of the common and easily recognizable types, you can work out the variabilities as you go, and as you learn. Essentially, the problem is one of teamwork among the general physician, the orthopedist, the neurologist and the neurosurgeon.

Arthritis of the spinal column, metastatic malignant processes, meningeal inflammatory processes, tumors of the spinal cord and its envelopes and hysterical states are encountered and must be separated out. The radiologist is the most helpful, and the most technically responsible of all. If he slips, the whole castle of stacked cards falls. He is not, however, infallible. Workmen's compensation cases are notoriously sources of grief, because of intrusion of their medicolegal problems into any given case. Finally, the keynote is careful history-taking, meticulous examination, and above all, extreme conservatism.

Comparing protruded lumbar and lumbosacral intervertebral disks with protruded disks in the cervical region, we find that there are many differences apart from the anatomic site involved. Protruded disks in the lumbar area can wait until all evidence is collected, and until the condition is carefully thought over, before we are committed to surgery. The question to be put to these persons is whether a surgical procedure, after its nature has been carefully explained, is one they want, and one they are willing to put up with, without promise of success. If there is any shilly-shallying on the part of the patient, conservative measures should be carried on in the form of a supportive lumbosacral belt, a hard bed to sleep on, and physical therapy, such as baking, massage and exercises. If the pain becomes intolerable, and incapacity to the point of economic disaster occurs, with increasing numbness and weakness of an extremity, the patient and his medical adviser are more than willing to go ahead together and throw the dice on the hazard of surgery, knowing full well that failure after operation may be worse than what went before.

Protrusion of an intervertebral disk in the cervical segment presents a more difficult problem. In so many cases wherein traction and physical therapy fail in a relatively short period, there is no going on with so conservative a regimen. Surgery then becomes imperative; the pain is too great, and the risk of waiting too serious, so that most well-developed protruded cervical disks must perforce be operated on early. There is, further, not the same risk of an unsuccessful operation when the condition is typical, and with surgery in competent hands, the results are quite good.

. . . *the sin they do by two and two they*
must pay for one by one.

—KIPLING: *Tomlinson.*

3

Good morning! I have a man coming here this morning who will show you his trouble. He is late. I think that this is being done purposely, because of his arrogance and pride of soul. He knows I want him here and now. He is an employe in a turf accountant's office, and he calls himself the "chief clerk." To explain further, he works in one of a chain of gambling and betting offices where the worship of the great god Horse is raised on high. He is chief clerk because he is the only employe in a mean little hole in the wall down on the quays. I pass there every morning on my way here.

He is a small, thin man with a bald head burgeoned by two carefully combed lateral locks of hair of a hue that is as red, and equally as gray, as that of an old fox. For this reason, his friends call him Foxy Macarthy, but also as a tribute to his shrewd knowledge of horses, and his ability to deal with his clients. It was only in recent years that I found out that his full and real name is Demetrius O'Flanagan Macarthy, and that he claims to have come of a long line of Irish nobility leading back to the ultimate source and pride of his ancestry, Red Macarthy, King of Munster.

He receives money in sullen silver or tarnished copper coins from those who bet either to win or to place on a given horse. He never gives advice; that is beneath him. If fools bet, that is their privilege. Once I asked him if he ever bet himself, and I got a smart reaction. It involved the factor that physicians never take their own medicine, lawyers never plead their own cases, and owners of taverns never drink their own wares. As he mentioned to me one day, "Man alive, I never bet, for not a thraneen have I got of the Holy Touch."

Strangely enough, in this predominantly Catholic country, Macarthy is a strong Presbyterian, and moreover, carries the plate in his church on a Sunday. I have attended his church and have seen him parade proudly up the aisle, with his plate loaded with the offerings of the devout. I noticed also, at that time, a peculiar, stamping, unsteady gait that puzzled me greatly. Here he is now, a staunch individualist and an ardent exhibitionist—at your service.

You will notice the gait that I have mentioned. It is unsteady because the owner does not seem to appreciate the lay of the ground under his feet, and he throws his legs out in all directions, with his eyes watching them as if trying to correct this grotesque stamping performance. He walks like a cat on hot sand, lifting his feet too high each time he takes a step. Nevertheless, he has never fallen and he reaches his destination safely.

I ask him, as I have done so many times before, what the chief complaints about himself might be. As usual, and in serial fashion, he says, difficulty in walking, pains in his lower extremities, and trouble in passing urine, or controlling its normal flow. Of less anxiety to him are impotence for sexual connection, attacks of nausea and vomiting, which are, however, rare in recent years, and a sense of numbness in his lower extremities, which, in turn, connects with his inability to feel the floor under his feet properly, and so affects his gait.

You have seen his unsteady gait. This is far worse when he is walking through poorly lighted streets, and after any debilitating influence, such as an infection of the upper part of the respiratory system, or influenza. There was a time in the past when it was especially bad after each attack of nausea and vomiting. Disturbance of gait was made much of by our predecessors, and the euphonious name for this disease was given by the French, as being, "ataxie locomotrice," or in English parlance, "locomotor ataxia." The Germans, fastening on the pathologic processes found after death, named it *"tabes dorsalis,"* representing a wasting away of the dorsal columns of the spinal cord due to syphilis.

Being shorter, the latter term has been universally adopted in recent years.

Mister Macarthy's gait has been bad for at least ten years but is not getting progressively worse. He has become adjusted to it, and even bears the collection plate bravely on Sundays. Being a professional collector on weekdays, he finds his plate always the most heavily laden, a sore point with his worthy colleagues.

Of all his troubles, his pains are the worst, and they stick to him like a throng of leeches. At the moment of his greatest happiness, a session of pain may start. It consists of short, sharp, sudden, lancinating jabs that hit him anywhere over his lower extremities, at his midriff, and infrequently, along either ulnar border of his arm. They hit him regardless of structure over bones, joints and muscles. The meanest of all is one striking him over the front of the thigh. Once a place is selected for pain, there it stays for that session.

Asked to indicate where the pains occur, he gently places a nicotine-stained index finger over various places. The area in each case is no larger than the smallest silver coin, and after a succession of these short, lightninglike stabs, the skin over the area becomes exquisitely sensitive. He can not bear to touch it, or to have his trousers press on it, yet he can grab this tiny area with his fist and squeeze it in a useless attempt at relief.

Apart from these spotlike pains, there are others running in strips, four to five inches long, and chiefly on the back of the thigh. Again, his index finger draws a line over the places where they occur. In the spot pains, the finger was placed vertically on the area, giving the impression that something was piercing the flesh; in the linear pains, his finger does a quick ripping or gouging movement along the long axis of the path of pain. After a period of suffering, the skin over these areas of pain also is sensitive.

Sessions of these pains last from three days to a week, night and day, and leave him exhausted from suffering and loss of sleep. A certain area is affected each time, and none other. The pains are so severe and sudden that they make him jump, cry out and curse when sitting or lying down; in walking, he has to stop, lest they pull the legs from under him and make him fall. He thinks they are worse on cloudy days and before a storm. They are partially relieved by aspirin; hence the diagnosis of "neuritis" and "rheumatism" which he carried for so long. He may be free from these pains for months on end; for this reason, in a free period he may deny that he has ever had such pains, by a conscious or unconscious wish to forget. The pains in his trunk zone may punch their way around his waist at various areas, usually in spots somewhat larger than the pain areas in his legs, but behaving in just the same way. The pains in the ulnar border of his hand also are of the spot variety, but are infrequent and not so severe.

These intermittent crops of pains, hitting only one small area at a time and being incalculably severe, represent his chief complaint as compared to the many others he suffers. They were the first subjective evidence of his disease nearly twelve years ago; they still appear at about the same intervals, and they are at no time becoming less frequent or less severe. There is no adjustment here in his ego; he dreads them and hates them.

We have spent a good deal of time in listening to Mister Macarthy's story; he does a brilliant act of description, for there is no imagination involved, neurotic display or self-pity. He gets down to stark realism when he tells you about this monster that has plagued him for so many years. The description he gives is typical of the lightning pains (dolores fulminantes) of tabes dorsalis. I have heard patients of every race, color and background describe them, and it is always the same story. I heard a Chinaman describe them, and even though I could not follow his language, his gestures were sufficiently dramatic, with the clinical findings, to satisfy me as to the diagnosis. More than that, there are no other pains in human disease that behave in just the same way. Diabetic neuritis, or the so-called pseudotabes diabetica, in younger patients, may mislead one, but the pains here are not the genuine article of tabes dorsalis. These tabetic lightning pains last indefinitely, even when results of serologic tests have been negative for years, when the disease has not progressed, and in the face of continuous modern and efficient therapy. They are essentially incurable, and constitute one of the worst incentives toward addiction to drugs.

I shall say this much about our friend of today: truly he is so glad at times to be free from these pains that he tries to forget that they will ever come again. He is getting to be a philosopher, and to recognize the fact that life is not life itself unless there are suffering and pain. You will note, however, that what I say of this man is a negation of my opening sentence on his pains. In the course of our talk, I have certainly developed, later on, a wish-expression—for someone else! The French say that to suffer is to become refined. Gold in the furnace, and all that sort of thing. I think that the French are a bunch of liars and pregnant with dishonesty, more especially when there is in being an aching molar at one end, and a rectal fissure at the other, to upset the equanimity of their corporate well-being, both at the ends and down the middle.

The urinary complaint of our patient is not intense, but actually it is the one disorder of function that leads to a premature death in a tabetic. It is, therefore, the most serious of all his complaints. Essentially, the problem is that of an anesthetic bladder, with all its reflexes for emptying deadened. The tabetic notes that he can go long periods without urinating, and during drinking sprees he may boast of it. He does not know that his bladder is inordinately full until it begins to leak into his clothing during the day, and into his bed at night. He may seek medical assistance then, and on catheterization, a large residual amount of strong-smelling, infected urine will be gradually withdrawn. There will be much pus in the urine, and the cystitis found to be present will have increased the neurogenic difficulty already there.

This patient watches his urinary output; if it is insufficient, he will press over his pubis and start contractions to empty his bladder; usually this is satisfactory. At regular intervals, through his physician, he checks for the amount of infection present and degree of residual urine. Should chills and fever appear, he goes to hospital, has a gradual drainage and lavage of the bladder, and receives antibiotics. So far he has a wise and competent urologist, who will see that his life is not jeopardized, and that his comfort is kept at a maximum.

Apart from Mister Macarthy's lightning pains, there was the

time, seven years or so ago, when I found him at the veritable nadir of his existence. It was a period he looks back on as something too terrible to visualize. All my sympathy and compassion certainly went out to this little emaciated wretch, as he was then, who was even meditating self-destruction. He thinks that I cured him then, but like Ambroïse Paré, I felt that I dressed his wounds, but that the good God had cured them. As I have said, he had reached his lowest point of adversity: he began to have tabetic crises!

He would wake up in the morning, feeling that something was wrong with his digestion, and before he could leave his bed, nausea would strike him. This was accompanied by extreme salivation, and he knew he was in for it! Vomiting followed shortly thereafter, and continued without remission for seven days and perhaps more. Everything he ate and drank was regurgitated, and fluids had to be given by vein.

What he called *pain* came on the second day. It was an extremely disagreeable sensation in his epigastrium, as if an iron hand were inside, wrenching and twisting his guts. It was present as a prelude to further forcible and persistent vomiting. It was nevertheless this vomiting of which he chiefly complained, and not the sensation of gut-wrenching in his abdomen; that seemed to be only part of the tendency to vomit everything inside his gastrointestinal tract, and to keep on doing so. Hot-water bottles or icebags on his abdomen were intolerable, and only added to his misery. During one of these crises, deep fist pressure anywhere on the abdomen produced no increase of pain. There certainly was no local tenderness, nor was there any chronic browning of the skin by a hot-water bottle continuously applied. Both of these observations are characteristic of tabetic crises, and show that there is no local abdominal lesion to contend with.

Suddenly, when he was down to his lowest ebb of strength and endurance, the crisis ceased, and he was able again to eat, drink and sleep. All drugs, including morphine, had had no effect. He usually lost from seven to ten pounds during these crises. He ate voraciously after they were over, and gained back his normal weight and strength. He felt reasonably well then.

In the beginning, these attacks came every few months; after a year or two, they came every month. At that time he was really bad, with these crises and his lightning pains. The only way in which I can congratulate myself on the management of this patient at that time is the fact that I kept him from becoming a dope fiend. In those dark days I came to know him better than ever before. During the last three years the lightning pains have persisted, but the gastric crises, by an act of God, have reduced themselves to the vanishing point. Deo gratias!

He has been impotent for the last two years. He has some vague desire, but erection and ejaculation are absent. His wife is somewhat difficult, but she can hardly complain, since certain eager gynecologists here have removed all her reproductive organs. Perhaps she thinks that things are not quite right, that she has still something coming to her from her spouse, and that she is being defrauded. Who knows? The vagaries of marital existence are known only to the contracting parties themselves. The clergy, medical advisers and legal representatives end up by knowing less than nothing as to what is intrinsically at fault between any given man and the wife he has selected to live with until "death do us part." We can never know their inner life.

The numbness of this patient's legs is due in turn to the physical findings that lead to his staggering gait. This we shall go into later.

Going into the very early history of this patient, before any symptoms of disease of the central nervous system had appeared, we are presented with not one blank page, but with many. There is no account of primary or of secondary syphilis, and at no time was there a satisfactory history of a Wassermann reaction in his blood and cerebrospinal fluid. Mister Macarthy would have none of that! According to his own story, he was in his premarital life devoid of the follies, impulses and the sexual irregularities of his day and age. He was, to his own knowledge, no less than a "plaster saint." How could such a product of a local Italian firm, in garish colors and set on a pedestal, climb down and be other than continent?

When I saw him first, his trouble had been with him for about four years. Results of the usual tests on the blood and cerebrospinal fluid had on many occasions been coldly negative, representing an uplift to his immaculate conscience. He had had, at the onset of his symptoms, antisyphilis therapy in the form of arsenicals and bismuth injections. They were not given consistently, but later on he had had many millions of units of penicillin, and in spite of all this, his pains, his ataxia and his urinary dysfunction continued. His gastric crises abated, but I had always felt that this was going to happen anyhow. As he is today, it is a question of a normal serologic state, with lightning pains in his legs, bladder trouble, an odd gastric crisis and ataxia, all of which, with his numb legs, can not but add up to a strong suspicion of tabes dorsalis. Historically, the diagnosis can be fairly certain, but of course we must await the report of the physical examination. The serologic tests have not helped us, but I feel sure that our physical examination will settle the problem.

4

I THINK the hour of eleven is approaching, when important persons in the City cease working and proceed to obtain the stimulating effects of coffee, tea and cakes, in order to spur themselves on to further efforts toward efficiency; naturally, they meet their business friends at the same time. We have heard much of Mister Macarthy's testimony as to his own sad personal affliction; it would be an act of kindness now to have him physically refreshed before we go on a little later to his clinical examination, and all that it entails. Accordingly, our ward sister has a tray ready for him, set with gleaming silver teapot, cream jug, sugar bowl, and a hot-water jug, so that he may pour his tea correctly, the way he likes it best. The tray is loaded with all kinds of sandwiches, muffins and cakes, and our friend is invited to partake, as a very welcome guest. As the Bible says, "Thou shalt not muzzle the Ox when he treadeth out the corn." In the meantime, we shall go to a bleak ward and work out the pathologic aspects of the presenting disease, that is, tabes dorsalis, and discuss the various scientific and philosophic factors involved.

Here is a rough sketch of the spinal cord in its mid-dorsal portion and in cross section. Attached are the anterior and posterior roots, and the root ganglion of the latter. I shall color in red the areas involved in tabes. The posterior root ganglion is partly affected, the posterior roots more so, and the dorsal columns have an extensive area of destruction. This is more marked in the lumbar region, and progressively less marked as the cervical region is reached, since normal incoming root fibers push the degenerated ones more to the midline. Careful microscopic studies have been made at the zone of the entrance of the roots into the spinal cord. It is there that pain fibers may separate out from those of tactile sensation, and these former fibers are much more damaged than the tactile. Hence, the dissociated sensory changes in the legs, wherein pain is affected much more than touch, and indeed earlier.

One can see at a glance that the disease is overwhelmingly one of the great ascending pathways of superficial and deep sensibility. It is predominantly a painful disease, and one interfering with co-ordination of bodily movement, balance, station and muscular control. Visceral functions do not escape; hence, we have bladder dysfunction, rectal and gastric crises. Amongst the cranial nerves, the optic nerve is often affected, producing optic atrophy and blindness; strangely enough, if blindness comes early, ataxia does not develop—a kindness on the part of nature. The fifth nerve may have degenerated, producing butterfly-shaped anesthesia over the face, and severe crisislike pains may occur in one eye and its socket.

The meninges around the entering roots are thickened, and by this compression of the dorsal nerve roots the characteristic lightning pains are supposed to be produced. The exact mechanism of production has inspired many weary pathologists to write even more weary, tedious and long-winded theses. We are still no wiser . . . . Our patient has finished his midmorning repast, has been undressed, is in bed and ready for examination. There is plenty to find, but it takes skill on the part of the physician, and hearty, intelligent collaboration on the part of the patient, to show it. Let us go back to him.

His pupils, exposed to bright light, are irregular and unequal, and quite small in size. The iris is muddy in appearance. On flashing the light on one pupil and then on the other, we find that no reflex is obtained; the pupils are fixed to light stimulation. When I ask him to look at my finger and so accommodate, the small pupils become even smaller: they are pinpoint, or miotic. The reflex to direct light is lost, but accommodation is preserved.

Here the irrepressible Macarthy intervenes with, "There was an ould mouldy cod of a Scotchman, called Argyll Robertson, who described these pupils and thought the trouble that hatched these pupils was in the spinal cord, only, Begod, he was wrong. Haven't I heard you say that yourself, many times?"

With that, he winks knowingly and belches loudly, as an appreciation of his wit and his as yet undigested collation.

The biceps, triceps and brachioradialis tendon reflexes are normal. The patellar and Achilles tendon reflexes are absent. The sound of the percussion hammer is dull and wooden, and these tendons respond like that of a fresh warm corpse.

I ask him to place his right heel on his left knee, and run this calcanean member down to his great toe, watching the movement carefully. He does this fairly well and cackles in triumph. Now he is to do it another time with his eyes closed, and if need be, bandaged. This time the heel wavers violently over the other shin, and ends up in mid-air. The same occurs on the other side.

"You know well I could not do that, anyhow," he glumly admits, but brightens up when I test the co-ordination of his arms. He touches either index finger to his nose equally well with eyes closed or open, and without even a tremor brings into contact both index fingers in front of his nose.

He has to leave his bed, that we may test his balance and his gait. He is asked to stand with his feet close together, heel touching heel, and great toe touching its opposite number. With some swaying he balances himself, with his eyes wide open and watching the floor. At a given signal, and with both my hands near his neck, he is told to shut his eyes suddenly. He does so, sways uncontrollably from side to side, and would fall headlong and violently to the floor, were I not holding his neck firmly, at the same time curtly telling him to open his eyes.

"That is that ould bloody German's, the Romberg's test. It is no good except in tabes," remarks the patient in a funereal aside to the class. "Anyhow, I have not got tabes," he concludes.

I ask him to walk the length of the ward in his bare feet, between a file of white-coated students. He does so bravely, but he staggers, with his feet striking high, stamping and shooting in all directions, and with his eyes glued to the floor. His gait is much worse than it is when he is wearing his shoes, for which I have no adequate explanation except that his shoes may give him confidence and represent a daily gait-pattern to which he has adjusted himself. I now ask him to walk a certain distance blindfolded, and get a sudden and firm refusal bound up with the fact that he does not want to fall and get a fractured hip, with a Charcot neuropathic joint, such as I described in previous lectures, in which he, of course, took an active part. He is wise, this friend of mine, wiser even than the little birds who feed along the Nile on the debris between crocodiles' teeth, and who keep just clear of their clashing jaws.

We are reaching by easy stages the last and most difficult part of the examination, and that is related to the patient's sensory functions, both as to deep and as to superficial sensibility. We certainly have a good subject.

We can assume that the upper extremities are normal in respect to deep sensibility, in that there are good function and no visible in-co-ordination. Accordingly, we shall concentrate upon the lower extremities, since they are seriously affected. We can test joint sensibility only in the toes; moving larger joints brings in errors that will take too long to explain. Taking the great toe between thumb and forefinger, and having the pressure equal on its upper and lower surface, we show the patient, with his eyes open, what we want him to do. Now, with eyes closed, he is to tell us, as we gently raise or lower the toe, whether it goes up or down. A refinement of the test is that he is to tell us the very second we begin to move the toe. Our patient here is useless, as you see; he does not in the least know what we are doing with either great toe. His joint sense of motion there is nil.

Placing a tuning fork while it is vibrating on either malleolus, we ask the patient to tell us when it has stopped. We calibrate the fork on our own extremity, and are able to tell, if necessary with a stop watch, when it dies down to our own sense of vibration. This patient feels the vibration not a whit, and with his eyes shut, he does not even appreciate the pressure of the tuning fork or its cold metallic contact. He feels just nothing. Compression of the Achilles tendon between the bended thumb knuckle and the fingers produces no pain, and pinching of the calf muscle equally is not resented.

All the textbooks talk of testicular sensation's being absent. We have, however, too valuable an organ here under our hands to risk injury by brutal pressure, even in an impotent tabetic. It has still certain cosmetic values, and should not be disturbed by a rashly produced hematoma. Malpractice suits have been engaged in for far less than that. May I simply repeat, then, that in this patient, in his lower extremities, deep sensibility is absent?

There is on the table a set of simple things with which to test superficial sensations. These are concerned with the feeling of touch, of pain and of degrees of heat and cold. There are an applicator stick with a wisp of long-fibered cotton stuck on it by means of adhesive tape, and another applicator with a collar of tape on the end, with a large-headed pin stuck through the collar at right angles. There are two small flasks holding hot and cold water. The temperatures should be reasonably far apart, so that hot is "hot" and cold is "cold," to even the most stupid patient.

A quick run over the face, neck and upper extremities here shows normal responses. We hit paydirt, however, in the region of the nipple. There is a band of anesthesia to pinprick within the fourth and fifth dermatomes. It is constantly present, both in the back and in the front. Above and below sensibility to pain is normal. Thermal sensibility is not felt in the fifth and sixth dermatomes. Above and below, it is normal. There are, therefore, two zones of anesthesia independent of each other, and taking in separately pain and thermal sensibility over the upper thorax. Tactile sensibility is not affected at all. In checking abdominal sensations, we find tactile sense to be normal and sensation of pain somewhat exaggerated, but it is of thermal perception that I would speak and which I would show you.

Mister Macarthy, knowing these secret rites, has developed an anxious and a more than apprehensive look. He watches me with gloomy foreboding, as I make the cold water colder and the hot water hotter. I have him bend over, and I deliberately place the cold-water bottle over his back at about the tenth thoracic segment. He lets a loud screech out of him, and now a higher, keener one when I place the hot-water bottle on his umbilicus, and saying firmly, "No more of that!" covers himself with the bedclothes and defies me to do more. I promise that I will not do so again.

In his history he tells you how particular he is regarding his bath water: how he measures its temperature with a thermometer, so that as he immerses himself, it will be only tepid. He can stand any number of spinal punctures, but not the preliminary cleansing of the skin with alcohol and ether. He used to like to bathe in the sea; being a nonswimmer he had to wade out, but when the water hit his midriff, he incontinently fled for the shore. He does not like heat or cold around his trunk, or between the ribs and groins, for he says it almost cuts him in two, and he definitely *does not like it.*

Going down to the lower extremities with pin, cotton wool and thermal bottles, we find that all is peace there. Tactile sense is moderately good, and is therefore in contrast to pain and thermal stimuli. Reaction to pain is pathognomonic. Below the knees, and in the feet, it is likely to be felt not at all. Higher up, there is this delayed sensibility to pain that is so characteristic. Prodding the patient in the thigh obtains no response, and yet, a split second later, and while we are going on to the next stimulus, the call of "Sharp!" is uttered. He may call a pinprick "Dull," and then almost immediately apologize that now it feels "Sharp!" to him. He says he feels the touch of the pinpoint, but that it gives no painful sensation until a short but definite phase passes, after which the sting is felt as it should have been when first he was prodded. This is delayed pain. It slows up the sensory pain tests, but it is diagnostic, in that there are few other diseases in which the phenomenon occurs.

Heat and cold stimuli are somewhat similar, but not so striking. It is the sensation of cold that is called "warm," only to be changed a second or less later, when the stinging character of cold is tardily felt. Down in the feet, where thermal and pain sensibilities are depressed almost to anesthesia, sensation of touch may be considerably reduced, but it is seldom entirely absent.

Tabes dorsalis is a disease of the *sensory* nervous system, in contrast to amyotrophic lateral sclerosis and others which are predominantly diseases of the *motorial* systems of brain and spinal cord. The former is a most painful affliction, but the patients suffering from it may live on indefinitely, if the urinary system is kept free from infection. On the other hand, the degenerations of the motor systems are painless, but sooner or later they lead to a fatal ending. They are not any more infrequent now than they were thirty years ago, whereas tabes dorsalis is becoming rare and scarce in our wards. Treatment in these cases of old, "burnt-out" tabes dorsalis is merely symptomatic. Tests of the blood and cerebrospinal fluid show no evidence of active syphilis, and therefore, there is present no active disease which could be modified by treatment.

I think we have done now with our friend Demetrius O'Flanagan Macarthy. I see him wince at his name, but it is an honorable and a noble one. When I first attended him, I treated him as best I knew. In all events, he had had everything elsewhere that might have been of value. I gave him a liquid medicine that goes back to our forefathers, and which consists of the simple formula of "Hydrarg: Perchlor: and Pot: Iod: for those who have left the ways of God." He did beautifully on this, and his gastric crises at that time were sore and sorry afflictions. *Post hoc ergo propter hoc*—they disappeared, and lo, I had a friend for life. The lightning pains continued, so that on that score my remedies failed him. He was willing to attend these classes in those earlier days, as the protagonist in a Greek play, but alas, he fell away. I had then to bribe him to come, since the supply of patients with tabes was fast dwindling. He is here now with a viaticum promised that will cover all expenses of travel and an honorarium to boot.

This time I have had, however, to explain to him the Law of

Diminishing Returns, and that tabes is becoming a dead and forgotten disease, not so important these days. According to his point of view, the situation is that other teachers in other hospitals have asked for him and his professional service. As he says quite logically, "If *you* can not give it to me, there's thim that will." Again I responded that he and his disease may occupy in future a glass case in our National Museum in juxtaposition with a reproduction of the dodo complete, as reconstructed from one hind leg. There are so many new diseases coming in that time moves on from the old tabes dorsalis to periarteritis nodosa, and further on, to the collagen diseases and myositides of unknown origin.

He is looking at me now, gentlemen, for all the world like a small boy, chastened and inwardly hurt. His nether lip protrudes, and his chin quivers as if he were going to cry. There are, in fact, tears already welling up in his doglike eyes. He does not know what to think, and his emotions are mixed. After all, he *is* an old friend of mine, and has kept me from gambling and wasting my substance on these unpredictable, mangy horses, with their suborned guilty triumvirate of owner, trainer and jockey. I have ready for him in an envelop a new, crisp, red bank note, bearing the portrait of the most beautiful woman Ireland has ever known, faithfully drawn by her artist-husband during her life that was only too short.

He is gone, Macarthy, like a deer wounded in our modern corrupt world. He clears the steps, appearing as if to fall at any moment but does not, and dashes headlong down the alley with his hard hat jammed on his bald dome, on his way to his place of business where he is always the wise man who consorts with fools, and savagely makes gain from their folly. He has paid dearly enough for his own, throughout the years that are past, although he will never admit it.

5

Good morning! In two more days you will be celebrating the fiesta of your patron saint, and there will be great activity on that day of all days in Ireland. There will be a nationwide call to prayer in every church that morning; at midday, a display of military might on parade, and all sorts of games and sports for the afternoon. The President himself will make a speech! It will be a long one, and in Gaelic, but you will be allowed a translation in the newspapers the day after.

There will be only one cloud over this otherwise pleasant seventeenth of March: the taverns, saloons, public houses, and all places where alcoholic liquors are dispensed will be solidly and firmly closed for the day. All back entrances will be closely watched by the Civic Guards, and whatever celebration there will be that evening will take place in the homes of the people, a good thing, no doubt, and reminiscent of Election Day in the United States.

In the fifth century, Saint Patrick, from the eminence of a high mountain, to this day called Croagh Patrick, cast into the sea all the serpents, venomous creatures and demons he could collect. They were many, and it took a long time to gather them together, and they have never reappeared in this saintly island since then. It stands to reason, Saint Patrick being a jealous saint, that not one of his protégés should ever see such creatures, even in a disembodied form around the period of his feast day. To see snakes and pink demons would be an insult to the holy and venerable saint. Is it not strange that in delirium tremens there appear no

204

angels, cherubim or seraphim to the hallucinated? . . . It is all to the good that this country retains its sobriety on its patron saint's day, where the twentieth century meets the fifth, and that holiness, abstinence and prayers are in vogue and solemnly celebrated. . . . But I see the ward sister beckoning me; our patient must be in the next ward down the hall.

This man aged forty-nine is suffering grievous pain. He has had it more than nine months, and it is located in his upper jaw, forehead, temple and occiput, behind the ear on the left side. It is definitely worse at night, when he finds himself impelled to walk the floor, sometimes from the time he retires until morning comes. At first, aspirin helped; later codeine, and now he is calling for morphine. It is a steady, nagging, severe pain, without any paroxysms, apparently made worse by nothing, except that it is more unbearable in those hours of the twenty-four wherein he hopes to get rest and sleep. It is almost as bad in the daytime, but at least then he can keep his mind occupied and partially forget it.

At first it was over his cheek and superior maxilla, but later it spread, as you can see, to involve almost the whole half of his head. Nothing relieves it now, except large doses of codeine or smaller quantities of morphine. He is altogether distracted with this pain. He complains also of loss of appetite, which he ascribes to his medication, and correspondingly there is a loss of thirty pounds over the previous nine months.

Six months ago he felt that his cheek was becoming numb, a sensation he describes as that felt when a dentist blocks the nerve of a tooth with procaine hydrochloride. This numbness spread to his upper lip, and into the teeth of his upper jaw. It seems now to be going also into his temporal region. During one of his bad sessions of pain, this numbness appears to be more intense. His forehead, tongue and lower jaw as yet feel normal to him. There is, however, a slow but continuous spread of numbness up to date, and it is becoming greater in degree.

About three months ago, he noticed for the first time double vision, mainly on looking to the left. The images have gradually separated farther, and even on his looking straight ahead, he now sees two of everything he looks at. His family have noticed that a squint has developed, and that his left eye is gradually drifting inward. He tried to relieve this by means of special optical lenses, but they had to be changed so frequently that the trouble and the expense involved defeated their purpose. He has had to resort to covering the spectacle lens over the left eye with a piece of paper, and using his right eye alone. At about the same time the diplopia began to bother him he noticed in his left ear a *full* sensation, as if the left eustachian tube were blocked. Hearing has diminished in that ear, and the stuffed sensation between throat and ear is extremely disagreeable.

Two months ago, while feeling around his neck, he discovered by accident a hard lump just under the angle of the jaw. He has kept close watch on this and finds that it is increasing in size; now it is visible, and is located in the anterior triangle, just in front of the sternocleidomastoid muscle. His local surgeon wanted to remove it, but the patient thought he would leave it for our examination. He thinks that there are now smaller lumps below it. He has had a bloody discharge from his nose this last month, for which there is no explanation.

He looks wasted, feeble and ill, and his color is bad. There is obvious paralysis, now almost complete, of the left external rectus muscle of the eye. Sensory tests of the fifth nerve show a blunting to pain, tactile and thermal sensibility, over a limited area of the left cheek. Sensory changes in his temporal region are entirely subjective, and the masticatory muscles function well. The corneal reflex is present and active. Examination is difficult because of his great pain, but he bears it as well as he can, begging only occasionally for codeine or injections of morphine. Nothing abnormal is found on examination of his mouth, tonsillar area or oral part of the pharynx. By watch test, his hearing on the left is reduced 50 per cent. His eye grounds are normal; also normal are pupils and their reflexes. Vision in both eyes is excellent.

Roentgen studies of his skull and thorax show no abnormal changes, and except for his generally depressed physical condition no physical changes are found in routine examination.

The lump in his neck is visible, hard and fixed to the tissues surrounding it; it is about 4 cm. in diameter. There are smaller lumps below it in the deeper tissues; these lumps obviously are enlarged, and seem to be indurated lymph glands along the cervical chain. A few days ago I had our laryngologist examine this patient's nasopharynx; a specimen of tissue for biopsy was taken. The results, including results of study of the section of tissue removed, and the report, I shall show you in the other ward where we first assembled. Let us go there now.

This man has an illness which we have followed step by step, and each gradation downward has its own meaning. His first complaint was of pain in the second division of the fifth nerve, on the left side. At first situated in only part of the second division, it spread later to involve the whole division, and was followed by half-sided headache suggesting involvement of the meninges of the skull. Destruction of the second division of the fifth nerve followed in the increasing anesthesia. Next the sixth nerve was attacked, as would be likely, since it is a long and vulnerable nerve on the base of the skull. Note that the death of this nerve was slow but progressive. The deafness and sensation of fullness in the ear have been caused by blocking of the eustachian orifice. The enlarged gland was another step on the progressive path downhill in this patient's history.

Can you not visualize once more then, this cachectic man, with, in his attitude, all the signs of pain, his appearance of being very ill, his squint, and the lump in his neck, and proceed to formulate a further examination by which we can know definitely what is behind all this? We have to go deeper; to date we have been merely playing on the surface, wasting our time thinking of unrelated things.

I have seen many good clinicians puzzled over this problem, for they did not have the assistance of those laryngologists who are accustomed to examining a nasopharynx, and who can dive below all superficial structures to find the pearls that give a final and proved diagnosis. I have seen surgeons remove the enlarged cervical gland, and finding it to be a metastatic malignant process, walk off, hands in pockets, whistling and satisfied that the problem had been solved. Neurosurgeons have explored the cranial cavity and have discovered nothing to explain the progressive morbid syndrome that you have just seen.

Our laryngologist has produced a specimen of the original tumor of this patient, and you can see it now for yourselves. Under the microscope you will find a minute section taken from a small bulge in the nasopharynx, in the fossa of Rosenmüller, and adjacent to the left eustachian orifice. This bulge had a tiny ulcer on top of it, and the section for biopsy was taken from the edge of the ulcer. Our pathologist describes the tissue removed as being a squamous cell carcinoma of high degree of malignancy. The laryngologist took half an hour to find it, and nearly missed it; he might quite possibly have sent back a negative report. Naturally, had that been the case, I should then have sent the patient back to him for another look, and would even have asked someone else to take up the search for this primary carcinoma, so certain was I that it was present.

So, from this hidden source, comes the evil we have seen today. This cancer arises away back in the dark nasopharynx and works up through the base of the skull and its foramina under the dura, and catches the cranial nerves as they penetrate the dural envelope. Usually, the fifth and sixth nerves are affected first; any of the other last cranial nerves may be later affected, such as the ninth, tenth, eleventh and twelfth. The original tumor may be a squamous cell carcinoma, as this one is, or, in young patients, a sarcoma from the nasopharyngeal adenoidal tissue.

The prognosis is hopeless, but for palliation we apply radium to the area involved in the nasopharynx, and deep roentgen rays to the affected lymph glands. The condition you have seen here this morning is *nasopharyngeal malignant disease*, with invasion of the floor of the skull outside the dura. It is a typical one, and I am sure that you will see more like it and recognize them in your stride.

In the final stages, the malignant tumor bulges now into the oral pharynx and displaces the soft palate downward. By inspection of the pharynx with a strong light, the tumor can be readily seen. By that time, the cervical glands are enormous, many more cranial nerves are involved, and palliative treatment is of less value. No matter what the cause is, or what the existing prospect for eventual cure, an early diagnosis has its merits in settling a problem wherein uncertainty may be worse than a death sentence. The patient and his relatives are entitled to know at the earliest possible moment what is essentially wrong, and what we can do about it, one way or the other. There is a merit in a scientific opinion based on facts and with an air of finality that proves to be true.

6

I HAVE here a lad in his twenties, clad in canonical black, whom I first saw a year ago. He was then a clerical student at a seminary which educates boys to be ordained for the priesthood, and then sends them far afield into missionary work. Most of them go to darkest Africa, to spread the Gospel and to Christianize the dusky natives. In such a life they must not only be perfect physically, but must be prepared to meet all hardships.

This boy, when in his third year of seminary, complained of a weakness in his right hand, and numbness in the ring and little fingers. The numbness was complete in the little finger, and occupied half the ring finger on the ulnar side. He found that the muscle between his thumb and index finger had wasted, creating an obvious hollow between the metacarpal bones of the right hand. There was corresponding atrophy of the muscles of the right hypothenar eminence. A few fasciculations were present.

He had found it increasingly difficult to separate pages of a book, to button his clothes, to hold a comb to part his hair, and to press together the snap fasteners of his gloves. Nevertheless, he could write, feed himself, and with his right hand do any hard physical work he was asked to do. His local physician had made a diagnosis of "progressive muscular atrophy," given a bad prognosis as to the spreading of this infirmity, and had advised that the boy be dropped from the Order, and returned to his parents to resign himself to a secular life. His career up to date had, however, been so excellent that his superiors asked for another opinion before acting hastily and harshly.

He is a tall, gangling youth of about six feet, two inches, and thin in the extreme. There was in his eyes the fire of an intense religious vocation, and a sharp punctiliousness shown in every step of our interview. He had no idea whatsoever as to why his right hand should have become weak and numb and why some of its intrinsic muscles should have become wasted. I had a great problem in working out the cause of his difficulty, and the suddenness with which it flashed on my consciousness must have been an act of divine guidance.

He had, in short, a moderately advanced lesion of his right ulnar nerve. There was the anesthesia of the little finger and half the ring finger, atrophy and weakness of the hypothenar eminence and its muscles, and a sunken, wasted adductor pollicis muscle. Moreover, a claw hand was beginning to develop. There were no other findings. The right ulnar nerve in its bed behind the medial epicondylar process was tender and somewhat enlarged; percussion of it increased the numbness of the little finger and ring finger, producing darts of pain in the same area. Nevertheless, the elbow joint was intact, movements of the forearm on the upper arm were unrestricted, and results of roentgen studies in that area were entirely negative.

Divine inspiration is not always available, and after much pondering of the problem, I was just about to give up all responsibility for the explanation of this clerical student's disability, when, as I mentioned before, I began suddenly to think more clearly and concisely about cause and effect.

I asked him what he did during his waking hours, apart from eating and taking the small amount of recreation he was allowed. In his earlier months in the seminary, he said, menial labors had been exacted of him, but later on he was buckled down to the essential functions of preparation for the priesthood. I gathered that praying and studying were then his chief occupations. And how did he pray and study, I asked. I provided a chair, a table and a book. Automatically, this overgrown, skinny youth, resting his head in his hands and with his elbows on the hard wood, entered into prayer. He was right-handed, and I saw that the corresponding elbow received most of the weight. In studying or reading it was grossly the same. He rested both attenuated elbows on the table, supporting his head with his right hand, and occasionally he lifted the *left* elbow to turn the pages of St. Thomas Aquinas' *Summa Contra Gentiles.*

This elbow pressure occupied at least three quarters of his hours awake. Studying and reading; reading and studying and praying, always with the elbow *and* the right ulnar nerve squeezed, compressed and painlessly traumatized by the weight of his head, arm and hand. If it had brought pain, he would have been on his guard, but in the concentration of his prayer and his study of the Scholastics, he had no concept at all that he was injuring himself and producing a *palsy of the ulnar nerve* that simulated, at least to the local physician, no less serious a condition than a "creeping paralysis."

The cause being found, the cure was effected. I advised him to pad well his elbows with cotton wool, and to stop resting his arm on the traumatized ulnar nerve. This he did, and my letter to his superior allowed him to continue his studies. He has just finished his course, a year after I first saw him; he is now ordained, gave me his blessing this morning, and is off to Africa next week.

He has been kind enough to consent to show himself to you this morning, and to tell you what his right hand, now normal, was like a year ago. There is still some numbness in the little finger, but it is minimal. The atrophy has filled in, the clawing of the hand has disappeared, the function of his right hand is perfect. All this foregoing story is so simple, the cause and prevention of the condition always so obvious, that I am almost ashamed to show you him, and yet, in my heart of hearts, l am not! Go thou, and do likewise.

As you have doubtless perceived, I feel rather proud of this diagnosis and of my handling of the problem. Had I failed here, this boy would have been returned to a lay existence in which he would have been neither "fish, flesh, fowl nor good red herring." Once having progressed so far into a priestly vocation, he would have found that there is no return to a life of worldliness that can be a completely happy one for him. A sense of frustration and embitterment forever dogs all the days of the lives of these men, who have almost reached the goal of becoming a superior being, and suddenly are plunged into the abyss of common clay. Every time they see a more fortunate one celebrate Mass, a fresh wound is inflicted on them. It is altogether understandable that some of them simply leave the Church, and embrace in matters of religion—just nothing. This is sheer waste of human energy, no matter in what channels the energy be subsequently directed, and it should, at all costs, be avoided.

Earlier this year I talked to you of tardy ulnar neuritis. In this condition, the elbow joint was so distorted by a previous fracture, or by more recent arthritis, that the ulnar nerve had an uneasy bed behind the internal epicondyle. It suffered therefrom, and had to be transferred to a more safe and comfortable location in front of the epicondyle. There at rest, and free from harm, it had a chance to regenerate, provided the previous damage had not been too great.

On the other hand, in these cases of ulnar palsy the elbow joint is normal, and injury to the nerve is caused by what the patient allows himself to do. I had one patient who had had an intensely painful iritis. To relieve his pain, he had sat for three days with his elbows on his knees, holding cloths soaked in hot water over his extremely painful eyes. When the pain in his eyes cleared up, he found that severe damage to both ulnar nerves had developed, which took at least two years to disappear completely.

Another patient, an elderly one, had a stroke over a weekend, and lay flat on his back on the concrete floor of a barn. When his family returned to the house, he was discovered and sent into the hospital. He recovered from his cerebral vascular disturbance, but was left with bilateral ulnar neuritis, caused by the pressing of both elbows on the concrete floor. When patients who have been operated on for abdominal conditions are allowed to lie flat on their backs, ulnar palsy may develop on one or both sides, because they have not been turned frequently enough in bed. This is something that is awkward to explain, after the patient has made recovery from a perfect surgical procedure. Happily, these ulnar palsies clear up in the course of time.

Finally, I have seen a patient with so bad a sciatic pain that he was confined to bed for ten days. The pain was in the left leg, and because of it he could not lie on the left side. Consequently, during his enforced confinement, he lay on his right side continuously, resting his head and arm on his right elbow, and in this position he read many interesting books, turning the pages with his left hand. At last his sciatic pain subsided, and he recovered from his invalidism, but he wondered, as he returned to an active existence, what had happened to his right hand that had made it numb and clumsy!

Many more examples might be given, but always there comes up the problem of a painlessly insidious appearance of ulnar palsy. It may even be bilateral, in which case the plural must be used. It is thrust under your nose for explanation, and there is *always* a reason for its being present. Try to find it! The cause is often so simple that it may, perhaps, evade your diagnostic acumen just because it *is* so simple. Having failed to spot it, you will be kicking yourself later on for want of common sense, and for missing the things so very obvious and so close to your face.

The trumpet of a prophecy! O, wind,
If Winter comes, can Spring be far behind?
—SHELLEY: *Ode to the West Wind.*

7

Good morning! Spring at last is coming in. The buds on the trees, that have been swelling the last few days, have burst their membranous birth cauls, and are now showing themselves as feathery tufts. There is a wisplike character to the trees at this time, reminding us of Corot, who loved to paint them as they appear now, against a dull, leaden gray sky. A few brave, hardy fruit saplings have put forth some timorous blooms, as if half afraid of a late and bitter frost. Beneath the hedgerows along the country roads I explored last Sunday, there were patches of deep brown turf blazoned with yellow primroses, while open glades in the woods were blue with wild violets. I saw robins and migratory birds coming back to the nests to which they had returned regularly every year. Most sweet of all, the turtledove was calling to his mate from many a dark patch of evergreen trees, sobbing out his love, and all the intense feelings that spring engenders.

The two signs of spring I had most counted on, however, were not present until I encountered them this very morning on my way to you. They are characteristic of life in a city. Far above my head were two tiny sparrows which had survived the winter here by eking out a precarious living from smoking horse dung, and scarce, vagrant crusts of bread. They were indulging in a frenzied, ecstatic, vociferous and determined consummation of their wooing, high in the sky, preparatory to building a tiny nest at some corner of a dull, stodgy civic building. The Lord surely loves each sparrow, for never have I seen one fall during their tiny but titanic efforts to procreate their kind.

Going down to earth, I found the other sign: two young boys, not yet ten years old, were rolling over and over in the mud of the street, locked in bitter combat, undeterred by any rules, punching, kicking and gouging each other. As a matter of fact, I had to stop my car, lest I run over them. As in the adventures of King Arthur and his knights, there should have been in the background a grubby little slum girl, with tousled hair and troubled eyes. I looked around and was disappointed to see no trace of a captive maiden to be rescued in accordance with the laws of chivalry. Hence, I assumed that the duel was one begot in their bones by spring, and the rising of sap in their muscles, unconscious in motive, and as primitive as the history of the terrestrial globe. A few coppers and a short sermon sent them off arm in arm, better friends than ever.

Today I am going to show you a very favorite patient of mine. You have passed her many times in this corner bed, no doubt without any notice on your part. At the times you were here, she was always asleep and motionless, and only the outlines of her body showed through the bed covers. During the previous six weeks, she has been as still as a half-submerged log in the backwaters of a river.

For this reason she has had to be fed. Her urinary and bowel functions have had to be taken care of, and at first she showed little or no response, either mentally or physically. She has been partly conscious, but has far preferred to be left alone in her warm bed, under many covers, and to assume none of the responsibility of wakefulness. Like a hibernating female bear, she has lived with her metabolism reduced to its lowest possible level of existence, while we, in spite of her attitude, have been pushing it steadily upward. We had hoped that after these gelid months of winter weather, now that it is spring, she would, with appropriate treatment, undergo a metamorphosis, and we are not disappointed in this respect. Hibernation is slowly ending now, and by late spring or summer we should see a completely different mental and physical specimen.

It will not be the kiss of a Prince Charming, however, that will finally raise this sleeping beauty to a normal existence in this world of struggle. More prosaic than that, it has been, and will continue to be, carefully calculated doses of little brown tablets, given regularly and in ever-increasing amounts.

First, I want to give you the story of how I met this lady, and the immediate *mise en scène* in which she, her best friend and I found ourselves. Later, the clinical history will be developed, and what was found when she was first admitted to this hospital. Finally, I shall show her to you as she is now, after weeks of cautious therapy, and shall finish with some remarks as to further treatment, prognosis and differential diagnosis.

About six weeks ago, late on a raw, rain-lashed afternoon in February, a colleague called me to announce that he was sending me a patient. There would be a friend along who could explain the circumstances. He apologized because the fee would be small, but the friend was paying it out of her own pocket, which, he said, was a very small receptacle. The issue was to avoid a summary commitment of the patient to the local mental hospital. Would I kindly take her into my own hospital wards where no stigma would be involved? She had been quiet enough until recently, but no doubt she would settle down and cause no trouble, once I had admitted her. The pattern of approach was so similar to many others that I gave the usual consent, but also with the usual amendment: that if she caused trouble, she would have to be discharged, and readmitted to a mental hospital, where greater facilities for disturbed patients are available.

With amazing alacrity, the two ladies arrived on my doorstep. It was getting dark, and my last patient had gone; I admitted them myself. They were an extraordinarily ill-assorted pair. The best friend, who called herself Mrs. Muldowney, was a huge, fat, middle-aged person, with brawny bare arms and a gigantic bosom, who exuded enormous, vital potential energy. I heard afterward that she had a curbstone market for fish in Mary Street, and she certainly smelled like it. Nevertheless, her face radiated such kindness and charity that I was willing to overlook the piscatorial aura.

Her friend, the patient, was so unobtrusive that I hardly gave her a glance as she glided into my room like a ghost, and seated herself quietly and passively alongside her friend. As in the ward here, you could have passed her a hundred times and never even noticed her presence. She took no part in the consultation, even though it concerned her recent behavior, her mental status, and what was to be done with her. She was as silent as Mrs. Muldowney was voluble. The latter arranged her hat, smoothed out her apron, and with her feet planted wide apart, started to deliver a lengthy oration. My dinner seemed to be further off than ever.

Madam, the fishmonger, produced without delay her opening gambit. In a torrent of words, she declared that her friend was a "quare one, and as quare as they can ever make 'em." She went on to say that for the last twelve months the patient had shown a loss of interest in her children, her husband and in what one would call her "home." I gathered that these paragons of behavior, her husband and children, had put up with a lot, but were now at the breaking point of human endeavor. The husband, poor man, was not with us because he had to work fourteen hours a day at the docks, unloading ships' cargoes. He, however, wanted his wife "mended," and returned sound in body and mind to him and to the little family of four "childern."

I was told, as I rose for air, that this woman, when well, was the finest on earth, and that no one could equal her devotion to her husband and "childern" in those years when she had normal health. She was, moreover, Mrs. Muldowney's best friend, and at that, our solid block of a woman burst into tears, and essayed to wipe them with the grimy apron she was still wearing, ever since leaving her home to bring her friend to the physician. She was a business woman, she claimed, and would not see her friend, for want of a little money, buried for life in one of "thim places." Call it womanly intuition, if you like, but she was not far wrong, as it turned out to be.

She told me of how bitterly her friend complained of the cold this past winter, hanging over a mockery of a hearthfire consisting of a mere handful of coals. In the meantime, she draped herself with all her clothing, and was not averse to using her husband's and some of the children's, whenever she could seize on them.

She would go to bed early, putting all that she had worn during the day under her and over her in bed. She usually slept until well into the forenoon. Now Mrs. Muldowney had her own brood, an exacting, dyspeptic husband, and, of course, her fish market, but, by some miracle, she found time to help out in the care of the patient and her family. If there is to be found true Christian charity, it dwells in these noisome Dublin slums, wherein poverty, misery and dirt may bring out the best in human nature, as is truly shown so often in these denizens of our squalid tenements.

During the last three months, things had gone from bad to worse. Mrs. Boylan, as the patient is called, suddenly took a violent dislike to the people living in the next tenement. The houses were once the town residences of eighteenth-century gentry, who had built their walls massive enough so that no noise could penetrate the heavy brick partitions. Nevertheless, Mrs. Boylan claimed that she could hear the people next door cursing her, calling her names, and attacking her character. At first, she would merely shake a fist in their direction; later she would rise from her crouching position over the fire, and beat with her hands on the thick wall, cursing her imaginary enemies loudly. She would then go back to the pitiful semblance of a fire, and for hours sit immobile, almost inside the grate.

Twenty-four hours before the visit of these two women to me, things had come to a startling climax. The tormented one now had gone over to the direct attack. Finding that banging on the walls produced no cessation of the persecutory auditory hallucinations, she sallied forth to take up her position next door, outside the windows of her supposed enemies. Here, Mrs. Muldowney interposed that these people were quiet and harmless, even though "the man of the house" was out of work.

"They would not hurt even a fly," she affirmed solemnly.

Mrs. Boylan yelled and screeched up at her neighbors, using words that even her friend did not know the meaning of, but they sounded bad enough! Swiftly going from words to action, the patient gathered up an apronful of loose paving stones, and with an unerring aim, flung each rock through the windows next to hers. She then retired to her usual place by the fire, showing neither emotion nor contrition. The Civic Guards were called, and while crowds surged around the street below, every window held a cautious head, protruding to find out what was happening. Red Cow Lane was in a turmoil.

When the Guards arrived, quiet was restored, and they began to make judicious inquiries. At just that time, Mrs. Muldowney came on the scene, and begged that her friend not be arrested, explaining that she was a nervous person, and "that her nerves had got the better of her." With tact and good judgment, these huge limbs of the law extracted a promise that as soon as possible this nervous affliction would be seen to by a physician, and that further assault and battery would forthwith be prevented. Mrs. Muldowney assured them emphatically that the very next day she would have the best "nerve doctor" in Dublin see her friend, and cure her of throwing stones into other persons' windows. A limited armistice was then declared, as of being from then on, between real and imaginary battling parties, whereupon the Guards departed, leaving Mrs. Muldowney in full charge.

When this stage of the story was reached, there seemed to be nothing more to say, and the kind friend had spun herself out with a final sobbing, all to herself. The dusk in the room had become darkness, and there was nothing to be heard except Mrs. Muldowney's final sob, ending in a wheezing centered around her opulent bosom. The patient remained silent, and in the darkness, could have been nonexistent. I was not happy as to what I should see when the lights were switched on. Already, I had so far branded her condition as paranoid schizophrenia, a potential trouble in my hospital, and her admission there only a makeshift until she was duly committed by law to the contiguous Grangegorman Hospital for the Insane. But, this seemed to be the very thing her friend was trying to avoid! My imagination led me to think that the woman, now silent and invisible in the dark room, was a wild-eyed, untidy character, with deep and dangerous suspicion in her glance, a tigress about to spring on her prey. I hesitated even a few minutes longer, and then turned on the lights in my consulting room. . . .

I saw a thin little woman sitting bolt upright, her hands folded in her lap, quietly looking at me. Her hair was neat; her cheap

dress was clean and newly pressed; she was as tidy as Mrs. Muldowney could possibly have made her. Yet, she looked the part
of a woman *naturally* tidy, and one who would have felt hurt to
be otherwise. Fortunately, Mrs. Boylan was still quiet, and in
the silence of the room now brightly lighted, this frail wisp of a
woman looked at me steadily, and in her eyes there was the
hunted, wounded look of a favorite domestic animal that is ill and
begging for help. She looked so very different from what I had
expected, that being troubled and mute, I simply kept looking
back at her, hoping to find the answer to this enigma before the
spell of silence was broken.

At last, I asked her gently what was wrong with her, and why
she had done such harmful things. The grandfather's clock in the
hall ticked off a full round of seconds before the answer, such as
it was, came. After what seemed centuries of time, in a harsh,
toneless voice, creaking like old leather, she said, "I do not know."
I put it to her that she was in serious trouble, and that I was willing to help her, if only she would give me some guide to her problem or problems. A sort of light came into her eyes, and again, in
that strange voice, she rasped out with great deliberation, "Only
the Lord Jesus knows how cold I am; can *you* ever get me feeling
warm?" I said that I would certainly try to do so, and made some
inane jest as to body temperature. After a gap of some seconds,
to my amazement she began to struggle at a smile. It grew, and
then passed over her face like a low-hung cloud over the earth, and
was as slowly gone. Evidently, this extraordinary woman, who
looked like an Egyptian mummy, had some glimmerings of reason,
as shown in her appreciation of my odd sense of humor.

It was at this time that a tiny bell started to ring in my head—
at first soft but insistent, and then growing ever louder. It was
calling me to something I ought to know, a diagnosis that was
easy, once one thought of the right channels of approach. It con-
veyed to me the realization that a physical examination, along a
certain line, would solve the problem. This I proceeded to do. All
thoughts of a primary mental condition were now rejected; the
patient was suffering from a physical disease with a mental
counterpart, but what was the disease? I had somewhat more

than suspicions now, however, as to the nature of this disease.

The room was well illuminated. I noticed that the patient's hair was coarse and scanty, and that it felt dry to the touch. Her lower eyelids were swollen, so that the puncta lacrimae could not discharge their function, and tears were occasionally running down her cheeks. Her eyelids, as compared to the rest of her face, were dead white. Her lips were swollen and bluish. Her eyebrows were scanty, and each outer third portion was gone. The color of her face was generally that of a yellow-white clay, except for a slight malar flush. Her body was cool—almost corpselike. The blood pressure was 90 systolic and 70 diastolic; her pulse was sixty beats per minute. Thermometer readings, taken orally, were 90° F.

Examining her Achilles reflexes, I found that there was a quick response, but an infinitesimally slow return. Unless watched for carefully, there seemed to be no return. This has been likened to the shock absorbers on cars, where, going over a bump, the body of the car dips suddenly, but returns gradually to normal, giving the passengers an easier journey. This pattern is not present in the patellar tendon reflexes, but it occurs similarly in the biceps reflex. Although the patient is miserably thin, there are pads of fat above the clavicle. The combination of swollen, bluish lips, the slow, creaking voice, and the edema of the eyelids in an otherwise thin face were very striking. Her hands were like dry chips of wood, and nowhere did I find evidence of sweating.

The bell in my head had long since ceased to ring—as a silent token of having guided me along the right path. I told Mrs. Muldowney that I would admit her friend that night to the hospital, and rightly or wrongly, promised to do her some good. The purveyor of fish was ecstatic, and somewhat spiked my guns by claiming that this was all due to her prayers to her patron saint, who, as far as I could see, was as yet not a registered physician. I ordered a cab, notified the hospital, and wrote a note to be given my house officer as to what should be done on the patient's admission.

At this point, the good friend approached me and placed on my desk a very small bank note. (I could swear it had fish scales on it.) She thanked me over and over again; then, speechless, and overcome by emotion and tears, she led the patient gently out the front door. There was no response from the latter, no inquiry as to where she was going, and as to what was to be done to her. Perhaps she is different today. I hope so.

Today is the twenty-second of March. Our patient came to stay with us on the seventh of February last. As reckoned by the calendar, she has been here six weeks, and has been treated continuously since she came in. She is sitting up in bed now and has given me a hearty handshake. In her blue eyes there is a look of gratitude and friendliness that I shall treasure forever. She gets up in the afternoon and helps around the ward, and everyone finds her a most agreeable and helpful soul.

She has a few things wrong with her still. She has no memory of events of two or three months ago. She has no recollection of her behavior in her home, nor of her seeing me that dark night in February, and after six weeks here, it is only of the last week or two of her stay in this hospital that she has any remembrance. Of all that preceded this last week or two, there is complete oblivion, covering many weeks and even months.

For weeks she has remained in this bed, oblivious to everything, and now she is beginning to wake up. I ask her if she remembers seeing me at my consulting rooms, and being admitted here. She shakes her head, and tells us that there is a lot she has forgotten about her illness, and adds that she is just as happy to forget it, considering what she has been told she did during that period. In other words, about three months have gone out of her life, of which she has not the slightest memory.

Even at present, her thoughts are slow, and because of forgotten words, she can not carry on a conversation as rapidly and efficiently as she would like. I asked her why she greeted me so effusively, and she answered that in her early return to consciousness, and in the struggle to orient herself, she had felt that I was a power for good, and not for evil. There are hazy memories with her in which I seemed to be fighting on her side, against the powers of evil.

On her admission to hospital, her pulse, blood pressure and

temperature were found to be below normal, as when I first saw her. Her basal metabolic rate was –30 per cent. The blood cholesterol reading was 350 mg. per 100 cc. of plasma. Her face is not so changed now as it was when she was admitted, but the lips and lower eyelids are still swollen, and the facial color is still like yellow-white clay, with a slight malar flush. Her voice is still rasping and croaking, but less pronouncedly so. Her hair remains dry, and she does not sweat, even with electric blankets or the baking apparatus. Her hands are more moist now, but her Achilles tendon reflex still shows the same phenomenon of a quick response and a slow return to a resting stage. The basal metabolic rate is now –15 per cent, and her blood pressure, pulse rate and temperature are more nearly normal. I would have you verify some of these findings, but most particularly, I want you to test this Achilles reflex, which is almost pathognomonic of *myxedema*. I think that in a few more weeks we shall have this patient as nearly normal as we can make her, but her basic maintenance dose will have to be determined, and she will have to take it all the rest of her life, while having regular, periodic basal metabolic readings.

The treatment of myxedema, as found in its early epoch, was quite as revolutionary as the use of liver in pernicious anemia, or of penicillin in bacterial infection. To change these hibernating animals into something approaching a human being was a tremendous advance in medical treatment. It had to be learned, however, that any sudden change from the patient's "frozen" state was a serious affair. The heart had been under a strain for a long time, and the kidneys did not take kindly to a sudden deposit of myxomatous material in their filter of the blood stream. Severe leg pains and muscle tenderness were complications of too quick an elevation of the basal metabolic rate, and all students of the problem of myxedema are agreed that the administration of thyroid extract should be slow, and subordinated to the degree of metabolic depression. At times, in the beginning, one must resort to homeopathic doses.

We gave this patient ¼ grain of desiccated thyroid extract twice a day, to begin with, and day by day the dose was cautiously elevated. There was no hurry; the majority of our patients take a long time to get into myxedema, and appropriately should take a long time to recover from it. A frozen hand should not be thawed too quickly! Our patient is getting at present 1 grain of thyroid extract three times a day. We insist upon using the desiccated variety, and it must be fresh and recently prepared. A strange thing about these patients is that they feel so wonderful on medication that they forget the cause, and become careless in their taking of thyroid. Inevitably they relapse, and then the paranoid reaction sets in, in that they assume that their physician has failed to "cure" them, and they desert him, go to another one, or into the hands of irregular practitioners, and end up just as bad as, if not worse than, they were before treatment was started. I do not think, however, that this will occur with this patient.

NOTE: This patient has regularly attended the Dispensary for nearly five years now, and gets her thyroid substance without question. She has been well all that time, and is able to do a full day's work.

Mrs. Muldowney has disappeared. I never see her now at the curbstone fish market in Mary Street. She has either gone to her eternal rest, or has emigrated to England, to sell fish on a larger and more profitable scale.

The differential diagnosis rests in the legal phrase, *res ipsa loquitur.* The patient *has,* or *has not,* myxedema. Looking at their facies, one either recognizes or misses the diagnosis. I have had numerous patients sent to me as afflicted with cerebral tumors, because of the apathetic mental reaction, the slow pulse rate, and the progressive dilapidation of the psyche. In each case, the typical facies and other corroborative signs of myxedema were sufficient to afford recognition of what was brewing. Pituitary tumors conceivably may cause trouble, since hypopituitarism may resemble myxedema, but roentgenographic examination of the skull and checking of the perimetric visual fields will settle this problem. The greatest difficulty, as I see it here in this patient, is the exclusion of a mental state *sui generis.* By the turn of a card, this patient might have been committed to a mental hospital, where she might have remained, unwept, unhonored and unsung, for the rest of her short life. Truly, the saints to whom Mrs. Muldowney prayed were potent ones.

And finally, like G. K. Chesterton, I *must* have my paradox. This patient has a condition that is *not* typical of myxedema. If you have seen myxedematous patients at other hospitals, or have seen pictures of them in a textbook, you will note a great difference. These so-called typical examples are fat, bloated monsters who have gained greatly in weight. This patient has been, from the time I first saw her, thin and scrawny. Actually, she has gained weight since she has been taking thyroid extract, because she is eating more, having now an interest in food. The heavy and bulky myxedemic patient loses weight under treatment, and he is a greater risk than this one, since there is an associated cardiac involvement, and the kidneys become overtaxed in getting rid of the myxomatous substance that has infiltrated all the tissues. I would be even slower in elevating the basal metabolic rate of such patients. Sudden death from pushing the administration of thyroid extract too rapidly is not at all unusual.

Relatively speaking, our patient here has been treated a little more rapidly and vigorously than many others. One does not usually think of very thin patients as having myxedema, but you had better do so from now on, lest you fall into grievous error in not giving a patient the very thing the body is crying out for, and is not getting.

8

THIS MAN is sixty-three years old and has ten children. He works twelve hours a day, when the run of business is brisk, cutting the throats of an infinite number of squealing pigs. He also drinks daily fifteen or more pints of black Dublin stout, with a white, creamy head and a fair alcoholic content. He had none the less enjoyed excellent health up to last Sunday morning, this day being Tuesday.

He had had a hard day on Saturday, when he finally retired from work, covered on the outside with the red, sticky gore of hogs, and well filled on the inside with the inebriating product of Messrs. Guinness & Company, Ltd. He was tired, and he went to bed soon after he came home, so as to be able to rise and attend an early Mass next morning.

His first conscious observation on awakening the next day was that everything he saw was double. He heaved himself out of bed, looked in the cracked mirror in the bathroom, and found that his right eye roved around in normal fashion, but that his left eye was turned inward, and could not be made to turn out. When he tried to look to the left, the double images were side by side, and they disappeared on his closing one eye. When he went downstairs, his wife noticed that he had an obvious squint, and he found a little later that by cocking his head to one side, like a chicken contemplating a grain of corn, he could suppress one of the double images. He also found that he was dizzy on going downstairs, and finally he put a patch over the left eye. Using but one eye, he had no double vision and no dizziness. He was very much upset by this sudden affair, and consulted his local physician, who sent him to me.

I found on detailed examination that the only thing wrong with this patient was *paralysis of the left external rectus muscle.* His peripheral vessels were somewhat hardened, but his blood pressure was not more than 170 systolic and 100 diastolic. The retina showed no changes suggesting a hypertensive encephalopathy, and his heart showed no enlargement, either by clinical examination or roentgenologic studies. The local physician had stated that he fears a stroke or pontine hemorrhage, and is uneasy lest a tumor of the brain be under way.

On examining this worthy citizen, we find that the only outstanding abnormal physical sign is, as I said before, complete paralysis of the left external rectus muscle. He thinks now that apart from having diplopia, he feels so well that he ought to go back to work with a patch over his left eye, and I am not at all sure that he is incorrect in this view. To take a man like this one, and coop him up in a hospital filled with bodily wrecks is certainly not good for his ego. When I saw him yesterday, his mustache was waxed on both sides, so that each end, tapering to a needle point, stood out like the antenna of an insect. Look how bedraggled it is this morning! He is like a woman deprived of her lipstick. Let him return to his normal life, wherein he is a lusty fellow, enjoying every minute of it.

These suddenly appearing palsies of the sixth nerve are somewhat less common than a Bell's paralysis. They have, however, a common feature, in that the prognosis is good. As a contrast, they occur always in the arteriosclerotic age. Some think that they are due to transient edema in the pons varolii, from a faulty circulation. Anything as gross as a hemorrhage is unthinkable, since the pons is so packed with important structures, and is such a vital organ, that grave and mortal results occur from its destruction. Besides, the seventh cranial nerve angulates around the pontine nucleus of the sixth cranial nerve, and both must inevitably suffer.

A cerebral tumor would be slower in showing itself, and while the sixth cranial nerve is the most common nerve to be involved in increased intracranial pressure, there would be headaches, vomiting and papilledema before such a manifestation occurred. This man shows no signs of cerebral tumor in his eye grounds, in the bones of his skull by roentgenologic examination, or in his symptoms or the general clinical examination.

It is more likely that a hardened arteriosclerotic vessel crossing the sixth nerve on the floor of the skull may give this nerve a squeeze, producing all the symptoms present in this patient. Anyhow, the diplopia clears up within a space of weeks or months, but it may recur, or it may appear on the other side in a similar, short-lived fashion.

I have a particular form of treatment, a sovereign remedy, that never fails in these cases. There is an ointment called Scott's dressing. It contains mercury, camphor and a greasy vehicle. It is very black, but it smells and feels good. The patient is instructed to rub into the temporal fossa on the side involved a piece of this ointment about the size of the terminal phalanx of his little finger, no more and no less. It must be rubbed in until all the ointment disappears, and this must be done conscientiously twice daily. There should be no cheating. The morning and evening inunctions should continue until all double vision disappears, and the patient, to all intents and purposes, is well again.

The most important thing advised with reference to this application is that the ointment be rubbed in clockwise. If question is asked why, a ready answer is most solemnly given: rubbing it in the *opposite* direction may cause the eye to become loose and fall out, such is the potency of the treatment, and such the danger of its misuse!

This is our last bedside demonstration before the Easter vacation. You will have leisure in which to see the fasting and the self-denial of Lent pass into the joyous Easter Monday celebrations. Easter comes early this year, and you have less than three weeks to wait.

Man is a highly integrated animal. At Easter time he may toy with the idea of getting married, but it is only the following June, or a June many years later, that he proceeds down the aisle to the church door, a bound and shackled man. Let you think of this during the coming weeks. In the meantime, I wish you all a happy Easter.

APRIL

"Damn that boy," said the old gentleman, *"he's gone to sleep again."*

"Very extraordinary boy, that," said Mr. Pickwick, *"does he always sleep in this way?"*

"Sleep!" said the old gentleman, *"he's always asleep. Goes on errands fast asleep, and snores as he waits at table."*

"How very odd!" said Mr. Pickwick. . . .

The fat boy rose, opened his eyes, swallowed the huge piece of pie he had been in the act of masticating when he last fell asleep, and slowly obeyed his master's orders—

—CHARLES DICKENS: *Pickwick Papers.*

1

Good morning! I have in another ward a patient from whom I hope to obtain for you the visual impression you would get, seeing his two greatest problems in action. I have placed him in a quiet ward, one containing few patients, and have instructed the Sister in charge and her nurses to leave him in peace there for the limited time I need. He had had no breakfast this morning, and he has just now been given a good one. I have seated him in a comfortable armchair in front of a warm fire, and have told him to relax. Finally, he has been given a newspaper, in which to read the most recent speech of our beloved Premier, who makes up for his lack of clarity of purpose by long-windedness and circumlocution. The experiment must have been complete by now, and it *may* fail. Let us go in, however, without any noise and softly on your feet, and see him.

All I had hoped you would see is present. Here is a fat little man of cherubic countenance, fast asleep. His head lolls back in the chair, his eyes are closed, his mouth is open, and he snores gently. His hands are clasped comfortably over his protuberant stomach, as if to hold on to the breakfast he has just had. His legs are stretched out, and the divine speech of our political leader has been dropped carelessly on the floor. In other words, this patient is sound asleep. But for my need to show him as clinical material, I suppose in all decency we should creep away and let him take his rest. There is, however, on the other side of the ledger, the fact that he is repeatedly falling asleep, and that, wherever he may be and whatever he may be doing, he can not fight the imperious demands of sleep. Let us wake him up.

A light touch on his shoulder and a gentle admonition to stay awake are sufficient. He is now sitting up, has arranged his spectacles, smoothed his clothes, and now awake, looks around somewhat shamefacedly. He will tell you that this is what he is doing all the time, and he is glad enough to have us see him in his predicament.

He is thirty years of age. In his 'teens, he first began to fall asleep at irregular hours. This tendency became more pronounced up to his twenty-fifth year; since then the condition has been stationary, and in some respects, better, for during the last few years he has found drugs that will keep him awake. Like many others suffering from this affliction, he is not satisfied with the effect of the drug, and rather than a palliative procedure, he wants a permanent cure.

He falls asleep at meals, while in company at a social function, and while traveling to a certain destination, he will often go beyond it. He sleeps standing up, and he has smashed numerous motor cars because of falling asleep while driving them. For a time he tried riding bicycles, but fell off them so regularly that he gave them up lest he break his bones.

He is married, but during his courtship he fell asleep so often that it is a wonder how he managed to propose. Apparently his wife wanted him, awake or asleep, and accepted this dormouse on his face value. On one occasion he helped his uncle paint his house. The two men were up on a wooden plank, thirty feet above ground, slapping on the paint, when to his horror, the uncle saw our patient drop his paintbrush, and then begin a headlong dive to apparent death on the concrete pavement below. He was caught just in time.

At about this time, he decided to study for the teaching profession, and here he made a terrific adjustment. He slept throughout most of his lectures, but his fellow students lent him their notes, and night after night, he studied them and his textbooks, walking up and down the room. Occasionally, he would fall asleep while standing up and reading, and then would fall to the floor, awakening himself violently. Often at meals in the college dining room he fell asleep, so that his face went into the greasy dish of meat and potatoes before him. In spite of all this, he finished the course of a rural schoolteacher, after which he married. Now he has a large family. He tells me that he fell asleep at each child's christening, and that eventually he had to confine his attendance at church to the bare necessities of his soul. As in the case of his teachers and fellow students, he found his spiritual advisers kind, understanding and even indulgent. Once he fell asleep at a graveside, and nearly fell into the grave where his relative was being lowered. This was put down to his fainting from grief!

In recent years he has planned his life to meet this serious problem. He leaves his home in the morning to drive ten miles to his school. Halfway along, there is a farmstead with a barn near the road, and a small lane leading up to it. He hides his car there, slips into the barn, and has a half hour's sleep, which he allows for, before leaving home. At his school, there is a back room with a bed. When the drowsiness begins to overtake him, he goes to this room, and again he sleeps. The class has been set a lesson to learn, and he has his favorites who go out in front on sentry duty to watch for an unannounced arrival of a school inspector. If such a one makes his appearance, the students wake up our patient to meet the invader. He is a good teacher, and nothing has ever been found wrong with his work. The children like him, are loyal to him, and there is no gossip. In the evening, on his homeward journey, he stops again at the barn, has a sleep, and latterly, by this means, has never wrecked his car.

Some years ago, another sign of his disease appeared. He had a hobby of raising chickens of the best stock he could find, and he was very successful. Now there was a neighbor's dog who also liked chickens, and who repeatedly raided his luscious white Orpingtons. Finally, one night, he waited in ambush for the dog, intending to kill him with a large stone. The dog arrived, and in a towering rage, our patient raised his hand to smite. Immediately the stone dropped out of his hand, his eyes drooped, his head fell on his chest, and his knees gave way. He fell to the ground, watching helplessly the rape of his best-laying hens. From then on, this pattern recurred whenever he got into a rage; as he will tell you, he becomes weak with anger.

Strange to say, when he is told a very funny story, even while he is laughing heartily, the same general muscular weakness will occur. He tries, therefore, equally to avoid rage or mirth. Let us try, this morning, to reproduce this phenomenon, which will occur only if he reaches the proper emotional level. I am asking him to take a ball of paper, imagining that it is a stone, and that I am a dog stealing his chickens. This will be hard, for the original canine marauder has been shot on another farm.

He has tried to work up a rage and hate against me, and twice he has thrown the paper ball at me, without result. But look, the third time has been effectual. Look! In a seeming nasty temper, he has hit me square in the face. With your watches, check what follows. . . . His eyes are drooping, his head is falling forward, and his arms are dangling by his sides. His knees crumple, and he is on the floor. This has evolved in about thirty seconds or less, and he lies helpless on the floor, although he is fully conscious. He gets up hastily, and brushes off his clothes, acting as shamefaced as he did when we caught him asleep. To all intents and purposes, he is again quite normal.

This tendency to fall or to collapse muscularly during heights of rage or mirth is called "cataplexy." The Germans call it the *Lächtslag*, or the laugh stroke, and leave out the similar effects of rage. This, with the imperious demand, under any circumstances, for immediate sleep, constitutes the main feature of **narcolepsy.** Sometimes cataplexy is the more marked, sometimes falling asleep is, but usually these two go hand in hand. There are a few other manifestations of narcolepsy, not always present.

In spite of the recurrent somnolence during the day, our patient sleeps restlessly at night, particularly on falling asleep, and again, he is restless before awakening in the morning. When he retires, he starts to fall asleep, when, in the half-sleeping, half-waking period, all sorts of hallucinations appear to him, which are always terrifying, and usually visual, in brilliant colors. Apparently, the terror of these horrible visions produces a form of cataplexy, for while seeing them, the patient becomes paralyzed, and can not move any of his muscles. He feels as if he were bound hand and foot, and all he can do is to groan in anguish. When with a supreme waking effort he jumps out of bed, he finds he can then move his limbs, and that the visions are gone.

One patient of mine, a priest afflicted with narcolepsy, when dropping off to sleep frequently had the vision of a huge, multi-colored cat, with enormous saucer-shaped eyes, who jumped on his bed and tried to tear his genital organs to pieces with long, sharp, cutting claws. He would groan loudly, whereupon his housekeeper would come into his room with an oil lamp in her hand. He could see her but dimly outlined, standing at the door of his bedroom, and yet, the great cat was still vivid and very busy. As the housekeeper approached him, she became more clear, and the cat started to vanish. A touch on his shoulder, and he would become at once fully awake; the cat would by then have disappeared, and he would compose himself for sleep. This vision might occur three or four times in succession, before he would drop off into an uneasy sleep for the rest of the night. This syndrome never occurs during the patient's waking hours, but may do so during the period of his awakening from sleep in the morning. The hallucinatory phase is called "hypnagogic," or "hypnopompic" hallucinations, and the resultant immobility, "predormitial," or "postdormitial" paralysis.

Many patients suffering from narcolepsy are overweight, as was the fat boy about whom Mr. Pickwick wondered; this is not, however, universally true. If one looks for it, in these patients with narcolepsy, he can see a drawn, tired look in the patients' eyes, as if they had been deprived of sleep night after night, nursing a relative who is ill, for example. They look always to be fighting sleep, which, of course, is just what they are doing, and that unsuccessfully.

The differential diagnosis in these cases is not too difficult. Thirty years ago, the condition was regarded as being of a psychogenic character. True, there are certain personality complexes involved, but I feel that these are a result of the disease, and by no means the cause. We shall discuss this when the question of treatment comes up. Narcolepsy is easily distinguished from petit mal. The narcoleptic patient is simply asleep, and can be wakened instantly with stimulation by voice or by touch. The patient with petit mal stares straight ahead, with open eyes, whereas the narcolept has his eyes closed in sleep, and his attitude is entirely one of somnolence.

The greatest difficulty in the diagnosis of narcolepsy is to distinguish between a pathologic sleep condition, and one that is just a little below normal. Almost all fat persons fall asleep easily, and tend to sleep in church, or during a dull lecture. It is our privilege to do so, even though the sharp elbow of one's spouse soon enough digs one out of hoggish slumber. The driver of an automobile may fall asleep and wreck his car; many do so, but not habitually. The narcolept reaches a stage at which driving a car, either in the daytime or at night, is impossible without accident. A man who goes to sleep on a scaffold many feet above the street, thus risking his life, or one who sleeps throughout a business conference which is vital to his professional and economic success, is an example which shows the matter of degree between a somnolent person and one who is suffering from narcolepsy. If undue sleepiness interferes with bodily safety, with economic advancement, or with social happiness, and dominates the life pattern of a given individual, it is then a matter of narcolepsy.

The associated cataplexy, predormitial paralysis, with hypnagogic hallucinations, and a certain facial expression and mental attitude, with imperious demands for sleep, certainly round out the picture. Obesity can be used as a corroborating factor, but gently at that. Given a patient who has tried position after position in the market of enterprise, and who has each time been discharged for going asleep on the job, one can readily sense a tragedy. This situation can be a tragicomedy or a comitragedy, depending upon how one looks at it. The patient we are seeing this morning is unusual in the respect that he has adjusted to his problem, and has profited by it. His life has not been greatly interfered with by his affliction, and he will do even better in the future. He is wise in his own way.

The pathologic aspects of narcolepsy are not clear. In the so-called idiopathic type, the findings at postmortem examination are nil. The electro-encephalogram is not helpful, inasmuch as there are many normal tracings, and the few pathologic recordings that are found are hard to interpret. Tumors of the tuber cinereum and of the hypothalamus produce somnolence, but not periodic or paroxysmal somnolence, as in narcolepsy, and there are no normal phases in between periods of sleep. Gunshot wounds and arachnoiditis of the sella turcica may cause sleepiness, but again, they do not produce the clear-cut syndrome which we saw here today. Tumors of the pituitary gland, or of structures around it, produce no such picture. In the end, we have to call narcolepsy a disease *sui generis.*

As to treatment: there is no cure. The disease, however, seems to come to a natural close in the early or the late fifth decade of life. Never is there seen a narcolepsy beginning in the fourth or fifth decades of life. It usually begins in young persons, and ends at their late middle age. There are, however, certain palliative drugs, which, when used properly, allow the patient a useful and active life.

The earliest drug to be used was amphetamine sulfate (benzedrine). It was given in doses of from 5 to 10 mg., three times a day, at the hours of eight in the morning, at noon, and not later than four in the afternoon. It is a cerebral stimulant and prevents sleep; hence, the last dose is taken early enough to avoid insomnia from its use. A more potent drug is methamphetamine hydrochloride (desoxyn or dexedrine). It is given in doses of 2.5 mg. increased as required to 5 mg., three times a day, at the hours just mentioned. The dose of both drugs must be kept below a certain level, and the local physician must supervise their administration. Otherwise, restlessness, delirium and even maniacal behavior may occur.

Theoretically, these drugs ought to be a great help in treating patients who have narcolepsy. They not only keep the patient awake, but in addition, usually help to diminish his cataplexy. They are less helpful in the hypnagogic hallucinations and dormitial paralysis. Under the influence of this medication, a patient ought to be able to get along and live a normal life, in expectancy of a final discharge from his burden later on, when he is still in the prime of his life.

The patient you saw this morning is one of those. In recent years he has found himself gradually able to relinquish his safeguards and subterfuges, and to carry on much better than formerly. I am reminded of a patient I had, a farmer afflicted with narcolepsy, who told me that he was so grateful for the medication because now he is able to drive his tractor without falling under it, and to work in his fields without having to go to sleep every few hours. The majority of these patients, however, from early in life cherish a grudge because they are not like other men, and they become mildly paranoic. They admit relief from the amphetamine drugs, but what they want is a cure, for ever and a day. They cease taking the tablets, relapse into all their former difficulties, and drift into a surly state of mind. They are generally a very unhappy and disagreeable group of patients to handle.

2

HERE IS a man who has trouble in writing. He is twenty-five years of age, and is an auctioneer's clerk. This involves working with his chief at auctions, writing down long columns of specified goods, the price bid after each item, and whether the article is paid for or not at the time of sale. He has to be swift, accurate and to the point. He has been doing this work for five years now, and he hopes to become a full-blown auctioneer later. Unfortunately, something has happened to his writing hand; in his case, the right one. He starts out at an auction writing freely, easily and legibly. Then something happens; the muscles in his forearm and the small muscles of the hand become tight. He becomes slowed up because of the spasm, which rapidly becomes a pain in his forearm. He holds his pen or pencil more and more tightly. His wrist becomes forcibly flexed, his shoulder is drawn towards the forearm, and his whole posture of writing becomes crumpled into a knot of arm, forearm and hand muscles, with each muscle fighting against the other for leadership. His handwriting becomes completely illegible. In the end there is an anarchy of all muscle groups engaged in writing, and in an extreme case, the pen is shot violently out of the hand, and all writing is at an end.

This patient took a month's rest, and then returned to work. He did well for three weeks until the trouble returned, bit by bit, but none the less, remorselessly. He complains bitterly of the pain in his forearm during the last phase, before writing becomes impossible. After a determined attempt to overcome his affliction, the muscles of his right arm remain sore to compression for days. The strangest thing of all is that, with the single exception of writing, he can use the fingers, hand, forearm and arm for any other activity.

He is a musician, and plays the violin and piano equally well. His affliction has not affected in any measure his ability to play these instruments. Moreover, he can typewrite without any difficulty, and at high speed, and he can shuffle and deal a pack of cards as well as, or even better than, anyone else. But he can not write for any length of time, and writing happens to be his source of living.

He has had a plaster cast modeled from the holding portion of his hand, and a pencil run through the cast, corresponding to the angle and direction of one held in the hand. The plaster cast was then remodeled, a light plastic material being used. The idea was for him to use his arm in writing, rather than his hand. The pen and pencil used had unusually large points. At first this ingenious device worked like a charm; it seemed to be the answer, but later it failed. Then he tried using his typewriter in the auction room, but that was not practicable, for the bids might jump a hundredfold just while he was changing his sheet of paper and carbon.

He is learning now to write shorthand; he can later transcribe his notes on a typewriter, if he allows for double the time in following an auction. There is also a machine on the market which he might try; one which will produce in phonetic symbols on an endless ribbon all that is heard. The symbols can be transcribed on a typewriter later, and delivered to the firm the same evening.

This patient is suffering from **writer's cramp.** It is a malady which was encountered much more frequently in days when there were no typewriters; when attorneys' clerks, for example, had laboriously to engross in a meticulous script innumerable sheets of hardened vellum with high-sounding verbiage. In those days it was called "scrivener's cramp," and it was just as incurable then as it is now.

Similarly, there are telegrapher's, milker's, cigar maker's, violinist's and pianist's cramps. Any rapidly repeated and complicated movement of the finer muscles of the hand and forearm may bring on a cramp. I have seen a barber with "scissors cramp." He was a gesticulating individual who, to every clip of the hair, would make several noisy, empty snaps with the scissors' blades. He ended by being in cramp halfway through every haircut. Cramp-afflicted persons seem to have a certain type of personality. For one thing, they are inordinately ambitious, and in all they do, strive continuously for speed and an ever-increasing volume of work.

Occupational cramp occurs only where the finer movements of the hands are concerned. A writer who goes into cramp when using a fine-pointed pen is able to write tirelessly on a blackboard because he is making a broad sweep of his arm. Telegraphers, at the turn of the century, had to use a fine, delicate sending key which necessitated the finer movements of the hand; telegrapher's cramp was extremely common then, but it has been very nearly abolished by the use of the "bug," an instrument which moves the sending key laterally, demanding the use of the entire arm. Now, messages are typed out, and are received at the other end in the same way in which they are sent.

Typing requires the use of the whole arm, and typist's cramp is relatively unknown. There are nowadays so few legal documents drawn up by hand, and typewriting is so usual, that scrivener's cramp almost ceases to exist. Bank clerks are using an increasing number of machines to make up accounts, and to add, subtract and divide. The large ledgers of former days, filled with meticulous copperplate writing, in banks and in large stores, no longer exist.

So much has been gained in the defeat of writer's cramp, that our patient should take courage. He can work elsewhere, in a position demanding a minimum of writing, and with his keen mathematical mind should make a success of whatever he attempts. Writer's cramp is incurable; once it has developed, it never leaves a person, but one *can* live without writing by hand, and earn an income without ever using a pen.

The cause of this trouble is unknown. The neurologists call it an "exhaustion of the nerve center"; the psychiatrists put it down to a submerged hatred for writing, and so forth. In the end, the cause is anyone's guess. At any rate, a clinical syndrome such as writer's cramp exists, and will continue to exist, *saecula saeculorum,* as long as a pen is used by too-ambitious writers. Let us all write less and less!

One need not be a chamber to be haunted;
One need not be a house;
The brain has corridors surpassing
Material place.
    —EMILY DICKINSON: *Time and Eternity.*

3

Good morning! We are well into spring now, and the month of April has supplied its usual gift of rain, so that there is a profusion of blossoms on the ground, on bushes and higher up on the trees. The rain ceased as I was coming here this morning, and from out a group of jagged, low-lying clouds, the sun poured down onto a sodden earth. Even the clouds looked wet. I was reminded then of the phrase, "Smiling through her tears," a most disgusting expression of thought. A psychoneurotic may do this, or a designing woman. They shed tears, either because of pain or of mental suffering, and yet they smile, showing a sweet resignation, and a bowing to the will of God. Indeed, in most cases, there is no real suffering, physical or mental, and the resignation is, to say the least of it, an acquired state of mind. Both smiles and tears act, however, as a powerful synergism, pushing up the emotional effect a thousandfold, and used at the proper time and place, they will gain much for the accomplished stage or domestic actress.

I am showing you today a woman who is forty-four years of age, a housewife, with three children. As you see her here, seated by the fire, you will observe that she is wearing on her left leg a brace of the type that dorsiflexes the foot, and stabilizes the ankle. Also, she has her head bandaged, and over these dressings she wears a little wool cap with a blue tassel. You may assume, therefore, that her head has been operated on in order to relieve a weakness in the muscles below her knee.

We shall give this woman's history, and later, consult our notes as to what was found before her surgery here, and how we arrived at a diagnosis and localization of the trouble in her brain. My preliminary remarks this morning had nothing whatsoever to do with this patient; she is stable and well adjusted, and if *she* sheds tears, there is nothing to smile about. I wanted you all here and in your places this morning, with no latecomers forcing their way in. I ask you to maintain an attentive quiet, with no shuffling of feet, or whispered comments about last night's orgies, for this problem has been a difficult one, and it has taken every means in our power to reach a correct diagnosis. We shall go through every stage in her examination, step by step, and for that, I want your complete attention and co-operation.

About eight years ago this patient fell downstairs. Apparently there were no severe consequences, since she remembered it only on our questioning her. Eighteen months ago she noticed that her left foot was becoming weak. She could not raise her toes from the ground in walking, and as a consequence, tripped frequently over rugs, objects and on rough ground. This condition had gradually increased in severity, so that within a few months her thigh muscles also became weak, and she found it hard to ascend or to descend stairs, unless in so doing she used only the right foot.

Next there appeared a wasting of the muscles below her knee on the left side, and the dorsum of her left foot felt as if it were "frozen" or "dead." Cramps appeared in both calves, more severe on the left side.

Then, twelve months ago, she consulted a neurosurgeon in regard to the increasing weakness of her left foot. He put an opaque medium into the subarachnoid space in the lumbar region, and tilted her under the fluoroscope, and as well, made stationary roentgen studies of her spinal column. He found, as he thought, a protruded intervertebral disk at the midthoracic region of the spinal column. He operated, and removed an intervertebral cartilaginous disk. In spite of this surgical procedure, the weakness of her left-leg and left-thigh muscles increased. She was then fitted with a steel brace to elevate her foot, so that it would not trip her so much, and also to support her left ankle, which was weak, and which frequently turned under her, causing her to fall suddenly.

Three months ago she began to have headaches. These consist of an aching pain across her nose and in both maxillary air sinuses. In addition to this, there were shooting pains in the occipital region, and an occasional aching in the frontal region. The episodes of headache were of short duration, but they frequently occurred between two and four o'clock in the morning, waking her out of a sound sleep. They were becoming more frequent and severe.

This is what we found on her admission to this hospital. She was a well-developed, well-nourished woman, stable and intelligent. On taking the brace off her left leg, we found that this limb seemed to be considerably atrophied; as we went down the leg, an increasing weakness was found. The thigh muscles were at least 50 per cent weak; the muscles below the knee ranged from a 75 per cent weakness to a total paralysis of the small muscles of the foot. For example, she could not wiggle her toes, nor could she dorsiflex or plantarflex the foot at all. The peroneal muscles were completely paralyzed. She could use her quadriceps, iliopsoas, glutei and adductor muscles only extremely poorly. The tone of the muscles was depressed, and the leg, when shaken vigorously, had a flail-like character. The right leg was weak, but not so markedly as the left.

Surprisingly enough, the tendon reflexes in both lower extremities were greatly exaggerated, more so on the left side. Babinski's sign was noticeable to a high degree on both sides, but it was most marked on the left. There were no changes in deep sensibility, and while she complained of a numbness over the front of the leg and dorsum of the foot, this could not be demonstrated objectively with pin, cotton wool, or hot-water bottles.

In testing the power of her left arm, we found that there was a slight but definite weakness. The tendon reflexes in the upper extremities were markedly exaggerated, particularly on the left. Hoffmann's sign, that is, twitching of the middle finger, thus producing flexion of the thumb, was present on both sides, and again, was more marked on the left. No sensory changes, deep or superficial, could be found in either upper extremity.

She was asked to walk. This procedure was difficult, but with her brace, and with her right arm around another's shoulder, she managed with great difficulty to cross the room. Without her brace she could not walk, unless she was supported by two persons. Her left leg was to all intents paralyzed and useless.

As to other tests applied to establish the diagnosis, there were first, the roentgen studies made of her skull. They showed that the sella turcica, in both the dorsum sella and the posterior clinoids, had become decalcified and eroded. The sella was not unusually large, but there was evidence here of increased intracranial pressure.

Second, examination of the eyes showed a blurring of the margins of both optic disks, more marked on the right, and the upper pole of the right disk had a certain degree of fullness. There was a suspicion of papilledema, but the swelling was not sufficient to allow us to be certain. Examination of the perimetric fields of vision was ordered, and this procedure was carried out four days later. As usual, the optic disks were again examined for evidence of increased intracranial pressure, before the visual fields were charted. A fresh, deep retinal hemorrhage was found above and nasal to the right macula; this was a new feature, and had not been present at examination four days earlier. There was found, as well, blurring of the margins of the optic disks, already reported. On testing with various-sized objects, the perimetric fields were found to be normal, and there was no enlargement of the blind spot. Again, our ophthalmologist revealed his suspicions as to early papilledema, but confessed that he could not be absolutely sure, one way or the other.

Third, electro-encephalograms were made. Here, the interpreter of her tracing, unlike the ophthalmologist, had no inhibitions as to his opinions of clinical causes and effects. He had reported that there were delta waves, grade 2, coming from the right sylvian area. There was also dysrhythmia, grade 2, in the right cerebral hemisphere, of more maximal effect in the right sylvian area. In his clinical interpretation, the electro-encephalographer claimed that these findings are indicative of disturbance of function affecting the right sylvian-parietal area. He has claimed that this type of recording may be produced only by a parasagittal lesion situated to the right of the midline.

At this stage, it was necessary to co-ordinate all our findings to see, as in a jigsaw puzzle, if they fitted any definite pattern. Before an operation here, we had to take into consideration the previous findings made concerning this patient, her operation in the thoracic region of the spinal column, and the removal of a protruded disk, and consider gravely whether or not all this was a strongly odoriferous, salty, red herring drawn across the path of our researches into the cause of this patient's illness, if only to annoy and frustrate us. Let us start with the patient's earliest symptom, which has persisted throughout, has become steadily more severe, and even now, is her chief complaint.

1. The first complaint was that of a weak left foot. This had increased to the stage of complete paralysis in that member and gradually the muscles higher up had become involved. It was only later that we found that, even though slightly, the left hand and arm had become affected. There was no evidence of facial involvement.

2. The leg had become flaccid and toneless; this might suggest a peripheral nerve lesion, but the reflexes were exaggerated, and Babinski's sign was quite marked. The tendon reflexes were also increased in the arm, and Hoffmann's sign was present, indicating an upper motor lesion in both arm and leg.

3. So far, the pyramidal tracts seem to be damaged at least as high as the cervical region. This eliminates the red herring *in toto*, since all activities in previous surgery were in the thoracic region of the spinal column. Where is the final location of the lesion?

4. The tendon reflexes are exaggerated on *both* sides, and Babinski's sign is bilateral. Hoffmann's reflex is feeble on the right, but strong on the left. The lesion is bilateral in the cord, brain stem or in the cerebral hemispheres. Remember that the foot and leg are flaccid and weak, but with exaggerated reflexes, and Babinski's sign. This suggests a cortical lesion. Where do the cortical leg centers come into close proximity, so that damage to one will inevitably hurt the other side, even if to a lesser degree? The great longitudinal fissure containing the falx and su-

perior longitudinal sinus, and both cortical leg centers close together, is a favorite site for meningiomatous tumors, with bilateral clinical signs.

5. Has the patient any evidence of increased intracranial pressure? She has increasingly severe headaches, coming on early in the morning and waking her. Roentgen studies have shown her sella turcica to be eroded and decalcified, as if by pressure inside the skull, and from above. The ophthalmologist, not knowing the diagnosis, has however, reported signs in the eye grounds which, if not conclusive, at least suggest very early papilledema, and therefore increased intracranial pressure.

6. What did the electro-encephalographer do for us? Plenty: he postulated the existence of a parasagittal tumor, more marked on the *right* side. At this point the neurosurgeon was called in for consultation. He followed with us this tenuous trail, but wanted more information, in order to make sure of a tumor's being present, and in that case, also to obtain a more exact location. With this end in view, he advised ventricular air studies.

These were done, with the patient prepared for surgery, if found to be necessary, immediately afterward. The first note in the diagnosis was then written. The ventriculograms showed that the right lateral ventricle was depressed and displaced to the left by a *right parasagittal space-occupying lesion* in the right parietal area. The patient was operated on at once.

Right free bone-flap craniotomy was carried out in the parietal area, so that the medial aspect of the flap was along the longitudinal sinus. The brain was under enormous tension. The dura mater was opened. A *meningotheliomatous meningioma* was found attached to the falx. A portion of this falx was removed, because the tumor had invaded through the falx. The tumor was completely removed, and the patient stood the operation well. The pathologic report on the specimen removed was that it was a meningotheliomatous meningioma, weighing 33 gm. and measuring 6.5 by 5 by 2 cm. The patient's convalescence was without complications.

As you see her now, you will, I am sure, appreciate why we feel very happy about our efforts. True, the weakness of the left leg persists, but a few days after surgery is too short a period in which to expect much change. One would even expect a worsening, because of the effects of dislodging so huge a tumor that has been in position a longer time than the history indicates. There remains an area of compressed brain that may or may not recover, now that the pressure is removed. Generally speaking, some recovery can be expected, and so often it is surprisingly more than one could hope for.

The localization of meningiomas is difficult because they engender so many distant symptoms. The tumor, by electro-encephalographic and ventriculographic evidence, was supposed to involve the parietal lobe of the brain. There were minimal clinical signs of this. The brain is not an exact structure for localization by clinical methods.

There are slides of the tumor for you to see. It is composed of large, pale cells, with a well-defined nucleus. These cells are in whorls, with many small, poorly formed blood vessels, in this particular type of tumor. It is a benign tumor, but it may recur after surgery. It is less likely to recur in this case, however, since the tumor, and its site of origin, the falx, were entirely removed. Altogether, we feel very happy over the results of the labor of many persons, working together as a team.

4

THERE IS a fine, strong lad of twenty-five to see me this morning. He looks well and healthy, and has but one simple complaint, and that is, that a week ago he woke up to find his hand dropped at the wrist, and he was totally unable to extend it. As a result, he can not use the hand at all, since, in such a position, the muscle flexors also have a very poor function, as well as the paralyzed extensors. Try it now, yourselves, and you will find that in grasping objects firmly, you have no power unless the hand is pushed backwards to acute extension. The patient can not extend his fingers or thumb, or his metacarpus and carpus on his forearm. He has what is called a *"drop-wrist paralysis,"* although it is the hand and fingers that are dropped, and not the wrist, which serves as a fulcrum. There is a tiny area of numbness, but not of anesthesia, over the roots of the thumb and index finger, dorsally.

The brachioradialis tendon reflex is diminished, but the triceps muscle reflex is intact. He has an obvious lesion of his radial nerve in the lower arm as it winds around the humerus, and is there lying superficially with the bone underneath. The triceps muscle is intact, for the reason that its fibers of nerve supply come off the radial nerve higher up. The brachioradialis is only partially involved, as is its reflex. It is the extensor group of muscles in the forearm, which supplies tendons to the thumb, fingers and hand, that is chiefly affected by this nerve injury.

This is a serious disablement. The patient has already been fitted with a cock-up splint, in order to lessen the drag on the paralyzed muscles, since the fallen hand tends to lengthen them. If recovery of the nerve ensues, there is still a taking-up of slack to be considered. Also, edema occurs in the dorsum of the hand that falls helplessly downward, and adds to the problems of rehabilitation.

The patient's statement that he went to bed well some few days ago, and awoke to find that he had a partial radial nerve paralysis, requires considerably more amplification before an opinion can be given, especially since facts we may learn may influence our prognosis. You may remember our mutual friend, Sherlock Holmes, in the case of the race horse, Silver Blaze:

Police Inspector Gregory asks him, "Is there any point to which you would wish to draw my attention?"

"To the curious incident of the dog in the night-time."

"The dog did nothing in the night-time."

"That was the curious incident," remarked Sherlock Holmes.

Here we have our friend, going to bed well and hearty, and waking with a paralyzed hand, totally oblivious to what might have happened during the night to produce this serious disability. It seems to me that this matter needs more inquiry; why did not this patient bark, or give some outcry? In cases in which a sudden or acute nervous system lesion occurs, one can not be too detailed in questioning. Every detail of the patient's life, directly before and after the occurrence of the lesion, must be inquired into, hour by hour, or even minute by minute.

When I went back to question our patient, I noticed that his clothes were hanging loose on him. I found out that, three weeks before the paralysis occurred, he had just recovered from an attack of pneumonia, during which illness he had lost twenty pounds. He had gained back a few pounds, but was still very much underweight, and I learned that he never had been plump or well nourished in appearance. It was then that, as the lawyers say, I got down to the statement of particulars.

The vague date of onset, a week ago, was established as a Saturday night, a fact suspicious in itself. He had worked until noon, and then had gone to visit a friend in a village three miles away. He went by omnibus, and took a return ticket. When he arrived there, he and his friend decided to go fishing. Our patient's friend is, I gather, one who makes his pleasure a business, and who works harder at it than he does in his office. The patient, still weak from his illness, covered miles of trout streams, and the fishing, he told me, was more than good. Late in the evening, the pair lurched wearily home, and being bachelors, set to cooking the fish themselves. Late as it was, they served up an enormous meal, which they devoured. Moreover, there were plenty of libations as toasts to their success in fishing, and by the time our patient even thought of his omnibus, it had long gone, and there was no other one that night. His friend soothed him, however, by assuring him that, having a spare bed, he could easily put him up for the night.

At midnight the friend pulled out a folding bed made of steel, and unrolled it. The mattress was sadly in default. The surface on which to lie was as hard as the hob of Hell, without the heat and flames. Our patient was thrown a few blankets, and exhausted by the afternoon's tramping and soporific from so many unaccustomed drinks, he put his underweight body on the nonresistant metal bed, and turned over on his right side, as he habitually slept. He fell into a dead sleep, almost a coma.

His friend, who had no thought of punctuality at business, aroused him late next morning. Our patient found himself lying in the same position in which he had stretched out the night before, but now he had a drop-wrist, or more specifically, a pressure paralysis of the radial nerve, as it emerges from its winding course around the humerus. You will, I think, agree that the details supplied us now are much more informative as to why this man has a drop-wrist, over and above the simple fact that he went to bed well one night, and awoke the next morning, paralyzed. Vulgarly, this is called a "Saturday night" paralysis.

Now for treatment, he should continue to wear a cock-up splint, and be given massage and exercises to the muscles operating around the wrist. Electric stimulation of the paralyzed muscles helps, beginning with galvanic, and later on, switching to faradic current, when the reaction of degeneration is diminishing. In these pressure palsies, the prognosis is very uncertain; it all depends upon how badly the nerve has been squeezed, and how much and how long the circulation of the vaso nervorum has been cut off. In the case of older patients, more especially diabetics, the prognosis is very bad, because of the poor blood supply to the nerves.

Finally, in any given case of pressure palsy, there must be many factors operating. Chief among them is a loss of weight, with lack of protective fat; atony of the muscles also is a factor in lack of protection. The toxic effect of alcohol, or of infectious diseases, is, I presume, only coincidental, but the most important factor of all is represented by a change in the patient's habits, a change of nocturnal and daily routine. Had our patient here fished gently, drunk little, and slept at home, as he usually does, he would not have a dropped wrist today.

MAY

1

Good morning! On Saturday evening last, being in my right mind and perfectly sober, I was coming back from a consultation in a rural district near here. The last rays of a setting sun were ending a perfect spring day, but were rapidly disappearing behind the treetops. The long Irish twilight was at hand.

I noticed that my water-gauge on the dashboard was showing signs of depletion, due to a slow leak in the radiator, and I had still twenty miles to go. It was in a sparsely settled part of the county, but a few miles farther on, I found a lonely cottage situated conveniently alongside the road and knocked at the front door.

The door was opened cautiously by a man who kept his foot in the door, and his head in the small aperture through which he allowed us to look at each other. I explained what was wrong with my car, whereupon he opened the door wider, so that I could see a group of men and women sitting inside, drinking what I took to be stout, and eating soda bread with butter. The fire seemed to be unusually bright, and all the available lamps and candles were lit. Everyone seemed to be startled by my appearance, since they all stopped eating and drinking. Although

255

I was not allowed inside the house, and the door was slammed in my face, kindness to a wayfarer asserted itself, for from the back of the house came three men carrying buckets of water.

Standing there, idly watching the operation of filling my radiator, I thought about how abruptly the door had been closed on me. With equal suddenness, a little girl in a spotless white dress, white stockings, and even white shoes, scuttled out of the house with a huge bunch of primroses clutched tight in her hands. Quickly she spread the golden, delicate, shining blossoms, with their light green leaves and stems, all over the doorstep and pathway leading to the front door, and in a semicircle across the front of the house.

Twice more she made her dash of exit and entrance, the first time carrying a porringer of buttermilk, and the second, a glowing coal of turf, clasped in a pair of iron tongs. She placed both items on the window ledge at the left of the doorway. Her final bolt home was like that of a rabbit pursued by a greyhound. The door slammed again, and even louder, for now she was at home, within doors, and safe.

My helpers, the bearers of water, saw me watch this strange rite, and doubtless heard me say, almost unconsciously, "fire, food and golden flowers." I remembered then that it was May Eve, when the fairies go trooping from house to house, and are placated by these offerings. I asked these men, Was it not so? They agreed, explaining that fire was for warmth, or to light an old pipe; milk was for nourishment for the aged; and the flowers were for the adornment of the young and more beautiful "good folk." By these gifts, the house was protected that night, and for the year to come.

By now the twilight was becoming dusk, and a speedy parting seemed the thing to do. My helpers indicated by gestures that they must return to the house immediately. Like the little girl, they rushed headlong into this sanctuary from fear, and the door slammed for the last time. There were still, no doubt, bright lights, a warm hearth, food and drink, and above all, a protective barrier outside this strong house that would protect them this May Eve from all the evil influences abroad. Cynically, I wondered how much credit they gave to that little girl for risking her immortal soul to make them safe to drink and eat on that May Eve. At the least, she would certainly have to confess to her pastor on the next Confession day, and receive a long admonition and a heavy penance.

I drove on, musing on this persistence in the belief in fairies, and the failure to eradicate pagan customs in a country so strongly religious and so Catholic in its outlook.

There are chapters in neurology that more than savor of the black art. You have seen, earlier this year, a patient suffering from Huntington's chorea. Do you remember his ridiculous, stilted, dancing gait, his many grotesque grimaces, and above all, his nasty, mean disposition? Across the Atlantic, in the seventeenth century, common ancestors of these our modern patients with this disease were seen in New England and in New York State, and such was their reputation, and so out-of-the-world was their appearance, that they were deemed to have supernatural powers, and many were hanged as witches.

During the epidemic of encephalitis of 1920 to 1925, that traveled around the globe, we saw some of the most weird clinical pictures of brain disorder that could ever have been imagined. It was as if Satan and his myrmidons had invaded our ranks. Movement disorders, or dyskinesias, in all possible variations of theme, were prominent.

Choreas, tics, athetoses, spasms, tremors, dystonias, and countless other unclassified explosions of pyramidal and extrapyramidal activity, came on us, thick and fast, only to assume other and different clinical shapes as each few months passed on. As the epidemic advanced, the current medical literature increased from a few bewildered reports to many thousands in each year of the cumulative index. It was a neurologist's paradise of description, and yet, a hell of too hasty a classification.

We had children who indulged in a noisy rhythm of hyperpnea, apnea, cyanosis and unconsciousness, repeated endlessly, day and night. One adult, I remember, who was a six-foot policeman, went through an identical performance each time, begging to be allowed just one more cycle! His mother thought he was bewitched, but no attempt was made with bell, book and candle, to exorcise his evil spirits, for by that time we were only too familiar with the syndrome as a nosologic entity.

In all these movement disorders of epidemic encephalitis there were two things confusing us. The first was the relative power, under certain circumstances, for the will to control these movements, at least temporarily. The second was the relative paucity of pathologic findings in the brain after death. Early in the epidemic it was a Tom Tiddler's ground, wherein the pathogeneticists fought with the psychogeneticists. There was a hint of disturbed physiology, bearing no signs, however, as to where it had acquired its being. I was reminded of Bishop Berkeley's famous aphorism, "What is mind? No matter. What is matter? Never mind."

Anyhow, this was no widespread form of national hysteria, for Parkinson's syndrome developed in a high percentage of patients later on, and they died some years after. It was found, among those who were traced at a later time, that the end results of these weird movement disorders were, in a majority of cases, paralysis, helplessness and often death. Psychotherapy was universally useless, and gradually the severity and magnitude of the disease were, through bitter experience, fully appreciated. We are now left with the usual phenomena of movement disorders so well described before the epidemic, and still present with us. However, it must be recorded that during the epidemic of encephalitis, movement disorders were more frequent, more severe, fantastic and crippling to mind and body than at any other time.

I am showing you this morning two patients who have **dyskinesia.** The first patient has a very common form, a quiet, gentle and unexciting performance, but one in which there are so many question marks as to the whys and wherefores, that my hand would be exhausted and the printer's type used up before I could fill out the full indictment of the ruffianly cause of this disease. The second patient is suffering from a form which is a riot, a rebellion of muscles, and a madder dance than is seen even in Huntington's chorea. Withal, this second patient is a kind, intelligent man who hates to give trouble, and who begs only to be inconspicuous, and not a subject for gossip in a crowded place. I have our first patient in another room, and the stage has been carefully set. We shall go to her now.

This woman is forty-three years of age and looks well and hearty. She is reclining in an armchair which is of the "contour" type, fitting the curves of her body, and holding her head and neck at a very comfortable angle. Her arms rest on the chair at a proper level, and her feet rest securely on the floor. This is the very antithesis of the chairs of the Victorian period, in which it was sinful to lounge, a bolt-upright posture being regarded as the only acceptable posture of a lady. The loose horsehair strands perforated her clothes and stockings, and by their sharp jags kept her awake and attentive to the sort of conversation prevalent in that period. . . . There is just nothing to see at this stage; our patient is far too relaxed and at ease with her surroundings.

She has told me that three years ago, without any obvious physical or psychic cause, her head began to turn to the left, especially when she was sitting upright or standing, and under no more than the usual tension of an afternoon tea party. She could, in those earlier years, control this turning of her head and neck, but the pull of her chin towards the left shoulder gradually increased in force. It became a continuous movement of pull, and correspondingly, of a compensatory mechanism to return her head to the midline, so that at times it seemed almost like a tremor, and therefore, the more conspicuous. She began to have less and less voluntary control of the head-turning movement. During the last year, however, she has found her own method of controlling it partially. If she places her left index and middle fingers lightly over the left side of her chin, it will return almost by magic to a midline position. No pressure is needed, simply the light touch of her fingers, and instantly, as if on command, the spasm will relax.

The patient is a very busy woman at home. Although her children are almost grown up now, she has gathered to herself one civic function after another to attend, and even at times to preside over. She is as well an active church worker and sings in the choir. Bit by bit, this affliction is making her more and more timorous of appearing in public. Now it has become almost a habit for her to appear nowhere without index and middle fingers of her left hand resting on her chin. During the last six months, the constant pull of the right sternocleidomastoid muscle is being rebelled against. At its attachment to the mastoid process, there has appeared a continual dull ache, as if at the fibrous insertion a chronic irritation had followed a persistent tugging movement. The muscle itself seems to have grown larger and more powerful.

At rest, as she is now, this patient is comfortable and without spasm. Lying flat on her back also eases her, unless she is unduly tense and nervous. Once she falls asleep, her sleep is never disturbed. She is at her best in the morning, but the spasm increases as the day goes on. Standing, walking and finer movements of her hands, requiring close attention, make her spasm worse; talking in public at her various societies does so particularly. Her condition is steadily becoming worse, and her range of activities gradually more and more contracted.

I have shown you our patient under circumstances the most favorable to her. It is morning, when the spasms are at their least. She is reclining in a chair, completely relaxed, with her back, shoulders and neck well supported. Further, she is doing just nothing to set her muscles in action. Accordingly, there is very little to be seen by you, but it is obvious that she can not spend the rest of her life in this fashion. Let us get her moving. I have had her clothing so arranged that there is a full view of her neck and shoulders—no more, however, than a strapless evening gown would show. I do not think that there is any one of you sufficiently striking in beauty to excite her, except in so far as your eyes, hungry for knowledge, stare at her.

Directly she moves from the comfortable relaxing arms of the chair, her head veers to the left, as shown by the new position of the point of her chin. Immediately up goes her left hand, and the index and middle fingers come to rest lightly and tenderly on the left side of her chin. The body of the right sternocleidomastoid muscle had become contracted, tense, and as taut as the wire hawser of a tug pulling a liner into dock. When the two fingers rest on the chin, the spell is broken, the head turns back to a midline position, and the neck muscles relax, so that each side of the neck seems to be under a similar and normal tension.

We stand talking to each other. Her fingers are resting on her chin, but as time goes along her hand grows tired, her emotions surge upward, and the torsion of her neck begins to return. Now, let us put her in the worst of all positions, and let this hellish visitation ride to its extreme degree.

I have her sit on an examination table without a back, and with her hands resting on her lap. I ask her to write a few lines in a copybook, then to sew a few stitches in a piece of cloth, and finally to tie up a small parcel. Her chin teeter-totters a few times from side to side, due to the pull of the muscles and her own ineffective voluntary efforts to overcome the spasm. Finally, a more gross contracture occurs, and her chin pulls far over to the left, and her head stays fixed in a position as if she were listening intently to a watch placed on the tip of her left shoulder. Now she is complaining of pain at the attachment of the rotators of the head and neck, on one or both sides. She is obviously miserable and ceases all activity, begging to be allowed to support her neck with her left hand.

By this time the muscles have run away with themselves, with the bit in their teeth. The hand-chin maneuver fails at first; later some obviously inefficient relaxation occurs, and there are frequent forcible contractions turning the head to the left, and spasms of irregular character can be felt in the neck muscles.

She is now allowed to lie down on the examination table, with a pillow behind her head. I sit at the head of the table, feeling both sets of neck muscles simultaneously and in alternate contrast. After a few minutes, all contraction dies down, and both sides feel soft, but there are occasional smaller bursts of muscle contraction present that do not, however, move the head. This last phase varies with the severity of the disease, when in a given case even lying down does not remove all contraction of opposing muscles, and the head still deviates to one side or the other, although not so forcibly as when the patient is in the erect posture and trying to perform complicated synergic acts.

Apart from the pain and embarrassment of this condition, there is an obvious disability directed toward our patient's daily acts. Her food must be placed well within the field of vision of the turning head. Bifocal glasses can not be worn, since forward vision in a turning head leads to an area of the eyeglasses where the positive inset lenses are not present. It is better to use plus lenses for reading, and other lenses for getting around. In eating, one hand has to steady the head and neck; hence there is but one hand with which to eat. In writing, one hand has to steady the paper that is being written on; with our patient, however, this hand is overbusy controlling the contraction. Books and papers must therefore be clamped rigid on a reading stand. Driving a car is extremely difficult, since under the patient's concern in avoiding accidents, the neck stiffens, the head deviates, and visual control is difficult. As I have said, our patient has now dropped most of her social and civic activities, partly from embarrassment, but mainly because she can not any longer address a meeting without suffering pain and nervous exhaustion from trying to fight her persistent disease.

Most of these patients have to do their important work in the morning, and must perforce rest all afternoon. I had one patient who called me at six in the morning from a sound sleep, and told me that I had cured him. Knowing my man, and his disease, I congratulated him and then scuttled back into bed. As I expected, he called again at about nine o'clock, saying he was worse than ever, and could he come to see me right then!

This patient you have seen has what is a typical example of *spasmodic torticollis.* I am asking her to resume her place in the chair by the fire. We can then go to another ward and discuss this weird disease further. You will note, however, at this moment, as she is crossing from the examination table to the chair, that her left hand is in close and loving contact with her chin on that side.

I am glad to have been able to show you a patient with moderately severe spasmodic torticollis this morning. It is a clear-cut syndrome, not uncommon, and one you will see many times in your professional careers. I may have spread the dissertation of spasmodic torticollis out too far and too thin, but frankly, I do not think that you can know enough about it, especially since so little is known aside from the clinical form it happens to take, which is fixed, and which varies so little from patient to patient, except in regard to the degree of severity. It is there for you to recognize, and to apply the appropriate treatment that goes with your day and age, which I hope to heaven will be better than it is now.

Throughout the years I have seen so many patients with this disease, coming from all ranks of society, with all possible temperaments, with nervous manifestations so widely different, and with yet the same intrinsic problem, that I have failed to see a psychiatric origin for the disease. Instead of the dictum that these patients are nervous and because of this their necks are in spasm, I feel that any emotional reactions or nervousness are due intrinsically to the disease itself. "My neck pulls to one side, and because of this I am nervous," seems to be a more nearly accurate interpretation.

Again, the increase of muscular spasm during muscular activity, particularly of a complicated type, reminds me of the small boy who sticks his tongue out while writing, or of the child with cerebral palsy and athetoses who goes into a riot of movements on attempting something calling for skill and emotional calm. These are well-known phenomena in which the release mechanism of unwanted, uncalled-for and abnormal movements is too sensitive. A small complicated movement performed with or without emotional tension may set loose a riot of unnecessary movements, conspicuous and embarrassing, subsiding in turn when the task is accomplished. There is nothing new in this phenomenon in certain well-known organic diseases of the brain.

If spasmodic torticollis is of hysterical or neurotic origin, it ought to be different according to place, circumstance and the emotional setup of the patient. Actually, and like trigeminal neuralgia, it is always the same clinical picture, and the same problem in respect to therapy. It attacks males and females in about the proportion of thirty-five of the former to sixty-five of the latter, and usually during middle age. Once started, it goes on indefinitely, with, however, occasional remissions. It may cease spontaneously, a gleam of hope we hold out to patients to mitigate their sad lot.

At various times the treatment was neurosurgical, psychothera-
peutic and neurologic, depending on the fashion of the day. To
date, all three have failed. The neurosurgical approach was section
of either the motor or sensory pathways in the neck. The spinal
accessory nerve was cut, and the first three or four sensory roots
(or motor roots or both). Section of the sensory roots produced so
much pain that this procedure was abandoned. Later, the motor
roots were the ones that were sectioned. As a further step, a bone
graft was inserted into the cervical vertebrae, so that movements
of the head and neck were very limited. Alas, all these procedures
were doomed to failure, and the patients were worse cosmetically,
physically and spiritually than they were before surgery.

The neck muscles may be regarded as the numerous fibers in
the thickness of a large manila rope. To cut one, or a few of
them, has but little influence on the mass of twisting muscles
left behind. Any that are left will continue to function, and being
unbalanced, will leave a distorted, hideous, weakened neck structure, with plenty of pain and discomfort for the patient, and a
permanent substitution for something that might have improved
spontaneously. It is then that letters of complaint come in by
every post to the surgeon who has committed himself. What
letters they are can not be imagined!

The psychiatric problem of spasmodic torticollis seems to be
plain enough to those who deal with psychologic complexes. In
the first place, the response to touching or supporting the chin
is prima-facie evidence of a hysterical reaction. Members of the
French school who emphasized tics, spasms and involuntary movements, in the nineteen hundreds, described many ways in which
a patient could relieve his affliction by certain movements. These
they called "antagonistic" gestures, and suggested that these
movements released another reflex movement, relieving or in-
hibiting the presenting complaint. I have never seen a patient
with spasmodic torticollis cured by psychotherapy. My friends
who are psychiatrists tell me that if one can work on such a patient
for one or two years, good results can be obtained. Remissions
occur sufficiently frequently, however, to make one highly suspicious as to cause and effect, operating over so long a period.

Treatment for this condition by a neurologist can, at the worst, be deemed ineffectual. It would consist of a planned program of rest, with periods of outside activity, so that the patient does not become cut off from all worldly life; mild sedatives, and daily neck exercises in front of a mirror, to try to overcome the spasm. For pain, physiotherapy in the form of heat, massage and an occasional stretching of the neck by block and tackle is helpful. At the same time, a philosophy of hope should be engendered in the patient, while he accepts at least temporarily the cosmetic deformity, with however, a resolute determination to achieve as useful an existence as is possible, especially in the early hours of the day when the condition is not so severe. The time element with these patients is indefinite, and they do not need to sacrifice their entire life to the disability, but should push on bravely toward a goal of economic self-support.

The differential diagnosis is not difficult; there is only one true spasmodic torticollis, such as that shown here this morning. Congenital wryneck occurs in children, but that is due to an injury and subsequent blood clot in the fibers of the sternocleidomastoid muscle at birth. There is a shortening of the muscle, but no spasm, and if taken early enough, it is amenable to surgery.

The pathology of spasmodic torticollis is entirely unknown. It may be a fragment of the massive phenomenon of dystonia musculorum or lenticularis, an example of which I shall show you later on this morning. Torsion spasms of the neck and the arm were not uncommon during the epidemic of encephalitis, but what I have shown this morning is different, since it seldom if ever goes on to Parkinson's syndrome.

When I first came here, I was consulted one day by a huge, ill-clad and smelly man, carrying a horsewhip. He had probably the worst form of spasmodic torticollis that I have ever seen. One sternocleidomastoid was as large as his forearm, and his head was twisted so far over that hardly any direct vision could have been possible for him. Moreover, during the time I saw him, the spasm did not once relax; it was fixed, and seemed to be a solid muscular distortion.

As usual in a hospital dispensary, I started to write a harmless prescription. He waved it aside, saying that medicine never did *him* any good. I suggested his seeing my neurosurgical counterpart. He would have none of that, since he stated that he had seen the results, and they were not good. Desperately, and with all my guns but one emptied, I asked him if he had ever seen a psychiatrist. His face took on an ineffable expression of disgust, and he told me that he had "argued" with such a man for months, and that no good had come of it at all. There was just talking, he said, and his neck was no better; if anything, it was worse. A silence settled between us, and I waited for it to pass.

He looked me as straight in the eye as his torticollis would permit, and touching his neck with a dirty, callused hand, said, "Then you have no cure for me at all, at all."

Another silence ensued, and then, very slowly I shook my head.

He bounced the butt of his whip on the floor, and with a "Thank you *kindly*, sorr," suddenly went on his way.

For my sins, I see this poor man every few days. He drives a flat-topped cart, standing up and holding the reins in one hand, and whacking his horse with his whip in the other. He steers skilfully through the heavy traffic around the auction rooms, hauling furniture knocked down to eager bidding customers. How he manages all this with his body one way, and his head and neck twisted to the extreme opposite angle, is impossible for me to estimate. I drive behind him in my car, and then try to sneak past him unobserved. I usually lose out, for in ringing tones above all the noise of the street, I hear, "Thank you *kindly*, sorr."

I had been abused and criticized for my care of certain patients who became well after days and sleepless nights of effort on my part. I had been thanked fulsomely for some slight services, and been rewarded far beyond what these services were worth, but never before had I been thanked publicly by a patient whom, by a motion of my head, I had consigned to the class of incurables.

2

THIS LAST patient you have seen is a perfect lady. Her affliction is of a quiet type, and not too conspicuous. It could indeed be regarded as something private, and not an affair that would bring an element of horror and pity into a large or small social gathering. As I promised you earlier on, this, our next patient, represents something terrific, and his malady brings a sense of dry-mouthed, scalp-tingling awe to all who see him for the first time. Later on, he makes friends so easily that we are inclined to forget or overlook his infirmity. Before he enters for your observation and study, I want to talk a little on the subject of the familial history of disease with respect to a given patient, and on the multiplicity of mistakes one can make in such a seemingly simple matter.

The student who takes a history from a patient is required to inquire into the morbidity and cause of death in at least the two preceding generations. People, however, move around so much these days that it is impossible to find out the health of various collateral branches. Galsworthy's *Forsyte Saga* was easy to write because his much-loved puppets stayed put. They didn't even think of living elsewhere than in London.

My man, who is coming to see us, is a very different sort. His father was one of a large family of six boys and three girls. The family was reared in the Joyce country, in County Galway, so that, as you know, all had the same name, and added to that, many of them were red-haired. Our patient's father, in face of so large a family of brothers and sisters, and so little land to support them, left to seek his fortune in America, where there are, in truth, many, many Joyces. He was almost illiterate, in that he could write just a few words, sign his name, and no more. Accordingly, he seldom wrote home.

It was a great excitement to at least this one tribe of Joyces, when the father of our patient wrote a laconic message to the effect that he had married a girl, and that she was going to have a baby. No address was given, nor was there any mention made of any of the members of his tribe in New York City, all of whom, for some curious reason, he had avoided.

The next letter, such as it was, told that a male infant had been born, and that the mother had died in giving it birth. There were some veiled references to trouble with his dead wife's parents. A few months later the child was sent home to the father's old parents in Galway, in the care of a couple of persons who knew nothing of the circumstances, and who were not even intimates of the father or wife. They had been given the child, and a monetary reward for bringing it across the Atlantic. When they delivered the child, if they knew anything about its parents, they were saying nothing, and holding their breath to cool their porridge. Shortly thereafter they left Galway to return to America, obviously relieved by the end of their mission, and close-mouthed to the end. Marriage certificate, birth certificate and copies of parish records were all conspicuous by their absence.

Some time later, an American social organization notified the grandparents that the father of the child had been killed in a railway accident. There was no mention of a will, no suggestions as to his effects, if any. All the family received was the bare notification of a death. Repeated letters to this organization brought no answers. The father of the child was dead, leaving no traces behind him.

The family lawyer was consulted. Having been informed that there was no monetary estate involved, and no pickings for himself, and even less for the family, he advised doing just nothing. The cost of following this family tragedy to its climax would have been colossal, and certainly would have produced no equivalent financial return. It was decided then to do nothing but to rear the grandchild according to communal custom, along with his cousins and second cousins. One thing they wondered about, however, and that was why this male child had been circumcised, especially since the local dispensary physician thought it had been a very crude surgical procedure, like as not, done by a lay surgeon with but little knowledge of anatomy! Circumcision is definitely not an Irish custom, and is very rare in the Joyce country.

Accordingly, I would say to this class that the "family history" is not "negative," but full to the brim with conjectures, fantastic ideas and a process of pure guesswork that may or may not have a bearing on the problem in question.

As I told you before, this patient whom you are about to see was at first reared by his grandparents. When they became too old for this added responsibility, they turned him over to his uncle and aunt who brought him up with their five children, of whom the middle ones were about his age. He seemed to be happy in that arrangement, and rapidly became adjusted to his new environment. He ate and slept with his cousins, and went with them to the same rural school, which was three miles away on the other side of a bog road. At all seasons of the year, the cousins could be seen walking together to and from school.

The first thing noticed about the boy that was unusual was that his right leg and foot did not seem to be normal. Even when he was sitting quietly there were continual spasms, mild in degree, but of a torsion character, pulling his right leg and foot in a contra-clockwise direction. With this there was a plantar flexion of the foot, and an accompanying eversion, so that the sole tended to look outward. All the toes were simultaneously flexed. The boy would rest his leg and foot continuously to stop this spasm, although it was not painful. For the greatest comfort, he sat on one chair with his leg, resting on another, flexed at the knee and ankle, with the toes flexed, and the internal malleolus lying on a cushion. In this position the sole was naturally more conspicuous, and his cousins always had great fun in tickling it. All the children went barefoot at that time. This movement of the foot was at first regarded as merely a personal habit of the boy's, and no suspicion was aroused as to what might follow. At times, his leg and foot were even quiet and seemed to be entirely normal; at others, they might bother him for hours.

The next thing noticed that seemed to be unusual about this boy, then at the age of eight, was his method of walking to school. It was then that the idea of demoniacal possession was vaguely thought of by the foster parents. *He walked to school backward!* Heretofore he had tripped along to school with his cousins, keeping well up with them. Later it was seen that he limped, that his gait was slower, and very often because of his infirmity, the children arrived late at school and were punished accordingly. They could, of course have left him far behind, but this they would not do. Suddenly, he found the way out. He discovered that he could, by walking backward, keep up with his cousins, enjoy all the precious talk on the way, and still be on time for the first lesson.

Needless to say, in a small community this was soon noticed and commented on. The local physician was consulted; he could find nothing wrong with the boy's leg and foot, except for the torsion spasm below the knee. The physician regarded this as a hysterical phenomenon, and prescribed an extract of valerian root and a porous plaster for his back. These did no good, and amongst many other measures, a holy medal, blessed by the Bishop, was hung around the boy's neck. It must be remarked here that his foster parents were kinder to him than to their own offspring, for was not this child, an orphan without kith or kin, more precious than their own natural children in the eyes of the Lord? As time went on, his disease was steadily progressing and taking in a wider territory.

The original spasm of foot and leg became more intense, and in the years that followed he could go less often to school, unless he was driven there by his foster parents. The leg became quite lame and distorted. The eversion of the foot at the ankle became fixed, so that he could no longer set his heel to the ground. The flexion of his toes increased, and sooner or later he began to walk on the dorsum of his toes and the inner side of his foot. Contractures developed, and a fixed *pes equinus* was the final result. Calluses developed on the dorsum of his toes, and were at times so painful that he could not walk at all on that foot and had to use a crutch or cane. The rate of downward progression was extremely slow, covering a period of years. For many months the condition had remained stationary.

At fifteen years of age he was obviously crippled, in so far as his right leg was concerned, but now some disturbance of the truncal musculature appeared. At table, in particular, the right lower extremity would go into its slow, twisting, writhing movement, except in so far as the distal contractures had sealed up the joints. The trunk would then begin to turn on its long axis, again contraclockwise, and he would almost fall off the chair. Putting him in bed would partially relieve the spasm. Marked scoliosis was only too evident. The spasms of his muscles were intermittent and relieved by rest, so that this poor, distorted caricature of humanity was able to help to a minor degree around the house. He suffered no pain, but school and the normal life of a boy were now at an end for him.

Judging by the nature of the disease as we know it, an inevitable involvement of the left arm was bound, sooner or later, to occur, and within a year or two more, his neck muscles were afflicted by this twisting spasm that was relentlessly increasing in severity and width of muscular territory. His face had not been affected, and his speech and swallowing also had escaped. This is in contrast to Huntington's chorea. By the time he was twenty years of age he presented a weird vision of muscular turmoil. Less and less did he go out, and neighborhood visits were discouraged. There were whispers as to the nature of his disease at the backs of taverns where women chiefly congregated, and inside houses amongst an elect few, before a glowing fire of turf. Old gaffers and their wives were strong to say that they had never seen "anything like *that* around this barony."

One afternoon, something very disquieting was revealed to the boy's foster mother, who loved him more and more because of his increasing helplessness. He had done some especially kind act in the house that morning, and had been so unusually affectionate, that she gave him a few coins to buy himself a gift in the village. His foster father took him along with him on his shopping tour, and the lad insisted upon going alone into a shop to spend his money for what his heart desired. They came home with their packages, and as usual, the boy climbed onto a couch, with almost every muscle of his body, excepting his face, pulling in every different direction. He stated that he was tired, and it was obvious that his trip to the village had wearied him excessively. He asked to be allowed to go to bed, and his parents carried him upstairs. A few minutes later there was silence. The father went back to his fields, and the mother applied herself to her household duties.

After an hour or so, the mother thought that he had slept long enough, and that possibly he would like a cup of tea. She went upstairs softly, lest if he should still be asleep she might awaken him unnecessarily. Outside the door of his room she stopped and listened, and set down the cup of tea and soda bread with butter. It seemed to her that there was a low, humming sound as of fairy music coming under the door. She pushed it open gently. The boy's bed was between her and the window, and his back was toward her. He was lying on the bed with a bag of coarse sweets beside him, into which he was dipping with his right hand, dextrously conveying the sweetmeats to his mouth. His left hand held open a magazine dealing with adventures abroad. His deformed foot was covered by the sheet, but the rest of his body was relaxed in repose, and as normal as it had been so many years before.

She watched him in amazement, and then, feeling suddenly faint, she stumbled against the chest of drawers, making a noise. He started up, and turned towards her a face that changed in a flash from happiness and composure to a look of anguish. All his muscles then went into violent spasm, and he became an even worse example of the hideously deformed, muscle-knotted helpless invalid she had put in bed an hour or so before. She stumbled downstairs, the cup of tea forgotten, and flung herself on her knees before the crucifix, and the smoke-blackened oleograph of Our Lady of Sorrows, to whom she had brought all her miseries and sorrows for so many years, in search of spiritual comfort. Next day the local physician was called in, and arrangements were made for the boy to be admitted to this hospital. You will see him forthwith. I have sent for him, and he is coming into the ward now. You must have heard him, since the noise of his footsteps is tumultuous, and to say the least, strange.

The first impressions one gets of this odd being are mixed. I suppose that the marble statue of the Laocoön, with the father and his two sons being strangled to death by snakes, is the earliest comparison that comes to one's mind. As a second thought, I remember seeing at a World's Fair a tiny gilt image made in France of a dancer, all arms and legs, dancing on a platform which revolved faster and faster by clockwork. The more rapid the revolutions, the more the arms and legs flew around in a grotesque fashion, and as if each limb would finally break adrift from its corporate attachment.

He has come in through the door of the ward like a wild young Spanish bull of Pamplona, in its first appearance in the ring at Seville. It seems as if he would take the door and its frame apart. Strangely enough, he avoids with skill all obstacles by a hair's breadth. Similarly, he has passed through your student ranks and has never touched one of you standing in his path. At my invitation, he takes with a bound a seat on the examination table, and now he sits there, with all four limbs, his trunk, and his neck in constant violent action. Note the enlargement of his muscles, except those of his left leg, which have atrophied. There is preservation of his speech and facial expression. I can count, in so far as my experience with him goes, on his being a friendly, agreeable and co-operative patient.

You will notice that he is of medium height, and built somewhat on a small scale. His hair is jet-black, his complexion swarthy, and his nose is of aquiline cast. The members of *his* branch of the Joyce family are known to be chiefly redheads or to have sandy-colored hair. They have high cheekbones, and either straight or upturned noses. Further, the males are all tall, more than six feet in height, and are slow-moving, taciturn individuals. This man moves like a scalded cat, and he has no inhibitions so far as conversation goes.

Studying his muscles, group by group, and their movements, we find that a certain number of fixed patterns appears. His right leg below the knee is now fixed, and immobile because of contractures. Above the knee, the thigh and hip muscles carry a ceaseless torsion movement. If that is contraclockwise, the knee flexes, is adducted, and the foot is kicked wildly outward. The foot by now resembles that of an aristocratic Chinese lady of the Ming dynasty, who had her foot bound to make it small. It is everted in the extreme, has taken on a curved, crescentic shape, and has the name of "the semilunar foot." Occasionally, spasms of clockwise torsion appear, in which case the foot belabors the right buttock incessantly.

His trunk muscles, working on their attachment to the pelvis, twist his body to either side. At times it seems a point of pure devilment in the disease that the body twists and contorts in an opposite way to any of the limbs. Accordingly, most bizarre postures appear. By now a marked and fixed scoliosis of the thoracic part of the spinal column is quite evident.

The hand and arm are the most highly developed portions of our musculature. It might be hoped that a careful examination of the spasmodic outflow into this musculature could give us some hints as to the ultimate cause of this disease. We have the hints, but alas, can not interpret them as to cause. . . . I have to wait, with our patient, until the wiggles and writhings come to a basic level, and then we can proceed.

I ask our patient to extend both arms forward, so that the palms of his hands face downward. At first he is fairly quiet; then, little by little, the hands begin to pronate farther, and each time, antagonistic muscles pull them back. The battle is soon lost; the pronation of the hands is rapidly growing, and more powerful jerks complete an extreme pronation, so that the palms face outward, with the elbows flexed. This reminds us of what we were told about those earlier years, when the right foot finally and in despair turned completely outward, and the cousins were wont to tickle the sole.

For the second test, I have him extend the arms with palms upward. This posture lasts no time at all. From the very beginning, the palms buck downward, reach the stage of the first position, as I have just described, palms downward, and then by a cunning series of torsion spasms, reach the last stage as you have seen, in that the palms fall outward, with elbows fully bent.

The third, and most important, test of all, as concerns the arms, gives us a negative result as far as any great muscular reactions are concerned. It actually suggests a position of rest. I ask the patient to put his arms behind his back. You may remember that this is the position he took when he first came in to us. It seems to be by far the most comfortable one for him. He bends his elbows, and then slips his hands behind his back, holding his hands palms upward, as far as he is able. All spasms of his upper extremities cease when he is in this position. The tragedy is that when he holds his arms just so, they are completely useless for any normal activity. It is no consolation that they are also useless in other positions, by virtue of the spasms, but at least the patient is more comfortable in this position. Further, the disappearance of his arm spasms when he is in such a position is pathognomonic of the disease.

Now, as to the disturbance in this patient's neck muscles, I am arranging a sheet that covers all movements below, and brings the neck spasms into high relief. His neck is twisting toward the left side. The muscles on the right side of his neck stand out under the spasm hypertrophied, and constantly producing a torsion of head on trunk. Is not this identical with the condition of the first patient we saw this morning? Her problem was an isolated one, and this neck-turning here is but one manifestation of a general disease characterized by torsion of the muscles of limbs, trunk and neck, along their long axis. Can we possibly escape the conception that spasmodic torticollis is but a fragmentary and non-progressive part of the full-blown picture as seen here of dystonia musculorum?

To sum up, this patient is suffering from *dystonia musculorum.* More recently, the disease has been called "dystonia lenticularis" because in microscopic examination of sections of the brain, the main lesions of the cellular systems are seen to be in the lenticular nuclei. The disease is seldom hereditary, but more commonly familial. As yet the most fruitful sources of the disease have been in the East Side New York Jews of Polish descent. It may, however, crop up anywhere amongst those of Aryan ancestry. Usually, one sibling of a family is attacked.

The disease begins when the patient is about eight years old, and slowly progresses over many years. It has been divided, as far as the clinical picture is concerned, into a kinetic, and its later-appearing static, type. The kinetic phase appears early, and freedom of motion is paramount. This is usually in the form of wavy contractions in a torsion fashion involving the extremities, the trunk and the neck. The face and bulbar mechanisms usually escape—hence there is an easy distinction between Huntington's chorea, Wilson's disease, or congenital athetosis. There have been cases described in which this disease is secondary to various toxic, inflammatory, traumatic and neoplastic causations, but most patients have a primary disease without any good explanation for its cause. The muscle contractions are more rapid in this disease than in athetotic diseases, and less so than in chronic choreas.

The muscle tone varies, as in those of the muscles that are contracting, and in those that are relaxed. This of course is nothing unusual, yet the term "dystonia" has been coined on the basis of this simple physiologic fact. This is not a practical help in diagnosis, since the movements are so rapid and shift from place to place so fast that we can not trace the course of hypotonicity merging on hypertonicity.

As I mentioned before, the earlier stages are kinetic, and the patient may wander as he or she pleases. This patient whom you are seeing today falls in this category, except in so far as his left lower extremity is concerned, which is now fixed permanently in contracture. Later on, more contractures will appear, and the patient, with all his limbs, trunk and neck stiff, and molded into a permanent fantastic shape, will become bedfast. Spasm is relatively now at a standstill, except in so far as feeble excursions are allowed around contractured joints. Only the face remains normal, marked, however, unavoidably, by the apathy of despair.

There is no treatment of any value in this spasmodic disease affecting muscles. This generally holds for many of the other dyskinesias. Certain drugs diminish muscle spasm, but have to be given in such large doses that both their side effects and current risks militate against such a form of therapy. Curare will diminish muscle spasm, but in severe forms of spasm it has to be given in doses that threaten life. The same is true of other antispasmodic agents. The milder sedatives are useless.

Section of nerve roots or of peripheral nerves only touches the surface of the disease, and as long as any fiber of a muscle is still innervated it will continue to contract forcibly. As seen in spasmodic torticollis, the whole neck has to be paralyzed, and to hang like that of a dead fowl in a meat market. A therapeutic result is thereby attained which is in no wise suffered gladly or received with gratitude by the patient and his relatives. This is true on a much more extensive scale in dystonia musculorum.

You and I must naturally feel very sorry for such patients as these two we have seen today. Paralysis, a negative form of incapacity, is much more easily borne than a constant tugging and spasm of muscles, which by their positive character render all other movements useless. The pathology of dystonia musculorum is found to be widespread degeneration of the cells in the motor cortex, the basal ganglia, and in the subthalamic nucleus—particularly in the lenticular nucleus. There have not been sufficient necropsies in cases of spasmodic torticollis to show where these lesions of cause and effect might appear.

The differential diagnosis of dystonia musculorum is not difficult, if and provided you have had some previous experience. The tendency toward remissions of weeks and months, when the patient is ostensibly well, and the sudden short cessation of all spasm while the patient is alone, leave suspicions of a hysterical complaint. Again, the strange ability to walk backward better than forward, and to have more peace in the hands and arms when they are behind the patient's back, may suggest a psychogenic quirk. The laws of movement in the muscles in this disease are not well known, nor are they known in spasmodic torticollis; but such a frequent occurrence of characteristic features in a given patient stamps the hallmark of organic disease on any case of movement disorder, and dissociates it from the ranks of hysteria. And yet this disease of dystonia musculorum was described originally by Thomalla as a condition called "torsion neurosis." The first word is only too apt; the second is outmoded.

Emotion, excitement and psychologic complexes increase the severity of the spasms. In the final and long-drawn-out stages, over many years, the patient sooner or later becomes bedfast. Contractures have developed, and the spasms still try feebly to work on joints fixed beyond repair. It is then that the patient dies from bedsores or inanition. It is, in truth, not a pleasant disease, and possibly in the end death is welcomed gladly.

In default of a full explanation of these dyskinesias, that certainly bear the imprint of the devil himself, all we can advocate is that one stay strictly within doors on May Eve! Earlier, a defensive barrier should be laid out in front of the house of masses of golden flowers, fire and food. To be sure, this is not in accordance with strict scientific research, nor is it in harmony with religious dogma, while the paganism in it is abstruse and far away from an established proved history of cause and effect. All I can say is, let us placate the hordes of his most satanic majesty. It is an easy task, and so far as I can see, if applied at the right time and place, infallible.

> But Hercules himself must yield to odds;
> And many strokes, though with a little axe,
> Hew down and fell the hardest-timber'd oak.
> —SHAKESPEARE: *King Henry the Sixth*, THIRD PART.

3

Good morning! I suppose it is not wise to attend a friend, in a professional capacity. In pouring out the bowels of our compassion, we may, and often do, miss significant signs and symptoms. Always there is present the wish expression that one's dear friend or relative may not possibly have anything seriously wrong with him. It is far better to have a medical attendant who is a stranger to the patient, and who is concerned only with handling a problem as he finds it, objectively, and devoid of any emotional affect. For a physician or surgeon to attend or operate on a member of his own family is now regarded as a crime in medical ethics. I would refer you to that fascinating group of short stories by Sir Frederick Treves, of which the first is "The Elephant Man." In one of these stories, a physician's young bride, with acute appendicitis, would have no one touch her except her husband, and he killed her on the operating table. She died thinking that he was the greatest surgeon of all time!

The patient I am showing you this morning is to me an old guide, companion and friend. Every year on Boxing Day, it is my custom to go to a small hotel in a wild, western part of this country, and I know that John Gaugan will be waiting for me there in the kitchen.

Some seven years ago, he was a straight, tall, belligerent man, with hair as black as a raven's wing, and with a pair of black, acquisitive eyes, set beadily close to a nose that was as aquiline as the beak of a mountain eagle. His skin was swarthy, and his figure was as lean as that of a coursing greyhound. He reminded one of a Goya hidalgo, just landed here from the Iberian peninsula. He could have come with the Spanish Armada during the time of Elizabeth the First of England, in the sixteenth century. Actually, however, his ancestors were more likely to have been smugglers of lace, brandy and dark-brown ale.

He was generally in rags and tatters, but I was always fascinated by the skill of his wife in patching, darning and sewing a pair of trousers so that they still served to cover his lower extremities decently. He acted as guide for fishermen during the summer, for wild-fowl hunters during the autumn and winter, and in between, he did odd jobs, poached and sold moonshine on the side. He was known as "The Diver," because there was nothing he would not jump for in the water or in the bogs if it brought him a suitable reward.

Each year during the Christmas-New Year period, he acted as my guide, and was a pleasant and informative companion. His imagination passed all understanding, and his conversation, bolstered by frank lies, could be very entertaining. He was the best poacher in the county, and knew ways of getting game when all else failed.

I went west last midwinter to my usual shoot. One naturally expects that the tide of things and men will always keep up its regular systole and diastole. It is saddening to find that a long, often-repeated and pleasurable anticipation has been curtailed, and that things will never be the same again. Some time before leaving, I had been advised by John's local physician in a letter that my guide had had a slight stroke six months before. It had been a sudden drag of the left leg and foot, he said, and had cleared up within a few days. A month before I left, my medical friend had once more written to me, to tell me that John had had a second stroke, that he had suddenly lost the power of speech, and had suffered a weakness of the right arm, but that again the attack had cleared up within a week. He added that John had aged considerably in a few months, and that he had severe high blood pressure.

Nonetheless, I left for my holiday. As usual, John met me in the hotel kitchen. He was stooped, his hair had become almost white, and he could barely control his voice. The next day, trying desperately to pretend that something had not taken place, and that everything was as usual, we went to the familial haunts of wild fowl. John's aim with his old shotgun was no longer good, and he missed more than he hit. His thought processes had slowed up, and his speech accordingly. What I missed most of all was that he could no longer tell braggart lies, with the facility and verisimilitude that he had always exhibited in previous years. I think now that what I had appreciated more than anything else he could give me in the past was his infinite capacity for drawing on his imagination, and for making unto himself a world of glittering, boasting phantasy. Sad at heart, I left two days after I had arrived.

One week ago, the local physician telephoned me to say that John had had another stroke, a severe one this time, and asked if I would take him into my hospital. He is here now, and you will be able to see what a faulty cerebral circulation can do to a strong man. It will bring up the very common problem of hypertension, with cerebral arteriosclerosis, and its treatment, more especially when cardiovascular accidents appear with increasing frequency and severity. The patient is in the last bed on the right-hand side. As I approach him, I am disturbed by the fact of his marked physical and mental dilapidation. He is only in his middle fifties, and yet he looks old and decrepit. His right arm and leg lie helpless by his side, and when he smiles or weeps, the left side of his mouth pulls up to the left side, distorting the right. He can raise his forehead and close his eyes almost normally, on the two sides. I ask him to use his right arm, and he merely picks it up as if it were a piece of wood, using his left hand. His right lower extremity lies partially flexed at the knee, abducted at the hip, and rotated outwardly, so that the outer side of his foot lies prone on the bed. I raise the leg with the knee bent, and the heel on the bed, and then take away my hand. The leg falls helplessly into the position described above.

The tendon reflexes are increased in the right lower and upper extremity, and Babinski's sign is present on the right, when the sole of the foot is efficiently stimulated with a sharp object.

I say a few kind and commiserating words to my old friend, and he immediately bursts into tears. A few moments later, at some sallies and quips I have made, he smiles broadly, each time with the face twisted to the left. He does not answer anything I ask him. He seems to understand partly what I say, but any effort to speak ends in grunts, and later in tears. He has obviously lost weight, and is skinnier than ever.

To sum up, this man has *a complete right hemiplegia, with an aphasia* so severe that we can not estimate what type it is. He shows also the usual emotional loss of control, such as spasmodic laughing and crying. This last probably is located in a release mechanism in the brain stem. Sensory tests were done, but were unsatisfactory because of his aphasia. Evidently he feels pain, for pinprick on the paralyzed side produces movements of defense by the nonparalyzed side against so disagreeable a treatment. It is impossible to evaluate his mental condition, but it certainly is deteriorated, because he pays little attention to things around him. From the history given by his wife, this condition, as in the other two premonitory attacks, came on in his sleep, and is present in full form as we see it now in the hospital. There has been no improvement in the condition during the few days it has been present.

I have a quarrel with my medical colleagues in regard to such cases. They are presented to me as a pure neurologic problem. The brain is damaged; therefore it is assumed that those who are interested in diseases of the brain should take over, diagnose, treat and state a prognosis. The fallacy lies in the fact that every one of these patients may be ill in some system of the body, other than the brain, and the hemiplegia, with or without aphasia, may be simply an end result. The first thing to find out is why this patient became paralyzed. Treatment must be directed to the underlying cause, and the effects of this cause can be taken care of later, provided the primary factor can possibly be cured, retarded or alleviated.

Why did the patient have a stroke? What kind is it, and how can we prevent his having the final one that ends his life? All these questions must be answered before any treatment is instituted. A complete general examination is necessary, taking in all the systems of bodily function. Mistakes that the pathologist will eventually burn you with are present all along the line leading to necropsy. Postmortem findings reveal, to our shame, neglect in clearing up possible cause and effect.

To return to our patient: as I have said, he looks ten or more years older than his given age. His hair is almost snow-white, his cheeks are sunken, his eyes are dull and show but little understanding. There is a marked arcus senilis. His face is a maze of wrinkles, and he is edentulous. As early as last year, I had noticed that his shoulders and back had become bowed, and that his gait was tottery; now he is very nearly helpless. His hearing is deficient, for I have to raise my voice to shout commands, which are but poorly responded to. His voice has the feeble, piping tones of premature senility. The skin on the dorsum of his hands can be pinched into a ridge that remains for minutes on end.

His pulse is rapid and irregular. The electrocardiogram shows auricular fibrillation, and the peripheral vessels are hard, and have the character of dense rubber tubes. The heart tones are faint and irregular, and roentgen studies of his thorax show a marked ventricular enlargement.

He is breathless on the least exertion, but there is as yet no enlargement of his liver or edema of his lower extremities or sacrum. His systolic blood pressure is 230 mm. of mercury; the diastolic blood pressure is 120 mm. of mercury. Such measurements are difficult to ascertain, however, because of the irregularity of his heart beat. His urine shows considerable albumin, and many hyaline and granular casts of the kidney tubules. The blood urea is 70 gm. per 100 cc. Nevertheless, tests of kidney function show less impairment than one would expect. There are no signs of passive congestion of his lungs or liver. Examination of his eye grounds shows marked narrowing and sclerosis of the retinal arteries. There are many hemorrhages in the retina, with exudates around the vessels, and my ophthalmologic colleague has suggested that the retina shows an old hypertensive retinopathy.

The patient is very restless; even though he is helpless, due to a complete right hemiplegia, nevertheless the intact left side of his body thrashes around all the time, as if in defiance to the other side that remains so still and impotent. He has worn away the skin from his elbow and heel on the normal side, and he is continually groaning and mumbling, as if in abject fear and despondency. The cold pressor tests must be used to exclude a tumor of the adrenal body, such as a chromopheocytoma, and an excretory urogram, to ascertain whether there is a unilateral kidney infection, with or without stones. These latter tests in this case yielded no further information.

Let us go out of earshot of this patient, who may understand more than we think. . . . He has had a stroke as a result of malignant hypertension that has gradually caught up with him, and like a convolvulus plant, it is squeezing everything within reach to death. Note the high diastolic readings. These have been persistent, according to his local physician, and according to our observation here, have remained so. The systolic pressure may vary, and in fact does so in hypertension, but in those cases in which the diastolic pressure remains high the prognosis is uncertain and bad. The heart never gets a rest, and tension never dies down long enough in the tissues. The vessels never are relaxed, and the incessant pounding through their branches is bound to produce damage, as in arteriosclerosis.

The next question is, whether the affair is a thrombosis or a frank hemorrhage. It is impossible to distinguish a hemorrhagic stroke from a thrombotic one. Generally speaking, the old-fashioned ictus hemorrhagica is a sudden, brutal affair, followed by immediate loss of consciousness, and with stertorous breathing. Also, the cerebrospinal fluid is bloody. Since thrombosis of a cerebral artery can produce an identical picture, we are never certain with which one we are dealing. Thrombosis is found to be, if and when it comes to postmortem, a much more common condition, but again, patients suffering from thrombosis are more likely to improve, go home, and die there, so that there is no necropsy. A patient with hemorrhage dies much more quickly, and presents so interesting a pathologic phenomenon on the hospital postmortem examination table, that the frequency and clinical importance of the condition are likely to be overemphasized.

This patient's strokes occurred while he was in bed asleep, and there was never the deep coma found with cerebral hemorrhage, so that the cause of the strokes is more likely to have been thrombosis in one or more vessels. More than that, if we could see his brain now, we should find it peppered with areas of infarction, some visible to the naked eye, and others seen with the microscope. He has probably had innumerable small strokes that had not reached a level of clinical interpretation. (The last stroke must have been a massive one.) It is this multiplicity of attacks that has made him become mentally retarded, prematurely old, deaf and forgetful. This diffuse brain damage has been called a *"hypertensive encephalopathy,"* and it carries an ultimately fatal prognosis.

Over and above this diffuse brain disease, he has sustained damage in other organs of the body. His retinas are damaged, and so are his kidneys. The heart is showing signs of beginning decompensation, but so far, the brain has taken the main assault, and is suffering severely. No matter what we do, this patient is going to die, and it is a gambler's choice as to which organ will fail first, and so cause his decease. I feel that there will be one more stroke—this time an apoplectic ictus. A cerebral vessel with damaged walls, lying unsupported in an area of softened brain, will rupture, and so the end will occur within a few hours. It is faintly possible that his blood pressure will go down, as a result of his living at a lower level, following this last stroke. He may then continue having a vegetative existence, paralyzed, speechless and helpless, for many months to come, and dying finally from hypostatic pneumonia. I shudder at this horrible thought. For a man of his kidney, he deserves a swift and clean death.

These long and lingering deaths from cerebral vascular disease commonly occur in more elderly patients suffering from cerebral arteriosclerosis, but without hypertension or associated disease in other organs. Dean Swift prophesied that his own death would be like that of a tree whose topmost branches had been struck by lightning. He was a long time dying, and it was his head, wherein the chief damage lay, that finally caused his end at the age of seventy-five.

It was only a few years ago that John and I were standing on the railway bridge crossing an outlet of Lough Conn. It was dawn, and Nephin Beg had evolved its strong, hungry, mountainous peak from the morning mist, and appeared as a pearly mirage reflected in the waters of the lake. We had not done well. The ducks were flying high on so fine a December morning, and our bag was empty. Suddenly, out of nowhere, a flock of widgeon came over low and almost in our teeth. We fired, and three birds dropped into the swift waters under the bridge. They were carried away, but lower down became caught in some bushes trailing the water. This could be only a temporary site, however, until the main sweep of water would again take them to its bosom, and they would be lost forever.

John called to his old red Irish retriever, below on the ground, telling him to get them. The dog was temperamental that morning, and afraid of the cold, swiftly running water. In spite of John's alternate curses and cajolements, the dog refused to budge. John rested his gun on the ironwork, and like an over-sized tailless ape, scrambled down one of the supporting pillars. Without waiting to reach its ground-end, he flung himself, twenty feet above, into the swift icy water. Fighting the stream, he reached the ducks, and a few strokes more brought him on shore, where he proceeded to give his poor dog a terrible beating, cursing him once more in a prehistoric Irish tongue. Rescuing the dog, his master, the guns and the widgeon, I got them all into my car and drove to the nearest place where a hot fire could be found, and a change of clothes for John, with many jorums of hot sweet punch.

This was the first time I saw how John had earned his local sobriquet, "The Diver," but there have been many similar incidents since. From dawn to dark he would constantly wear me out in the pursuit of game, and never quit until the odd lost bird was found, by fair means or foul. You have now this morning seen that pitiable wreck that was John Gaugan. Could this continuous profligate waste of energy in a poorly sustained body have worn him out, and thus caused this breakdown? I do not know. All I can say in sorrow is, "So let it be with Caesar."

4

I HAVE a friend here who is willing to show himself to you this morning. Like ourselves, he is a disciple of Aesculapius, and a good one at that. Last night he came to town, to have me check him over. We had a small hot bird, and a large cold bottle for supper, and I prevailed upon him to come here, as a true scientist, "on exhibit," as it were. I am glad that the glories of a May morning have not dispelled his promise of last night, a promise based on roast chicken, and the bubbling glamors of the Widow Cliquot.

He and I were graduated at about the same time from different universities. We were both medical officers in His Britannic Majesty's Army at the time the enemy attacked in the spring of 1918. My friend had many wounded to care for, while luckily for me, all of mine had been evacuated. I ran so fast that I escaped capture, but my colleague was made a prisoner of war. To escape somewhat from the tedium of such a life, he started to read the novel, *War and Peace,* by Tolstoy. It was in three volumes, and it takes a lot of reading to finish this monumental work. He told me later that he had just finished the first two volumes dealing with war, when the armistice of November 11 was declared, and he was ultimately repatriated. He never did finish the part of the trilogy dealing with peace; he was much too glad to live it out as he found it, and enjoy it in the later postwar era.

He had built up a large general practice a few miles north of here, and he did everything in medicine that he was qualified to do. With surgery, obstetrics and general medicine, he had very little spare time. Often he worked around the clock. Vacations have been few, short, and totally inadequate. Like most physicians, he had no sense of business, and most of this gruelling, high-tension work of long hours, both night and day, was poorly paid for, if at all.

Ten years ago he suffered from a nosebleed on the left side. It was not copious or alarming, but persisted for three days. He consulted one of his local colleagues, who rightly took his blood pressure. It was 230 systolic, and 110 diastolic! Aloysius, as his name is, was then fifty-four years of age, and his work was becoming increasingly heavy. One of my friends here in the city was consulted, and he found that apart from this hypertension, there were no other signs of organic disease. He was nevertheless told in no uncertain terms that he should immediately take a vacation of three months, away from all his duties, and rest his mind and body as far as he was able. Later he was to return to a schedule of work very much less than that which he had done in the past and was doing at the time. In spite of this advice, and as in the old Latin tag, like a dog he returned to his vomit, and as a sow to her wallow. He did just nothing to change his life, and consulted nobody about his health until a more serious turn in his affairs took place.

Five years ago, after a very busy week of night and day work, he was called to attend a patient at his hospital which was close by. It was ten o'clock at night, and he had not yet gone to bed. He went on foot, and found a patient with a minor injury which he took care of, and in a few minutes he was ready to go home. It was then that he noticed that his right leg was not normal; it seemed to be weak, and dragged, and it had not the normal sensibility. He walked home, undressed, and went to bed, hoping that things would be normal again in the morning. He slept soundly until 5:00 a.m., when his telephone rang. He found that an obstetrical patient had been admitted, and that he was needed immediately. He dressed and walked back to the hospital, and on the way found that his leg was no better, but he arrived safely and took charge of the birth. Happily for him, it was an easy one, for now his leg was becoming more weak and numb, and his hand and arm had become affected. The patient had a slight perineal tear, and he tried to stitch it up, but could not manipulate the needle and its holder, and had to give up trying.

This time he had to be carried over to his house by a hospital attendant, for his right leg was by now useless. He was put to bed, and his local colleague was called. His speech was somewhat mumbling; he mixed up some of his words, but in general he was able to make himself understood. A decision was reached that he should be sent to this hospital, and by 9:00 a.m. he was here.

On admission, it was found that his blood pressure was 140 systolic and 100 diastolic. His pulse was sixty beats per minute. Results of urinalysis, blood counts and roentgen studies of his head and thorax were normal. The indications of an electrocardiogram were normal, and all tests of blood chemistry showed nothing informative. He had hemiparesis involving the right arm and leg, but to a lesser degree, the face. His speech was indistinct, but evidence of aphasia was very small. One time he called a fountain pen a "pencil," and then immediately changed to a normal terminology when he noticed his error. He was not unusually restless or depressed, but was quite understanding and ready to accept advice. He was of normal weight, and looked no older than his given age. His temperature was normal.

Careful studies of the patient at that time showed a normal cardiac activity; the kidneys were unaffected, edema of the lower limbs was absent, and the retinal vessels were within normal range. Going back to his hemiparesis, all muscles in the right side had some movement. His hand was the worst hit, for he could not move his fingers rapidly, and while he could flex his fingers feebly, dorsiflexion was impossible. His grip was weak, about 10 per cent of normal, but he could move his arm at the elbow fairly well, and could partly elevate the shoulder girdle. He could not write. Similarly, movements of the lower extremities at the hip joint were well done, at the knee less so, but movements around the ankle joint and in the toes were almost nil. When he smiled, his face pulled to the left side, but forehead and eye muscles were normally active. Tendon reflexes on the right side were exaggerated, and Babinski's sign was found to be present on stroking the sole of the foot. He could not walk without being supported, and could not use the right hand to dress himself. He could empty his bladder and move his bowels without aids.

He was kept in bed four days while the various tests were done, and then he was allowed to sit up in a chair. Daily readings of blood pressure showed but little change from normal. Within a few days, movement in his right arm and leg improved. He had been given histamine intravenously, and inhalations of an oxygen and carbon dioxide mixture. Whether these were responsible for his improvement is problematical; nevertheless, he did improve, and a week after leaving his bed he could walk around, dragging the right leg. His hand, however, did not participate so happily in this improvement, and he had to be dressed, and could feed himself with the left hand only.

Considering the personality of our friend, it would be understandable that as soon as he found his feet, he would turn resolutely, like a homing pigeon, toward his place of abode, and fly to it fast. This he did. He has, however, in the five years that have elapsed, come back for re-examination at nearly regular intervals, and for that reason he is here today, to have a going-over. I can guarantee, however, that no matter what we advise, he will sleep with his family tonight. He states that he feels very well, and he can demonstrate to you how nearly normal is his gait. The increased reflexes and the Babinski sign remain, and he can not hop well on the right foot, which, after all, is a very severe test at his age. During the years he has been checked by me his blood pressure has varied from 230 systolic and 120 diastolic to, months later, 180 systolic and 100 diastolic. Today it is more than 200 systolic, and also more than 100 diastolic. We can find no evidence at this time of cardiac, renal or retinal degeneration.

I have kept the condition of his hand to the last. It is the most highly specialized organ controlled by the brain, is the earliest to be damaged, and the last to recover. His finger movements are not good; he is definitely clumsy in finer acts, especially those requiring considerable dexterity. Although he shakes me by the hand, I know that organ can not now play a piano or bow a violin. And yet, he tells me that he does a certain amount of surgery, and as well, attends a small number of patients. He is now sixty-four years of age, and should be ready for retirement. In his record there is filed a letter written about four years after his stroke; that is, about a year ago. There are others, written before. In between, there are some written by members of his family, at his dictation, bewailing the fact that his hand has not improved enough to enable him to write.

With the greatest of satisfaction, therefore, I am now passing around this poor scrawl written last year; will you compare it with this letter he had written to me before he had his stroke, when, to all intents and purposes, he was well, and before his hypertension got the better of him? The even flow of his preictus period may be contrasted with the irregular letters and interweaving lines of his writing, done four years after the stroke. *But*, I would draw your attention to the fact that the letter is legible, is to the point, has the right words used in the right sense, and that it is far better than much of that which you careless, slovenly, lazy brats of today put out to annoy an examiner of written theses. This patient can now write, can express his thought legibly, and certainly he shows no agraphia, nor extreme clumsiness of the right hand.

I shall ask him to write now, this time a short sentence. The task is slowly done, but the result is even better than that written a year ago, as you can all see for yourselves. He is able to tie his shoes, and can do this with slight effort. I have a piece of ham here, with a thick rind. There is in it, in a certain place, a four-inch cut simulating a wound. A surgical needle and needle holder are supplied, with rubber gloves. My colleague dons the gloves, engages the needle in the needle holder, and in but little time an orderly row of stitches appears. It is not perfect, but so nearly so that it takes away your breath. As he walks away, you notice that there is a slight halt to his right leg, as if there were some trouble there, or he with a painful corn!

He used to play piano and violin. He can do neither now, but on certain parades of the Sons of Ireland he is near the head of the procession, playing the bagpipes, which require but few movements of his fingers. Moreover, the bag is under his left elbow. He keeps steady time on foot with the marching men, and more than that, when the skirl of the pipes rises to a high, patriotic, heart-rending scream, he will frequently do an impromptu dance, in his kilts. I have seen him do it, and it *was* stimulating.

Mentally, he has been entirely normal, after the shock of the vascular accident had passed off. His judgment is sound, his emotions stable, and his grasp of what is possible, and of what is the best to do, with regard to a medical problem, is as good as ever. He can fish, and shoot wild game, and he does both, to the best of his ability. Accordingly, both in his work as a country physician, and in his play between times, he has reached at least 50 per cent of normal, but for reasons of safety, he is not using all that percentage of normal. His relatives see to that; they watch him continually.

My colleague, Aloysius, therefore is in full pursuit of happiness. He is at last doing some medical work that may rejoice his soul. It was a touchy business, deciding whether to call him a permanent and total loss to the insurance company, that was bound to aid him financially, or whether to risk the cancellation of his policy by his resuming work. Fortunately, the representatives of his company were wise and considerate, and a deal was made whereby a certain amount of disability payment was withheld, based on terms of his present limited earning power. A generous sum was awarded monthly, because of his continued disability, and the risk of more to come at any time.

He still has evidence of hypertension, severe at times, but he is holding up under it well; his bodily organs as yet show no signs of deterioration under this terrific, heaving, expansile thrust, expressed in every part of the body by virtue of the blood vessels of supply. The blood vessels contract down to a tiny channel represented by their individual lumen. Is not this last a defensive mechanism, or is there a primary contracture of blood vessels, producing hypertension? The same old chicken produces an egg, and the egg produces a chicken, and then again, which process comes first?

Nevertheless, I am glad to have shown you this morning two patients with diametrically opposed clinical courses. The first, a younger man, is breaking up into a helpless, hopeless state of impending death from hypertension, hypertensive encephalopathy, cardiac disease and an early renal breakdown. On the other hand, my colleague and friend has had just as severe a hypertension for many years. He has had *a relatively severe cerebral vascular accident,* from which he has made a surprising recovery. As long as five years ago he was advised to profit by his warning. In regard to this warning, however, and in the vernacular, he did not give a hoot about it, but pursued his own sweet way. His blood pressure should have dropped to normal after the stroke. It did, but within a few months it soared again to as high a level as, if not to a higher than, he had had before the stroke. As every slight improvement occurred, he seized on it in order to regain, if possible, the life he had led before, and now he is ministering to a few patients, both medically and surgically, in so far as his health will allow, guided always by the judgment of his wife. It is, therefore, not the hypertension that counts, with respect to these two patients, *but what resistance their bodily organs can put up to such a strain.*

For this reason, the prognosis in an individual case must be carefully weighed out, since so many times all calculations as to the future fail utterly to give the correct answer. It is with these patients that most careful choice has to be made as to the use of long, tedious and expensive courses of physical training, re-education of movements, and all therapies leading to rehabilitation to an active, useful and wage-earning life. I suppose that within the first month or two after a stroke, this can be decided, and experience on our part, with courage on the part of the patient, means everything. The patient may die after further strokes, or from complications; he may become a helpless log, a care to his family for many years; or, by great good fortune, he may be able gradually to take his place again in the circle of those persons who count in his determination to overcome any obstacle impeding a return to normal or near-normal. He may even live to an advanced age, and then die from the bite of a rabid dog!

To return to this, our second patient, who is now beginning to manifest a look of hunger, with an obvious strong desire to escape from this esoteric group, I have but a few more words to say. He is slowly getting better, and is again doing a part of his work, so rudely interrupted five years ago. He travels abroad with his family, enjoys life, and is mainly concerned now with watching the development of his grandchildren. True, he has periods of severe hypertension, and may feel as if he has the sword of Damocles hanging by a tiny hair, ever over his head. Yet he realizes, as we should do, and so often fail to do, that this is the common fear of us all. Even you young and heedless sprites may go down to a horrible, searing, smashing death when next you take out the family car, and drive it too fast around the very corner that you have been explicitly warned about.

Only time can show which way the cat is going to jump, but it is well to be prepared for this feline saltatory response, and to travel with it. Never allow things to become static, except, perforce, in the case of death, which cancels all obligations, moral, monetary and merciful. Every day a patient lives under your care, you must keep thinking and praying, "Are we doing enough for this poor, stricken, helpless, wretched person?" These patients of ours are so glad for so little, and an active physical therapy department attached to a hospital means a lot to them. For one thing, pain over the joints of the paralyzed side adds so much to their misery, and heat, massage and exercises can do much to relieve it. They are well justified, even when affairs are hopeless.

Paraphrasing John Donne, there is the Bell that Tolls, and for whom does it toll but for you? In the ward, you see these poor persons who may be dying, and it quite certainly never occurs to you that you may be the next to go—or perhaps, in a month, a year, a decade or more from now. I admit that this is morbid thinking. It is far healthier to dream that you will live to a ripe old age, surrounded by members of your family, and covered with the honors of a lifetime's glorious achievement. We older ones are content just to *live*, and to enjoy the simpler philosophies of life which we picked up along the way.

Doctor Aloysius John Maguire and I are proceeding now to Jammet's Restaurant. I shall take the rest of the day off as a tribute in honor of his presence among us. A table has been ordered for luncheon. We shall have Galway oysters in the shell, jellied calf head and brains with sauce ravigôte. Crêpes suzette will follow, and a cold, brown, long-necked bottle of Steinberger Kabinett Spätlese of a good vintage will wash it all down.

We shall talk of "shoes and ships and sealing wax; of cabbages and kings," and of how we won World War I. I can assure you that hypertension and strokes will be as far from our conversation as the diatribes of Swedenborg, and all his kind. As medical advisor to this morning's Patient Number Two, I regard all this as an excellent form of therapy. He will go home, feeling even better than he did when he came, and he will continue to feel better, even up to the next yearly occasion of the comprehensive examination and physical evaluation that I shall choose to give him. I shall certainly look forward to seeing him at that time, if both of us are spared.

By telling of it,
Made such a sinner of his memory,
To credit his own lie, . . .
　　　　　—SHAKESPEARE: *The Tempest.*

5

Good morning! On the way here, and just before I came to you, I had to pass the church of the Capuchins. It was here that Joyce, in his *Portrait of an Artist as a Young Man,* made a soul-stirring confession that should have changed his whole life, and landed him in the kind hands of the Jesuits. In that event, we should never have had *Ulysses!* I am now wondering if that would or would not have been a great loss. Time will show.

Church Street crosses North King Street farther on. This latter street leads from the Smithfield Market Square, where, in the early hours of the morning, hay, potatoes, and small grains are sold at auction. There is a tiny nubbin of a lane that leads into North Brunswick Street, on which a few yards away, on a left turn, this hospital faces. In the lane there is a large public house with a huge neon sign, visible from afar on black winter mornings, announcing, "Drinks served here from 7:00 a.m."

I have often wondered why this tavern was opened so early in the morning. I *should* have thought of Covent Garden in London and of Les Halles in Paris, where farmers and raisers of produce come in to the markets at five in the morning to sell their products to the local jobbers for distribution in the cities.

It is quite probable that these poor persons who come in to Smithfield Market leave their homes in the country at about midnight. Their produce is carried in a cart drawn by a horse, and the speed can not be more than a few miles an hour. The poor tired horses, with their halos of steamy sweat, jog on, mile by mile, until the Market is reached. Then, a quick sale, with money in the fist of the farmer, and nothing else to do but to adjourn to Moriarty's in the lane. There they drink pints of black porter, with a white creamy head on each libation, and begin to feel almost human again, until the time comes for the slow journey back. In the meantime, the quiet, patient horses are up some back lane, each with a nosebag of satisfying oats.

By the time I pass Moriarty's on my way to you on a Tuesday morning, all the market sellers have departed, and are on the way back to their homes. It seems terrible that a human being should have to drink alcoholic beverages so early in the morning. There are, however, no arrangements for feeding these poor rain-sodden, tired-out creatures, except with flyblown ancient sandwiches. Yet, what these sellers of hay, potatoes and small grains want is a potion that is food and drink together, and in such a category can well be put Dublin's dark brown stout. . . . I have always prayed devoutly that for each of these countrymen there is, on his return, a good woman waiting, who will greet him affectionately, provide him with dry clothes and good wholesome food, even though meantime she is rummaging in his pockets for what is left of the sale!

We have here this morning a foreigner to meet you, one who has been washed up on our shores, an unusual guest, and therefore, we must be especially kind to him. He is indeed worthy of this kindness, since he never complains, and Sister here will tell you that he is an ideal patient, doing everything which he is told to do—except one thing, and that is that he will not change his ideas of the past, or of the present. To the future he pays no attention, and he is, in truth, quite oblivious of it. He is a Scot, and his name is Ian MacGregor. His native city is Glasgow, and he has the rich brogue of that area where the letter *r* is not squandered, as it is in England, but used judiciously and with full effect.

He is at least fifty-eight years of age, looks well nourished and seems to be utterly content with himself and with his surroundings. The only trouble I find at the very beginning of the taking of his clinical history is an important one, and that involves the question as to what he really complains of, and why he is here in the hospital, and further, why he is in bed with a cage over his feet to keep the bedclothes off them. The answers to these questions are short. He has *no* complaints, and he is here because the physicians have ordered it. Moreover, he is not at all sure that this is a hospital, and more specifically, he is in doubt as to the nature of the female saints who minister to him: they might be nurses; then again, they might not be; he does not know for sure. And yet he looks at them as they pass his bed, with affection and gratitude. He says that his legs are sound and well, as he can prove to us by a meticulous account of his activities yesterday and last night. Here the history and presentation of the case are becoming nebulous, so let us turn to the facts of the case, as related by others. The patient will not object.

MacGregor came to this country ten years ago as a forester. He had done this sort of work for a noble lord in Scotland, who, having eventually to sell his land to pay his taxes, passed him on to a friend in Ireland, who had large holdings in timber of various kinds. The pay was good, and MacGregor, being single, Scotch and of a saving disposition, was able to accumulate a warm nest egg of savings. He lived in a country hotel, and every day he went around the demesne cutting trees, planting new ones and protecting the rest from natural pests and dry rot.

So far as his social life went, he was not very communicative, and for days on end would speak to no one; often as not he sat at the bar of his hotel, gloomily looking into a drink that was consumed only after an hour or more had passed. He never treated anyone, or accepted a treat, and he was looked on as a moody, taciturn, solitary drinker, harmless withal, and always avoiding trouble.

He retired early to bed, but the curiosity-mongers noticed that his last act before retiring was to buy a small bottle of whisky to carry up with him to his couch of slumber. Nevertheless, he was up betimes in the morning, and out in his woods, when everyone else was asleep. There he seemed at his best. The men who worked under him talked of his leading a gang to work at a double trot, with which they could not keep up, and then reaching the place of active work, shaming much younger men by his drive, energy and attention to duty. Once a tree that was being felled commenced to fall over a heedless, lazy worker and MacGregor dashed forward and threw the man bodily out of the line of the falling mass. He succeeded, but one branch crushed his foot, and he was under the local physician's care for a long time. It is for such an episode as this that his men worshipped him, although at the same time they hated him for being a hard taskmaster.

Time went on its way, and our patient's habits changed little; if anything, he became more seclusive. He never went to the local picture theater or to dances, and certainly not to a church of any kind. He was polite and kind to the female staff, re-membered their birthdays and never failed to send a wedding present when it was due. At the same time, he never took a girl out to an entertainment, nor was he ever seen with one outside the hotel. If anything, he was more communicative with the male staff, and he seemed to have a passion for having his shoes shined properly in the morning. He was most critical of the preparation of the food served him, but contented and quiet when it was as he had ordered. Every year he went on a journey to Scotland to see his brothers, and usually came back more cheerful and slightly more talkative.

I suppose in human affairs there is seldom a state of absolute balance, but rather a swing to one side or the other, certainly as time goes on. I have heard of men, however, whose habits of living had changed but little over a course of many years. But in the case of MacGregor there had been an almost imperceptible change in a downward direction, a year or more before he has come to us here. He became even more silent, and the volume of his nightly potion became greater by slow degrees, as he left the bar each night. Moreover, he went to bed earlier and was getting up later in the morning. There were times when he would press the bell button in his bedroom to call the night porter for a further supply of drink. His interest in his food slackened and often he would sally forth to the woods without any breakfast at all, and eat only at night, without appetite or discrimination. He no longer cared whether his shoes were polished or not, and the hotel "boots" was the first to take advantage of this disinterest.

The climax occurred six months ago when he went to the bank and came back to the hotel with a stack of banknotes, approximating three hundred pounds. He had an interview with the hotel manager. The money, he said, was to be placed in the hotel safe and drawn on as he saw fit. He had that day resigned from his position as forester and as excuse claimed that he was very tired and wanted a complete rest. Now, nothing surprises people in this country, particularly hotel managers, more than the request that strong drink be sent up to a room, if and when the bell button is pressed. This service MacGregor requested, and that food should follow, and he would remain in bed. He asked particularly that all calls, messages and letters to him be ignored. He assured the manager that being a nonsmoker, he would not set his bedclothes or the house on fire. One more thing he asked for, and that was that an ample stock of the whisky he drank, a lesser known Scotch blend, should be kept on hand at all times.

This retirement of Ian MacGregor took place some time in October, and he completely disappeared from all ken. The habitués of the hotel thought that he had left town. The day and night porters knew better, for every so often, night or day, a bell would ring, and the box in the office would show a small red indicator trembling over a number, and whether it was midnight or midday, a bottle would go up to a room whose door was always kept closed. He was never noisy or troublesome, and was always polite when the bottle was brought to him. In the beginning he ate regularly and read the daily newspapers. Later he ate less and less, and remained just lying in bed, gazing at the ceiling, seemingly content that he had reached the happiness of being able to achieve the state of "the world forgetting and by the world forgot." That happy state could of course not last forever.

Several factors began to operate. His stock of money began to diminish rapidly. Additionally, the hotel manager could not see himself taking the responsibility of keeping this man in food and drink forever. Also, the brothers in Scotland began to press for information as to MacGregor's physical and mental state. Both, by then, were in a precarious condition. The brothers came over from Scotland and found him very confused and unable to walk. By this time the hotel manager was all too glad to get rid of him, for his financial assets by then were assessed as being just nil. There had been, however, no attempt at bookkeeping, with respect to the original fund delivered to the hotel—it was just gone!

He was admitted to this hospital a month ago, at the request of a local physician, a friend of mine, and here he is, for your delectation, scientific inspiration and advice as to what we should do for him. He has what is a classic example of a disease described by Korsakoff, a famous Russian neurologist, and known as *"Korsakoff's syndrome or psychosis."*

He co-operates well in his general examination. His systolic blood pressure is 125 and his diastolic pressure 90. His heart seems to be normal, as do his lungs to ordinary examination. His urine shows considerable albumin, with many casts of various kinds, but the value for his blood urea is within normal limits. His liver is not greatly enlarged, and bromsulphalein tests of retention of dye show a surprisingly small amount of damage to the liver. His legs are weak, in an increasing degree from the hips down. His thighs are about 25 per cent below normal strength, his legs below the knees are 50 to 75 per cent under normal power and the intrinsic muscles of his feet are completely paralyzed. He can just barely wiggle his feet and can not move his toes at all. The final position of his feet in bed is that both fall downward and need a back splint and a cage to keep the weight of the bedclothes off, and to retain them at right angles to the legs. The skin of his feet is white, smooth and glossy, and tinged with pink.

There is a diminution of subcutaneous fat and sweating is profuse around the toe endings. The calves of both legs are exquisitely sensitive to pressure, and such a procedure is greatly resented by the patient, who, however, forgets this intrusion into his comfort almost immediately afterward. Tendon reflexes in the lower extremities are completely absent. Joint and vibration sensibility in the knees, ankles and toes is also gone. Superficial sensitivity to touch, pinprick and thermal stimuli is almost normal in the thigh zone, but is about 50 per cent absent between knees and ankles. His feet below the ankles are almost anesthetic. He does not know the position of his feet in bed, or whether one is lying across the other, and the test of running one heel down the other shin, with the eyes shut, is almost impossible for him to perform. His arms, hands and cranial nerves are by contrast entirely normal. Let us get him out of bed.

The usual slippers and dressing gown are provided, lest we shock the amenities of the ward. Two strong students lift the patient to a sitting position on the edge of the bed. All support is now retired to a near and watchful distance, and he is asked whether he can walk. It is then that there is noticed a marked atrophy of his calves, his anterior tibial muscles and those of the peroneal group. His thighs are shrunken, but less so in comparison with those muscles below his knees.

He consents readily to step out from his bed, and as one would expect, when both feet are on the floor and he tries to stand upright, he is about to fall precipitately when his two guards seize him, and lift him bodily into bed, out of further harm. He has muttered something about his feet being asleep, but seems to be in no way perturbed that he can not walk, let alone stand.

He has full control of his urinary and bowel sphincters. I would have you feel this man's lower limbs, gently, since they are very tender. Atony, or flabbiness, is present, and when a leg is held above the bed, the foot and toes dangle downward helplessly. Also, I would ask you to try the reflexes: the touch-and-sound of the percussion hammer is at one with the total lack of response.

This patient, as you have seen in our clinical examination, has a well-developed and advanced *alcoholic peripheral neuritis.* His arms, trunk and cranial nerves have escaped. He has more than that, however!

You may remember my drawing your attention to his pleasantness, his agreeableness, his attitude of self-satisfaction and his general smiling happiness. The fact that he can not walk or even stand does not upset him. If he has pain, he does not complain. As a patient he co-operates well and does everything he is told to do. His voice is low, but cheerful, and he keeps up his appearance by shaving himself, keeping himself clean and brushing what hairs he has left. He is most approachable and gives a good history of a certain sort, one, of course, that is all his own story. There are many missing elements, but he supplies others to make up for this vagueness.

The only difficulty he has created in the ward was to tell one of the younger nurses a story which was so plausible that it sent her running to the Sister in charge, since it involved a serious dereliction of duty in the hospital. It amounted to the fact that MacGregor had been out of the hospital unaccompanied and had been drinking all night. Further, this paralyzed man had *walked* out!

Sensing something of interest on hearing this story, I had many interviews with the patient, with a stenographer present, taking down questions and answers. Also, I got a large-scale map of the city of Glasgow, a few picture postcards of the city buildings and the like, and his brother supplied me with an old family group photograph. I have a projectoscope here, and as far as time will permit, we can further investigate the mind that is still left to Mr. Ian MacGregor.

I ask him what day of the week it is, and he answers "Monday." This is close, since the day is Tuesday, my morning to teach. The day of the month he does not know. The season and month of the year he arrives at very slowly. His eyes wander over the trim lawns which he can see well from his bed, the many flower beds blazing with color, the blue sky with great fleecy clouds so low over the hospital, and the emblazoning sun glorifying everything. His answer then is that it is summer, and either June or July, which, after all, is close enough.

We are now going to get a shock. I ask him what year it is, and promptly he replies, "Nineteen hundred and ten." That would be thirty years ago, when he was a young man of twenty-eight. No matter what I suggest, he will not change his idea of time. He tells me that a few months ago, in a Presbyterian church, he attended a memorial service for the death of the late King Edward the Seventh, and that this year is the first one of the reign of George the Fifth, King of England and Emperor of India. He remembers attending coronation festivities a few months ago, and that he became very drunk. Here he leans back in his bed, and cackles with merriment, with an impish challenge to his listeners.

I outline to him World War I, the uneasy years since then, and the beginning of World War II. He looks bleak, and suggests that we are ahead of ourselves. I remind him of his life in Ireland these last ten years and of his tragic downfall. He hoots me to scorn, always with a big smile and in a low and tender voice. Finally, in exasperation, I ask him where he is *now* and what he is doing. It is then that a veil comes over his face and he stammers a reply that he does not quite know where he is. Next thing, he volunteers to tell me what, to his knowledge, he has done the last few days. I can promise you a fascinating tale. I have heard the story several times already, and it is always the same.

You remember the episode of the young nurse who sincerely believed MacGregor's story, and in all haste reported him to the Sister in charge. I do not doubt that before he is finished, you will be similarly impressed with his seeming veracity. Again, about what is he talking? Is it about an episode that occurred thirty years ago, which has been burned into his brain forever? Remember that all memories after this real or imaginary period of 1910 have been erased, and that he lives, quite happy and content, from minute to minute. Or, is this story a complete fabrication, built up out of whole cloth? I have heard it repeated so many times so convincingly, and with such exact and plausible detail, that I do not believe the latter, for I can not conceive of more than two forgeries' being completely the same. You may all sit down. Since the patient's voice is very low, and especially for the benefit of those in the rear, I shall repeat the story as given us today, and be his interlocutor.

He says that yesterday, which was Monday, he took a street car to Glasgow, and at a well-known tavern met his friends and spent the day. How he managed to leave the hospital and reach another country, with his limbs paralyzed, he does not explain, and on being tackled with this incongruity, he becomes simply confused, so we give him a free rein and let him tell his story according to his lights. It must be observed that at this stage his story largely takes in and emphasizes the one function utterly denied to him, and that is the ability to walk.

We have here on the screen a map of Glasgow and its environs, and the tenuous path of his itinerary drawn in red. This was worked out from previous interviews. Let us see whether it will be the same today. I am sure it will. From time to time as his journey progresses, I shall pass him the picture postcards, with the names of places erased, for his recognition. Up to date he has not failed to recognize them.

He says that at the tavern he met three friends; according to his memory they were Baldy Craig, Ross Stuart and Henry Mac-Gillvray. According to the patient's brothers, these erstwhile boozing companions have, as a result of War, Pestilence and Drink, long since died. And so, *yesterday* these three ghosts, with my living but stricken friend, started out on what is known as a "pub-crawl." From their meeting place, we can follow the red line, step by step, correlating it with the pictures of whatever famous buildings they passed.

At noon they stopped at a restaurant in Sauciehall Street, which is identified on the map, and on a picture postcard which he recognizes. There they got food and sustenance for further wanderings from tavern to tavern. The only point of difference here is that they picked up some girls to enliven the party. Mac-Gregor does not remember their names, but he smiles tenderly at the memory. They were sprightly and gay, eating all they were given and drinking all they were offered.

By this time the red line is beginning to wiggle all over the city. It is amazing how a man almost *non compos mentis* can give in such detail a drunken party of more than thirty years ago. Is it true, we can ask ourselves once more, or is he making it up? It is strange, however, that he has a complete possession of place, time and circumstance, checked so far as we can go. His ghostly friends, alas, we can not recall to life; his girl friends gave no names! But, he identifies street after street, and they all lie along this red line.

By ten o'clock, the girls, being presumably virtuous, departed for home. To replace them, the four musketeers made a beeline deeper into the city, to the slums, brothels and abodes of sin and shame. MacGregor recognizes the district as called out from the map and the straight course of the red line. Here, because of his

Calvinist conscience, he is seen to blush deeply. The line ends there, indicating shame, regret and a desire to forget. His ability to forget, as you have doubtless noticed already, is his strongest virtue. This affair of the four comrades in the brothels of Glasgow reached into the early hours of the morning. By then, MacGregor felt the imperious need to return to this shadowy place where he now exists, in peace and quietude. How he traveled back here, and arrived, is no one's story, except in that he is here now, and very glad to meet all of us.

He is here now to see you because he thinks that the Sister in charge has so ordered. Actually, he complains of being tired, and says that he can well take a day off from his peregrinations, have a full night's sleep and be ready for a twenty-four hours' spree tomorrow! He knows that his three friends will be waiting for him, and that is all he cares for.

Psychiatrists tell us that when a patient has reached a stage of nirvana, with a happy though useless adjustment, it is unwise to shock him out of it too suddenly. I have a hellish temptation, nevertheless, to avoid this ruling. There is in my hand a group photograph of MacGregor and his family. From this there has been made another photograph in which MacGregor has been taken out, enlarged and suitably mounted. The group picture was taken around 1910. I am dropping the group picture and will use this other piece of evidence of what our patient looked like during the era of all his stirring experiences. Let us hand it to him, as an experiment; it may cause untold anguish and rebound on us in a tragic fashion.

He has the photograph now, and looks at it long and earnestly. He even turns it over and looks at its back.

"This is some mon I ken well, but I do not ken him now. I can not remember where and how I met him," he murmurs, as he adjusts his spectacles for a clearer view. He has placed the picture on the bed, then picks it up again and studies it.

"That Glengarry bonnet is verra fashionable today," he notes, and then the picture drops to the floor, and seemingly his interest ceases as he lies back on the bed, smiling at the ceiling.

This experiment is a complete failure. Let us adjourn to another room to discuss the pathologic aspects of the disease, its prognosis and treatment.

We are all in the corridor leading to Ward No. 4, which is almost empty. A nurse pushes her way through, and tells me that Sister wants me to come back immediately. Kindly go on to where we are going to meet next, and I shall tell you later of any problem that may have arisen.

     ❋   ❋   ❋   ❋   ❋

I arrived back in the ward, and was faced by a highly indignant Sister, alongside MacGregor's bed. The photograph still lay face down on the floor. The man himself had both hands over his face, and through his long, bony fingers a continuous flood of tears gushed forth. He was sobbing as if his heart were ready to break. He would not answer me, and my every appeal was followed by an even louder exhibition of grief. Accordingly I left, the Sister and I first removing all the paraphernalia of the morning's clinical discussion. The photograph was the first thing to be taken out of the room! I presume that later in the day, the patient will be his usual satisfied and contented self. It teaches us a lesson, however, showing that if more than 90 per cent of insight into one's psychic content is gone, what remains, no matter how small, may, when once aroused, act as a bomb with a terrific explosive force.

The prognosis here is bad. In such cases as this, when death has occurred, pathologic studies have shown widespread and irreparable damage to the cells in the brain and to the fibers of peripheral nerves. Treatment consists in feeding with diets high in vitamin B. Synthetic vitamins, particularly of the B family, are administered in large doses by mouth and parenterally. Ultimately, most of these patients drift into homes for chronic disease of the central nervous system, and eventually die.

6

Good morning! I have two patients this morning to show you. Both have a sensory and motor paraplegia, with some involvement of their sphincters. They are both about the same age, and have about the same degree of disability. There all resemblance ends, for the history of each is completely dissimilar, and in turn calls for a very different idea as to causation. In your junior years, it seems to you that to recognize that a patient is paralyzed and numb from the waist down is so sufficiently brilliant a stroke of nosology that no more need be said. You may even go so far as to work out the exact level of the spinal cord where the damage has occurred, and then sit back, satisfied with your tremendous accomplishments. I can assure you right now that you have left still undone the essential factor that should bounce back and hit you in the face, and that is, "What is the *cause* of this phenomenon?" On this cause may rest the vital problem of success or failure in treatment, or even more, the factors of life and death. Worse still than death, there is the ghost of permanent invalidism.

I would further draw your attention to the fact that with respect to these two patients, the importance of a carefully extracted history of events leading up to the present clinical picture is paramount. This is, I think, more true in neurology than in other

308

medical specialties, since a disorder of anatomy tends to be so sensitively responded to by disorders in function. This is more marked in diseases of that soft, mushy, white, dead-looking material called the spinal cord. The brain, in contrast, has many of its own secrets of response to disease or damage as yet not known to us. The spinal cord is a more delicate structure, and suffers a dissolution of its continuity very poorly, from the very beginning of the disease.

Again, I must emphasize the time element, as given by the history. A similar end result has been attained in each patient, but the speed of downward progress is a vastly different one. This speed determines diagnosis and prognosis.

* * * * *

This patient is a woman aged forty-three. Seven years before, she had begun to notice a dull, nagging ache over the top of her ninth right costal cartilage in front. As weeks and months went on, the pain spread to involve the corresponding ninth thoracic intercostal space, and gradually approached the spinal column behind. She has never had, however, any backache in that region. The pain was continuous, worse at night, but never were there any paroxysms of pain, such as are seen in disease of the gallbladder. There were no digestive symptoms, and repeated roentgen-ray studies of the gallbladder showed it to be without stones, and always functioning normally. Nevertheless, cholecystectomy was advised, and, for one reason or another, refused. The patient found that a sitting-up posture was helpful, and often at night she slept in a high chair, with her trunk flexed. Occasionally, when the pain was quite severe, she knelt alongside the bed, and slept with her body lying across it. Up to date, this pain has become progressively more severe, and she has been taking codeine with aspirin in increasing doses for relief at night.

She noticed also, as the pain became more severe, that the skin in the area involved had become increasingly sensitive, and that light touch, or a closely fitting girdle, was intolerable. She could no longer use an electric heating pad, since that was irritating, and, if anything, it made the pain worse. The nocturnal character of her pain became more marked, but pain did not greatly interfere with her daytime activities. She dreaded her nights, particularly the early hours in the morning, and craved early daylight and its concomitant periods of relief.

Two years before, physical signs had begun to appear. She liked to wear high-heeled shoes, but had to discard them because she found her right ankle becoming more and more unstable. At one time she fell, and fractured a bone in her right arm as she used it to break her fall. At this time she had first noticed a progressive numbness in her *left* foot, which month by month ascended into the leg, the thigh, her groin, until finally at this present date, it occupies her trunk up to, and at about, the level of her original pain on the opposite side. It was only one or two thoracic segments below the pain level, but on the left, the opposite side of the body. The weakness of the right leg increased steadily, and she had finally to use a cane in order to get around.

About a year ago, her sphincters gave her trouble, in that there was a precipitancy of urination which she had to reckon with, to avoid wetting her clothes. She was very definite that the right leg was the weak one; the left was the one that had abnormal superficial sensation. As proof of this, she stated that she had burned the left leg last winter with an electric pad which she was using because the leg felt so cold, and moreover, the burn that took so long to heal had been a painless one. She complains of jerking in her legs at night during the last few weeks which, with her chest pain, keeps her awake. She thinks that the right leg, like its fellow, is now also becoming numb, and as if asleep.

The examination is easy, if you know what to look for. The patient has spastic paraparesis, more marked in the right leg. On walking, she drags this leg, with the toe scraping the floor. The left leg moves nimbly enough, but she can get around only with the aid of a cane in her right hand. When she is back in bed, all neurologic manifestations are normal above the waist. She exhibits one sign of considerable importance, and that is that while she is raising her head and trunk off the bed, her umbilicus moves upward. This means that her abdominal muscles above the tenth thoracic segment work normally, and pull against those paralyzed below that segment. The navel must move with the *tense* muscles.

Both legs are spastic and weak, but the right one is more so. Babinski's sign is prominent on that side, but is also present on the left. The tendon reflexes are disproportionately exaggerated; again, more active on the right side. Ankle clonus is present on the right. Try it yourselves.

Her left lower extremity is not normal. Touch sensibility is slightly reduced, but pain and thermal sensations are gone out of the limb. The only response is at a level as high as the tenth thoracic segment on the left. I would have you note that at that level the response to pain and temperature is overactive just where normality is reached. There are, therefore, above the numb area, a few segments of hypersensitivity. With an ethyl chloride spray, moving upward from the foot to the tenth thoracic segment, no discomfort is claimed until that area of hypersensitivity is reached, when there is a sudden cry of pain and discomfort, and both legs jerk upward. Superficial sensation in the right and weak leg is almost normal. Joint and vibration sensibility (called "deep sensation") are definitely lower on the right side; these sensibilities are fairly keen on the left.

To recapitulate, the patient's right leg is very weak, and it is on this side that her earlier girdle or root pains first appeared. Her left leg is numb, mainly to pain and temperature sensation; there is a sharp level at the tenth thoracic segment wherein sensation appears again, conversely going down the body, and at about that level, suddenly sensation becomes lost. The difference between the loss of sensation and its reappearance going up the body, with its disappearance going down, is only one or two cord segmental areas. It is there that there is a marked hyperesthesia to pain and thermal sensibility. Joint and vibration sensibilities are diminished or lost on the paralyzed side, and where the root pains occur. These pains from the beginning were at the segmental areas supplied by the ninth thoracic nerve root on the right side of the body.

These complex data represent *the syndrome of Brown-Séquard,* the Anglo-French neurologist, whose other claim to fame was that personally he had an overflow of sweat on the skin zone supplied by the second division of the fifth nerve on one side. It was usually produced by chocolate, which he never ate in public. The Brown-Séquard syndrome means a hemicord lesion on one side, compressing a spinal root, the pyramidal tract on that side, the crossed spinothalamic pathways of pain and thermal sensibility, and the uncrossed pathways by which joint and vibration sensibilities are perceived. The lesion is focal and painful and may be *a tumor involving the spinal cord.* It may arise in the cord itself, from the meninges or nerve roots, or from the bones encasing the main pathways of motor and sensory function.

Let us turn her over in bed, lest shame strike us for missing a Pott's spinal disease in this land riddled with bone tuberculosis, or a giant-cell sarcoma, which would be even worse. I had one such patient in this ward for six weeks, undiagnosed because the members of my illustrious staff were satisfied to accept the effect and ignore the actual cause—Pott's caries!

Her back is free from blemish. Fist percussion produces some pain over the tenth thoracic vertebra, but there is no gibbus. Roentgen studies of the thoracic part of the spinal column show no pathologic changes. As an aside, why do house officers do roentgen studies in the *lumbar* segment of the spinal column when the trouble is obviously in the thoracic region? The spinal cord ends at the upper border of the second lumbar vertebra, and a lesion in that area can not and does not produce a clinical picture such as this! I suppose they do so because paralysis of the legs means to them a lesion in the lumbar region. Lesions which can produce such paralysis can occur, and do more commonly, in the thoracic and cervical areas of the spinal column, and even going further in the brain hierarchy, up to the parasagittal region of the brain.

To reach a state of precision, we start with the pronouncement that this woman has a progressive lesion involving her thoracic spinal cord on the right. With this long history of root pain, it must involve the right ninth or tenth dorsal nerve roots, probably the former, since sensory decussation in the cord is slow and involves many segments at a time. It is compressive in character, hence the nocturnal pains of this lesion and the resultant maneuvers of the patient to obtain relief, which, at the best, is small.

Can we pinpoint this process more accurately, and surgically explore that region with a minimum of destruction of bone, and a minimum of time on the operating table? At this stage we can do spinal puncture, and immediately thereafter inject an opaque medium and do further roentgen studies with the patient on a table that can be elevated or lowered as required.

Yesterday spinal puncture was done. The cerebrospinal fluid was light yellow, as you see it here in the tube. The protein estimation was more than 150 mg. per cubic centimeter. At the time puncture was done, and with a water manometer attached to the needle, compression of both jugular veins produced no rise in the pressure level in the manometer. Coughing or straining produced a quick response in the level of pressure. From that, we assume accordingly that there is a complete block in the subarachnoid space somewhere along its course in the spinal canal. There is something along the neuraxis, shutting off the circulation of the cerebrospinal fluid.

To be more specific, and to localize this blockage more definitely, we injected a fluid substance opaque to roentgen rays, having made room for it by withdrawal of a generous quantity of cerebrospinal fluid. The patient was then placed on a table that tilted up or down, and in a dark room, the course of this fluid opaque to roentgen rays was observed under a fluoroscope.

The opaque medium had been injected at the second lumbar interspace. It progressed up the spinal canal until a thoracic segment of the spinal cord was reached. It then stopped. Roentgenograms were made and developed immediately. A column of opaque medium was seen suspended at the ninth thoracic segment, and a characteristic cup-shaped upper margin was seen, due no doubt to a rounded mass in the spinal canal, compressing the spinal cord.

About all the facts are in now, in regard to this patient, and can be correlated. Clinically, this patient has a slowly progressive process squeezing her spinal cord on the right side, and at about the ninth dorsal segment, where it also irritates one or two spinal sensory roots. Our mechanical tests, with spinal puncture and the introduction of a medium opaque to roentgen rays, narrow this process down further, to a tumor arising in the spinal canal and compressing the spinal cord.

At this final stage, I am showing you what should be an easily recognized and typical instance of a tumor of the spinal canal, benign in character, accurately localized and easily removable. These cases of tumor of the spinal cord constitute the most elusive and difficult problem in neurology. Like criminal problems, the steps from the indictment to the verdict of "guilty" are infinitely multiplied and infinitely crooked. The final proof of guilt is one fraught with many difficulties.

The pathologic characteristics of tumors involving the spinal cord are multifold. They are usually divided into extramedullary tumors, and those arising in the substance of the cord itself, or the intramedullary tumors. The common extramedullary tumors are those arising from the nerve roots, neurofibromas. Those arising from the meninges are meningiomas. There are various rare kinds, such as lipomas, cystic tumors and gliomas. There seems to be no limit to what has already been described in the literature.

Arising inside the cord itself, there are ependymomas, with or without associated syringomyelia, and more rapidly growing gliomas. Tables have been constructed to show the differential diagnosis between extramedullary and intramedullary tumors. In a given case, however, no such differentiation is possible. Chronic inflammatory lesions, such as chronic arachnoiditis circumscripta, arise to bother us, and above all, there is ever the problem of malignant metastasis from an unknown primary source. Lymphosarcoma may give a clinical picture of a benign tumor, and depress us sadly when it is found at surgical exploration.

Suffice it to say, then, that the clinical picture may be one which merits surgical exploration of the cord. To the relatives must be given the message that almost the last word is said when the surgeon explores the cord at a given segmental level. Something is found and is examined by the pathologist at the time of the surgical operation, and a surgical and pathologic diagnosis is made on the spot. No promise can be given beforehand as to the success or failure of surgical intervention.

You are fishing in deep waters, my masters, when you approach disease of the spinal cord with a view to surgery and cure. The clinical examination must be meticulous, to the nth degree, and include a general examination of all organs, before focusing on the site of the lesion. Your roentgenologic studies of the spinal column must be done by competent observers, and followed if necessary by the assessment of spinal hydrodynamics, and the use of media opaque to roentgen rays. Above all, in cases of disease of the spinal cord, do try to avoid the wish-expression of *always* finding something amenable to surgery, just because the results therefrom are so good, and because naturally you are loath to send your patient home to linger, paralyzed and helpless, for the rest of his days. There are plenty of problems of disease of the spinal cord that seem so hopeful before surgery that prove to be hopeless when the spinal cord and its envelopes are exposed. Always, therefore, leave a substantial margin of failure when discussing the problem with the relatives before the final test of surgery is evoked.

One word more, which will be exemplified in the second patient of this morning's endeavor. Any pathologic clinical entity involving the spinal cord, if it comes on rapidly, and in a space of days or weeks, is bad. Tumors of the spinal cord amenable to surgery take their own time, as with this patient, where nearly seven years were involved. There is a stage of ripeness in these instances, when the patient is as yet not bedridden, or completely paralyzed, with incontinence of bowels and bladder. It is then that surgical removal can produce its best results. Such a case, taken in its tide, leads on to fortune for patient and physician. As a contrast, a rapid, sudden and brutal destruction of a spinal cord means only that one must stop, look and listen, inasmuch as the prognosis here is apt to be the worst in our ken of evil diseases.

NOTE: This patient was operated on a few days after this lecture was given. A neurofibroma was found. It was about 1 by 2 cm., and was found arising from the right ninth thoracic nerve root. It was completely removed, and there were no complications. The patient's convalescence was quite satisfactory.

A year later she was seen and examined. By then she had almost completely recovered all her functions. Very few signs of neurologic changes were found. She was doing all her housework and shopping. She walked without visible signs of difficulty, but most important of all, she was *free from pain.*

7

WITH REGARD to our last patient, it was apparent that it took months, and even years, to reach her final state of disability, as we saw it here in the hospital. Progress of her disease was slow and orderly, and could be followed anatomically and physiologically. This second patient whom I am going to show you has a much shorter history of illness, with greater damage to her spinal cord, and that damage is of a brutal nature, without regard for anatomic structures, except in an overwhelmingly destructive fashion.

This patient whom you are going to see is a woman, aged forty years. She complains of an inability to use both lower extremities. They are numb, and this numbness goes as high as her waist, in the region of her umbilicus. She can not at present control the functions of her bowels or bladder.

Three weeks ago she was on a trip here by motor car with her husband. It was a long journey from the Southwest, but they had many friends along the way. For economic reasons, they carried a small tent and a mattress with a waterproof sheet, and slept out in the open each night. Like gypsies, they cooked their meals in the open air. Unfortunately, they ran into bad weather, and the first few nights of the journey it rained incessantly. They became soaked inside their tent, mattress and ground sheet notwithstanding. Their friends were still far off.

The husband was of the gay, carefree type; the patient was merely a long-suffering piece of goods that put up with him and regarded all his utterances as saws of Holy Writ. They had no children, a matter to be thankful for now, considering the economic issue of her future health.

After the first two or three days of rain-soaked traveling, she timidly suggested going to a hotel in order to dry out, for some pains had recently developed around her waist, and she regarded them as being rheumatic. Her husband scorned this idea. The next day she felt feverish and had a chill. Her husband loaded her with whisky and aspirin, and she confessed to feeling somewhat better. The third day, however, the pains around her waist had become increasingly severe, and she found herself stumbling over the tent ropes; her legs felt heavy as lead, and her knees gave way, so that on a few occasions she fell down heavily. It was then that her husband conceived the idea that she was neurotic, and roundly abused her.

The late afternoon of the third day was dry and sunshiny, and rather than start an argument, she pulled herself around on her hands and knees to do the simple tasks of cooking, washing the dishes and packing, in order to leave early the next morning. This seemed to dispose of the problem, as far as her husband was concerned, and that night he criticized her very little. He felt that she was getting over her neurotic reaction to the miseries of the trip.

On the fourth morning she could not leave her bed, simply because both lower extremities and the lower portion of her back were completely paralyzed. Worse still, she found herself lying in a pool of urine, of the passage of which she had no knowledge. Later, her bowels emptied themselves incontinently, and she lay filthily in her feces and fluid excrementa. She was at once terrified and mortally ashamed, and even at that horrible moment, apologized with bitter sobs to her husband for having soiled their bed.

The lowest form of human species may ultimately realize that he has made a grave error. The husband was no psychologist, but he had enough sense to call a physician immediately, and the patient was forthwith brought here by ambulance, where she is now, in another room awaiting our examination.

As a matter of psychologic interest, the husband is now extremely solicitous about his wife's condition. He takes his hurt feelings badly, and works out the conflict by being critical, demanding and very disagreeable to all of our staff here. Last night

I discussed the problem with him. I regret indeed that I was not so smooth and even-tempered as I should have been. Like Achilles, today he is licking his wounds, and sulking in his tent. It is better thus, for we can now go ahead without interference, and find out what is wrong with this poor woman, how serious it is, and what to do about it. She is in the second ward on the left.

My gifted house officer has made a careful examination, and I would have him demonstrate his findings. More important is it, that you should verify them with your eyes, your ears, your nose and your sense of touch. The only way in which your sense of taste would be involved would be in a figure of speech: that you have the savor of bitter tragedy and almost irreconcilable loss.

As you may note, the patient has complete paralysis of both lower extremities, equal on the two sides. Beevor's sign is present, in that the umbilicus moves upward when she attempts to sit up. This means that the upper abdominal muscles are intact and the lower ones paralyzed; hence, the umbilicus moves upward. Further, it is significant of a lesion in the region of the tenth thoracic segment of the spinal cord.

The paralysis of her legs is a flaccid one; the limbs are cold to the touch, and as she lies on her back, both feet are in eversion. Raising each leg passively in turn, we ask her to hold it up, and then we let go. Immediately the limb falls helplessly onto the bed, with a sullen thud. She has an indwelling catheter, since otherwise the bed would be continuously soaked. Pads have been placed on her sacrum, trochanters and heels, to prevent bed sores. The only way her bowels can be made to move is by enemas, and that is not always wholly satisfactory, since impacted feces frequently have to be dug out from the rectum by a rubber-gloved hand.

She has no feeling at all for sensations, superficial or deep, up to a sharp level at the tenth thoracic segment crossing the umbilicus. Above that, sensations are normal. We are happy to note that during the few days she has been here, this level of anesthesia has not climbed upward, as it so often does in these abrupt instances of infection of the spinal cord, indicating an extending process that will end inevitably in the death of the patient.

The tendon reflexes in her arms are normal and active; in the lower extremities they are abolished. This suggests a state of spinal shock. There is some response to stimulation in the upper abdominal reflexes, but in the lower there is none. Anal reflexes are absent. She can not feel when her bowels move. In passing water, she has no sensation of its passing. She can not feel the catheter in her urethra, nor can she feel an enema nozzle in her rectum. She can not sit up in bed without a bed rest, and then only for very short periods. She can not stand or walk, even with support, for her legs crumple under her at the knees and hips, and she falls immediately support has been removed. Apparently, all her functions have ceased below the tenth thoracic segment, and she is a total loss from there on down, in regard to the spinal cord and the body it serves.

We call this condition an *"acute transverse myelitis"* or *"myelopathy,"* by virtue of its sudden onset, and the concomitant complete cessation of all the functions of the spinal cord at a certain level. We assume that the lesion is confined to a few segments, but we do not know how many segments are involved below the clinical evidence of damage: it may be the whole spinal cord below the tenth thoracic segment, or only one or two segments. While the condition of spinal shock prevails, it is difficult to tell what the segmental involvement is. Later on we can be more certain, especially if the reflexes return, the legs become spastic and some voluntary movement appears below the level of the lesion.

I suppose that the cause of this patient's illness must be attributed to an unusual exposure to cold and damp, in which she lay all night on wet and chilly structures, while she lived a life to which she was totally unaccustomed. As a contrast to this, however, her husband slept alongside her, under identical conditions, and had no symptoms therefrom. Considerable debate could be indulged in under this heading, but the fact remains that this woman is now totally paralyzed from the waist downward, and she is not as yet showing any signs of recovery. Further, this paralysis followed immediately on a period of exposure to cold and dampness, and while she was lying down.

Spinal-puncture examination of the cerebrospinal fluid helps us here not at all. Readings of the pressure of the fluid on compression of the jugular veins show normal responses; the fluid itself is normal in every respect, including the reaction to the Wassermann test. Roentgen studies of the thoracic part of the spinal column show nothing abnormal. The general physical examination shows no primary disease, such as tuberculosis, leukemia, lymphoblastoma or cancer.

Most careful inquiry into the patient's history gave us nothing to suggest that, as in multiple sclerosis, this was just another episode of the disease. Actually, the patient insists that she had been very well until this trip was undertaken, and that during the trip and under its unusual conditions she was struck by this serious affliction. We use the word "transverse" in the diagnosis to indicate that at a certain level *all* structures in the spinal cord have been damaged. As I mentioned before, we hope sincerely that it is only a certain segmental level that is involved, and not the whole cord below that level.

The classification of these myelitides, or acute myelopathies, is chaotic. It merely results in trying to bring into order a Hydra-headed group of diseases of the spinal cord that up to date are poorly understood. The classification itself is at fault. Sometimes it is based on the clinical history and findings, unsupported by pathologic investigations; often it owes its origin to observations made either at surgical exploration or by examination at necropsy. In a great many instances we just do not know what is behind the problem.

The prognosis for these unfortunate paralyzed persons, such as we see here in front of us, is at the most a guess. Take the case of the so-called acute benign infectious myelitis that may be epidemic, and which will certainly clear up miraculously in a few weeks or more, as may be the case here, and compare that with acute necrotic myelitis. In this latter disease, the spinal cord is reduced to a dark, formless, pultaceous mass, and this process of destruction may ascend, day by day, even higher, until *exitus lethalis* takes place. I am glad that this is *not* the case here.

This patient had no history of an acute infectious illness antedating this acute myelitis. Even the bullying methods of my junior counselor-at-law could not extract any damaging evidence. It is known, however, that every exanthematous disease we know may have a complication referable to the central nervous system during the illness, or as it is subsiding. More usually it is a meningo-encephalomyelitis and not a pure disease of the spinal cord, such as we see here. Scarlet fever, measles, mumps, typhoid fever vaccination and so forth may produce damage to the spinal cord as a complication. Such damage is, however, mixed in with all sorts of other complications in the central nervous system. Acute septicemia, arising from amongst other things, may produce a myelitis, abscess of the spinal cord, or an extradural abscess. Clinical investigation ought to settle this problem.

Acute demyelinizing diseases, such as multiple sclerosis and neuromyelitis optica, may strike suddenly, but again there are so many other signs of a diffuse, rather than a focal, disease of the spinal cord. One or more vertebrae may be undermined by tuberculosis or cancer, and may collapse suddenly, impinging on the spinal cord. This sudden paralysis may suggest osteomyelitis of the vertebrae, but roentgen studies of the spinal column will settle the nature of the mechanics producing sudden paralysis.

In the final estimate as to cause, with respect to a given case of acute transverse myelitis, it may be largely a matter of opinion. Syphilis was a notorious cause of sudden destruction of the spinal cord, due to a syphilitic endarteritis obliterans of the blood vessels supplying the spinal cord, but syphilis itself, due to many factors, is gradually ceasing to be one of our major outpatient and hospital ward problems. We may say *"Ave atque vale"* to it, but I for one miss the stimulating clinical effect on students of that old rascal, Treponema pallidum, and the diagnostic problems it presented every week or oftener. Remember, however, there is always an exception, a sporadic case. A suspicious mind in neurology, as I have said before, is as valuable as gold.

Involvement of the spinal cord in pellagra, sprue and pernicious anemia is slow and insidious in onset. These diseases do not, therefore, enter into the problem. Vascular diseases of the spinal cord, apart from syphilis, are very rare, and besides, they appear only in the aged and arteriosclerotic patients. Sudden onset of paraplegia may occur in cases of dissecting aneurysm of the abdominal aorta, shutting off the blood supply to the cord by occlusion of the intraspinal vessels of blood supply. Often enough, roentgen studies will show the dilated, calcified walls of the descending aorta. Abdominal exploration, inspection of the aneurysm, and injection of an opaque medium will clear up the question of whether the aneurysm is the whole cause of the paraplegia.

The prognosis here of course depends on the cause, if it can be ascertained. Possibly those patients with myelitis that occurred during an acute infection, or followed it, have a slightly better chance of recovery. The acute demyelinizing diseases have their remissions, and the acute septicemic processes can be attacked by antibiotic agents and brought to a standstill.

It is, however, in such cases as this one, wherein the actual primary cause is unknown, that difficulty arises. We have no knowledge of the organism or virus which was introduced into this patient's central nervous system, as a result of exposure to cold and bad weather. Therefore, at this stage we just do not know how things will go, but we shall certainly watch the patient carefully, day by day. In the meantime, she is being protected against decubitus ulceration and her urine is checked daily. If it shows signs of infection, and organisms are present, antibiotic agents will be given. The catheter is removed for certain periods of the day, and the patient is encouraged to try to void her urine without help. An anticonstipating diet has been prescribed, with mineral oil, and again she is being encouraged to try to evacuate her feces.

The physical therapy department takes her in charge twice daily. Her lower limbs are massaged, put through passive motion in order to prevent contractures, and movement, if it returns at all, is encouraged by cheers and enthusiasm. Even with the worst prognosis, she will be graduated from the bed to the wheel chair as soon as possible.

Then her arm and shoulder muscles will be strengthened tremendously by exercises aimed at hauling around her useless nether extremities. She will be taught to exercise on parallel bars, supporting her body, and also projecting it along. Later, a "walker" will be used, in which she will push herself along like a baby who has not yet learned to walk. Next will come crutches, of a kind that rest on the arm rather than in the axilla, and finally, double walking sticks may help her to get around.

Mark you, all this is for a completely paraplegic patient who has not shown any signs of recovery. What must the results be with a patient who has regained 30, 40, or 50 per cent of walking capacity? More than that, among these patients with "benign" myelitis under treatment, recovery ensues much faster than in leaving it to Nature and the patient's caprice.

With our modern departments of physical therapy, no patient should be allowed to rot in bed and die of toxemia, if and provided that the patient is mentally normal. The urinary disturbance can be taken care of by the urologist, who resects a portion of the bladder's neck, provided there is a marked retention of urine. Thereafter, a program of urinary control is taught, and at regular intervals the patient goes to pass water. The bladder develops a habit, and, aided by suprapubic pressure, empties itself. Many of these patients in this way keep themselves dry. Accordingly, and at the worst, patients with these focal lesions to the spinal cord, of traumatic or inflammatory origin, have a chance in the future for a useful and happy existence. It is only those cases of progressive diffuse disseminated diseases of the nervous system that seem to defeat our purpose, and yet, even many of these patients can be helped to do better than lie in a bed of hopeless surrender.

With this our patient, first we have to hope for a recovery, small or large, in the part of the spinal cord involved. The pathologic findings are simply a loss of structure, with few signs of inflammation, or none at all. We see only the necropsy specimens, wherein the extreme course of the disease has attained. We can not tell what has happened in an individual case, and possibly conditions may be less grave than they appear to be.

This patient, and our friend, may have only an apparent, rather than an actual, damage to the spinal cord. Her face lights up at this message of hope, and her hand seeks mine, grasping it convulsively. I can assure her that we will do all in our power, all that is possible in this day and age, to get her back on her feet, walking normally. She, however, must work with us, and for us, using all her strength and will power, and co-operating with us to the very last fiber of her being, regardless at all times of temporary discouragement.

Further, this is possible, and I hope with all my heart that it may actually occur. In the ghastly gray hours before the dawn, in this public hospital, a Presence may be felt, who will lay His hand on my patient, and in a low voice, showing infinite pity and grief for all the pain and sorrow in this world, will say,

"Rise, take up thy bed, and walk."

> *Master, this is Thy Servant.*
> *He is rising eight weeks old.*
> *He is mainly Head and Tummy.*
> *His legs are uncontrolled.*
> —KIPLING: *His Apologies* (SCOTTISH TERRIER).

8

Good morning! I saw a police arrest this morning, and for that reason I am late. The wretched victim had apparently been up all night drinking, and had thought to finish off his orgy by a few hours at Moriarty's, which opens at 7:00 a.m. I pass the place every day, coming to the hospital, from which it is separated by only a few hundred feet.

My man emerged unattended from Moriarty's, and by all appearances, he was footless. He staggered down the lane, rebounding from one side to the other. I noted that his legs were far apart, that his eyes were on the ground, and that his hands were clutching for whatever support he could get from the walls around him. At one time he held lovingly onto an ass's head, but the creature bit at him surlily. It was then that Law and Order arrived, characterized by two huge Civic Guards. The usual crowd collected, and enjoyed the ceremony with great glee. Rhadamanthus produced a large notebook and a tiny stub of a pencil, which he sucked judicially. By that time the drunk was headless as well as footless, and fell into the straw on the donkey cart. A few minor movements, and he was on the cart, reaching swiftly a state of oblivion.

This was a serious infringement of discipline to Rhadamanthus, and to Minos especially, since the owner of the ass-and-cart just then dived out of Moriarty's, protesting vigorously against the usurpation of his *lares* and *penates* for an illegal purpose. Aeacus arrived suddenly, and the three judges of the lower world discussed the matter gravely with the owner of the ass-and-cart. There were some very tricky and debatable points of law involved, but common sense prevailed. The owner contracted to lead his ass-and-cart the few yards necessary to reach the nearest Guard's Barracks, without reward, and as an act of civic responsibility and justice. The three Guards flanked the cart, the crowd dissolved, and the drunk slept on. What the donkey thought, he did not say; anyhow, he had had his bite into the corpse he was carrying.

✿   ✿   ✿   ✿   ✿

This patient we have here is a man of forty-five years. His chief complaints are headaches and inability to control his gait.

Fifteen years before, he had noticed a noise in his right ear that sounded like frying fat. From that time on, the ear slowly became deaf. The patient had to switch the telephone receiver to his left ear when receiving important messages. Repeated examination of the affected ear showed no cause for the tinnitus or deafness, and he learned to live with the condition and to put up with it.

Five years before, his wife had died. At the funeral, which was in the winter time, he noticed at the graveside, a numb, frozen sensation in his right cheek and right side of his nose. Returning from the funeral, he noted that his gait was unsteady and that he had trouble in getting in and out of his car. His unsteadiness was such that he lurched mainly to the right side. He had no vertigo or dizziness.

In the years that followed, the numbness of his cheek spread to involve his lower jaw, his lower lip and the right side of his tongue. He had become more and more unsteady on his feet and there was some awkwardness of his right arm and hand, particularly in writing, buttoning his clothes and dealing out a pack of cards.

One year before, his condition had rapidly worsened, and new complaints came thick and fast. His swallowing was interfered with, and on his drinking out of a fountain the water came through his nose. A mean and steady pain came to him then, involving chiefly the mastoid and posterior occipital area of the skull. It was usually worse early in the morning, and was inclined to wake him up. Sometimes this pain made him nauseated; occasionally he vomited. His vision became double, chiefly on looking to the right. He noted that the double images were getting farther and farther apart. This made him even more uncertain on his feet, and from then on he seldom went out alone. It has been noticed that the right side of his face is inactive, that the eyelids stay far apart and that he seldom blinks on that side. The numbness of his face has now spread to the forehead, which prickles and tingles incessantly.

He is here in bed for us to examine. Note the wide-open right ocular fissure, and that it seldom blinks during conversation. As a matter of fact, his face is immobile and pulled to the left when he talks. His right corneal reflex is abolished; the left is intact. Movement of the eyes horizontally shows a wide, swinging nystagmus on looking to the right; on looking to the left, there is also a rapid nystagmus, but not so wide and forcible as it is on looking to the right. He has a weakness of his face muscles on the right, almost a complete paralysis of the seventh nerve, and the external rectus muscle of the eye on that side just does not work at all.

Checking sensations of the area of the fifth nerve, we find that there is a 25 per cent reduction in the third division, a 50 per cent reduction in the second division and about 10 per cent reduction in the first division. This is for all forms of sensibility. The motor functions of the fifth nerve are as yet preserved on the right.

The soft palate and pharyngeal muscles pull over to the left, indicating that the ninth and tenth cranial nerves are weak. The eleventh and twelfth are still intact.

His eye grounds show definite papilledema in both optic nerve heads, equal on the two sides. Roentgen studies of his skull show very little, but special studies in Stenver's position show an enlargement of the right porus acusticus. Please look at these films; they are here for you to study and to learn.

The patient is out of bed now, and holding on to the headboard in a fearful manner. When he is walking without support, there is a typical titubating cerebellar gait, legs wide apart and lurching to the right. Note the head tilted toward the right, supposedly a vestibular pattern response. There are no changes in his reflexes and plantar response is normal on the two sides. Finger-to-nose test is well done on the left, but there is a definite in-co-ordination on the right. His handwriting is not good, but it is still legible. His speech is thick and drunken, a matter of grave suspicion to his local Civic Guards. If they would spend as much time on him as I do, they would know better!

My friends in the otolaryngologic department have indeed been helpful. The audiographic machine shows complete loss of hearing on the right side. Caloric tests, that is, syringing cold water into each ear consecutively, show the usual response of vertigo, nausea, vomiting, and nystagmus on the left side. On the right side, just nothing occurs. On the right side, his eighth nerve is dead, both in its vestibular and in its cochlear portion. This concludes the whole damning indictment that this man has a tumor arising from the eighth cranial nerve on the right, and from nowhere else. It is affecting other contiguous parts of the brain. These are so close together that they make this indictment all the more surely resting on a firm foundation.

As to differential diagnosis, I am afraid I can not see any difficulty here. We see a tiny nidus of tumor starting in the portion of the eighth cranial nerve that lies just inside the porus acusticus. It starts to grow and thus brings other structures into its horizon. I have described this foray of extension; it is for you to follow it up anatomically. . . . Every step has an anatomic and a pathologic meaning, which it is up to you to understand.

The patient is to be operated on tomorrow. Our present technic is to take the tumor and nerve out whole and intact. The old timorous intracapsular enucleation left a sizable mass in front of the pons, which, because of postoperative edema, led to death some forty-eight hours afterward. Now we get the tumor out, regardless of difficulties in surgical removal. There is a cure, then, that is most satisfying and the patients are not necessarily upset after the operation. Within my experience of thirty years, the mortality rate has dropped to a small 10 per cent and the final result is not simple alleviation, but what one may call a "cure." I have to hand this to my surgical colleagues, who have done the seemingly impossible.

The tumor has involved the seventh and eighth cranial nerves. In order to remove it *in toto,* both nerves must be sacrificed, since all parts of the tumor process must be cleared from the internal auditory meatus by bony débridement. The eighth cranial nerve will not regenerate, but the patient can get along with only one nerve of hearing, if it is intact, as it is here. The seventh later can be attended to by an anastomosis of the spinal accessory nerve, and the facial nerve on the same side. In this particular case, a result therefrom is problematic, since the seventh was dead even before surgery. In the case of other patients, in whom the seventh cranial nerve was intact or only partly destroyed before the operation, an attempt to recover facial expression and movements may be made within six months of surgery by spinal accessory-facial anastomosis. The patient loses the power, temporarily, of elevating the shoulder. Other muscles, the levator scapulae, for example, may be taught to do the job, so that by practicing before a mirror, the patient may switch his shoulder movement to his face, by concentration and dissociation of muscular movements. This takes time and effort, but it seems to be worth while. At one stage, if he tries to smile, his shoulder wiggles; at another, if he shrugs his shoulders in Gallic fashion, his face jerks. Finally, however, he smiles when he wishes to, shrugs his shoulders when he feels like it and each movement becomes independent of the other.

Removal of an *acoustic neurofibroma* in the 'twenties and early 'thirties of this century had a shocking mortality rate, and a patient who survived represented even a worse wreck than he did when he went to surgery. Now, taken early, these patients are a credit and a heartfelt satisfaction to those who operate on them. When the tumor has been totally removed, there is a cure, and consequently, no recurrence.

Going back to clinical observations, it is not widely known that an acoustic neurofibroma can produce facial neuralgia so exactly like tic douloureux that they can not be separated clinically. This facial pain is usually on the same side as the tumor, but most puzzling of all, it may occur on the opposite side. When it occurs early, it is very confusing in the differential diagnosis of trigeminal neuralgia.

9

HERE IS my friend, yclept Bartholomew. I do not know his other name or names. He is a little, short, stocky runt, but remember, so was Napoleon Bonaparte, who conquered nearly all Europe. Our patient's business is farming, but his hobby is raising pigs—pink ones, black ones, and those who seem to be the color of heliotrope, and who smell as sweet.

It is apparently the custom to castrate the younger males, leaving enough for seed for the next batch. The patient was engaged in this engrossing ceremony about twelve months ago. He held between his knees a somewhat more powerful and well-grown specimen than usual. With his left hand, he held the sources of that particular porcine dynasty, and with his right, he held a sharp, triangular-bladed knife, which he has here now in his hand to show you.

At this stage, the little pig rebelled. He had no complaint regarding being held between constricting knees. He disliked having his organs held and pulled on, but when he saw the flash of a steel blade, he determined that now was the time for action. As our friend here made his pass over the target with his knife, the pig went forward, carrying his owner's left hand with him. Accordingly, instead of severing the spermatic cords of the piglet, the knife entered the volar surface of the patient's wrist, making a deep incision which bled freely. Immediately after being cut, our friend Bartholomew noticed a numbness in the ball of his thumb, and the volar surfaces of the index and middle fingers. He also noticed some numbness in the palm of the hand, at the base of the thumb, index and middle fingers.

His local physician gave him an injection of antitetanic serum, cleansed the wound, and then sewed it up tight, in order to stop hemorrhage. The understanding was that later it could be opened, the median nerve exposed, and secondary suture done, if deemed advisable. It is thus that we see brother Bartholomew almost a year later. As to the pig who resented being "neutered," he is at present a champion boar, whose services are called for incessantly, since his offspring to date, even in so short a space of time, have won many blue ribbons.

The wound healed readily, and but for the disagreeable numbness in the thumb and index fingers, Bartholomew thought that he had escaped lightly. There was some weakness in opposition, that is, bringing the left thumb over to touch the corresponding little finger. There was also a wasting away of the muscles of the thumb, which you can see even now. The slip-up in castrating a pig did not show its serious side until a month later, when the wound was healed, and when he still had a relatively useful hand. Let us look at him now, and see what has happened in the interim.

He is a most co-operative patient, but there is one thing that he will not allow you to do, and that is, touch or manipulate his left hand. He holds his left arm flexed at the elbow; the forearm is semipronated. The elbow is adducted firmly toward the trunk. As a result of this, his left hand is held in a guarded position, with thumb and fingers partly flexed, so that the hand is cupped. At no time is the palmar surface of the hand allowed to touch his body, or anything else, for that matter. The right arm, forearm and hand move easily.

Note his expression of long-continued suffering. He is nervous and jittery, and starts violently at any sudden noise or movement. I make a pass at his left arm, as if to examine it, and he pulls away violently, long before I could even reach it. I give him a cigaret, and he takes it in his right hand, places it in his mouth, and lights it with the same hand. His left hand is virtually useless.

At this stage he complains of a constant, burning, hellish pain in the palm of the left hand, clustering around the bases of the thumb, index and middle digits but also radiating into these fingers. He can not allow this hand to touch anything, as I have said, or to be used in any way, since every stimulus given to the area supplied by the median nerve is responded to by violent, burning, insufferable pain. Emotional reactions increase this pain, and even a wrong note in music will bring it forth strongly. The hand seems to crave warm, moist applications, and constantly there is a small pad of cloth in the palm of his hand. Your textbooks will tell you of men who, when nothing else was available, used their handkerchiefs soaked in urine for that purpose.

Now we have to pin him down in regard to this strange complaint, and if necessary, open Pandora's box. He is asked to place his left hand palm upward on a small table. The palmar surface of his hand is swollen, red and glazed, and there are small pinpoints of white flecks on the surface. The area involved is, as I have mentioned before, in the volar surfaces of thumb, middle and index fingers, and also occupying a small zone of the palm at the bases of these fingers. The maximal area of pain and hypersensitivity is in an area between the base of the thumb and middle finger. Because of constant soaking with wet pads, the skin is also sodden.

Touching any of this area is resented violently; but with patience, care and diligence, we can ascertain that there is a partial sensory loss in respect to pain, thermal and tactile sensibility. Some of these responses are of the thalamic syndrome character. The stimulus is poorly felt, but when once appreciated, is exaggerated in character, and a far greater response is recorded than occurs over normal skin. There are some trophic changes, in that the fingers are clawlike, and the nails curved and split. No matter what we do with this patient, there is always, always this burning, intolerable pain.

The wound where his knife entered is well healed, and the scar is not excessive. Pressing on this scar gives no evidence of a traumatic neuroma. I have asked him to take his hand off the table. You will note the alacrity with which he obeys this command, and resumes his previous posture of his hand held close to his belly, like a poker player with four aces. He has not, however, the same expression! His is that of a dying, disease-riddled duck, alone in a rain-spouting thunderstorm, full of misery, madness and death.

From the facts of this case, the patient cut his median nerve. He did not sever it entirely, but partially. Better had he cut the nerve *in toto,* for then he would not have suffered for a twelve-month this ungodly pain. It is these partial lesions of the median or the tibial nerve (usually incorporated in wounds of the sciatic) that produce this syndrome of *causalgia.* With "little Latin and less Greek," you may be able to translate this causalgia into "burning pain." It is an apt title, and remains fairly distinctive from case to case. However, there are occasions when doubt is held as to the diagnosis, particularly when patients do not respond to established methods of treatment.

The tibial and median nerves are so much more often involved, because it has been claimed that these nerves carry more sympathetic fibers than others. They are more *painful* nerves, and respond to trauma wherein the nerve is *not* completely severed very poorly, and with great pain of a causalgic type. Treatment in the past has been neurolysis, that is, dissecting out the nerve and removing the scar tissue. The nerve has been severed and resutured. Later, sympathetic plexuses around large vessels have been removed. Finally, under the assumption that these causalgic syndromes were caused by sympathetic influence, the sympathetic pathways and ganglia have been ablated.

There is a sympathetic ganglion in the cervicodorsal chain which is composed of elements comprising the inferior cervical ganglion fused with the first thoracic ganglion. It is called the "stellate ganglion," and it lies just in front of the base of the transverse process of the first thoracic vertebra, hugging closely the anterolateral portion of the body of that vertebra. It is part of the chain of sympathetic ganglia descending into the thorax. If it is destroyed, there is a cessation of sweating over the face, neck and arm, on the side cut, and to a variable degree, below the arm. Horner's syndrome also appears on that side. This is a contraction of the pupil (or a miosis), an apparent recession of the globe of the corresponding eye and a narrowing of the ocular fissure. This is sufficiently conspicuous to indicate that the stellate ganglion has ceased to function. All pain of sympathetic origin ceases, and that is the point of importance in these causalgias, for we believe that it is from sympathetic involvement in wounds, tumors and other lesions that these burning pains arise.

Accordingly, with respect to this patient, our treatment would consist first in an injection of the stellate ganglion with procaine hydrochloride. The needle is inserted above the clavicle and directed toward the base of the first thoracic transverse vertebral process. We hope to enter the ganglion and soak it thoroughly. If the procedure is successful, Horner's syndrome appears, and sweating ceases in the face, neck and upper extremity of the side injected. All pain should then cease immediately, but it will return in a matter of hours. Some enthusiasts claim that if this injection is repeated, relief of pain will occur for longer and longer intervals, and that possibly, after numerous injections, the pain that is relieved will not come back, and the patient will be cured.

More conservative workers state that the pain may not be relieved, even though Horner's syndrome appears, indicating a successful injection. Again, the ganglion may be missed entirely, and there is no evidence of its being chemically damaged. This same group of surgeons uses the injection only for the purpose of prognosis when total surgical removal of the ganglion is suggested. In a satisfactory block, with relief of pain, more promise can be given to the effects of surgery. Should the chemical block of the ganglion fail, surgery is undertaken without promise.

Anyhow, ablation of the stellate ganglion in a high percentage of cases relieves this misery, for which in previous years we had no cure. In those instances in which relief of pain is not achieved by ablation of the stellate ganglion, there is still the possibility of cordotomy, or cutting the spinothalamic tracts on the opposite side in the upper cervical region of the spinal cord.

Finally, there is the last resort of lobotomy, or cutting the corticothalamic tracts in the frontal region of one side or both sides of the brain. In cordotomy the patient should have no perception of pain in his arm; in lobotomy, what he feels of pain is unheeded by him and is laughed at merrily.

Women patients find that Horner's syndrome is somewhat disfiguring; therefore, to obtain a better cosmetic effect, some surgeons remove the head and vertebral end of the first rib and remove the *second* thoracic sympathetic ganglion with success similar to that attending removal of the higher placed stellate, but without a "queer-looking" eye as a final and permanent result.

With respect to this patient, the chances are that ganglionectomy of the cervicothoracic sympathetic system, whether it be the stellate ganglion or the second thoracic, will give him relief from pain and a new lease on life. True, it is a destructive operation, but he stands only to lose his sweating in the area involved, and in the stellate operation, to have the disfigurement, which is extremely slight, of Horner's syndrome. He sacrifices little to gain a lot. The risk of surgery in expert hands is extremely small. One complication to be dreaded is that in the digging for his sympathetic ganglion, his *somatic* nerve roots may be damaged, and severe pain of somatic nerve-root origin may persist for months afterward. This complication, however, is becoming less frequent as the operation is being improved, and even at present it is rare.

Pain is something we all wish devoutly to avoid. If it is present, we want it cured, and even if no cure is available, there is still a continuous demand on the part of the sufferers that their last few years, months or days of life be made reasonably comfortable. Drugs are seldom the answer, unless death be swift. Addiction is a terrible price to pay, and moreover, toward the end, the returns from this price are inadequate.

The pathways of pain from the sensory nerve to the thalamus and its cortical connections have been severed to stop the conscious, feeling brain from receiving such hurtful stimuli. This is destructive surgery, and it has its own boomerang in altered physiology and corresponding psychologic reactions. A positive cause does not always produce a negative result. In the section of sensory pathways *something* results which may be more distressing than pain. "Pain" may be felt thereafter in a different form, more disagreeable than that which it was planned to relieve. The last resort is in surgery done at the highest level that one can reach; namely, that in the frontal lobes of the brain.

Lobotomy produces a patient who feels pain but does not worry about it. He may, in some instances, become a brilliant green cabbage, and we know so little of the psychology of a cabbage. Does this leafy vegetable have a better life on this planet than we have? I fear so, and I hope so, but I do not know. This is our last answer to pain relieved by surgical methods; we can go no higher in the central nervous system hierarchy. The only step beyond that is death. As far as we know, all pain ends there.

JUNE

Take us the foxes, the little foxes, that spoil the vines:
for our vines have tender grapes.

—THE SONG OF SOLOMON.

1

Good morning! The teaching year is shortly coming to an end.
I have some clinical problems saved up for you, and therefore I
feel that we should indulge in a final period of extravagance, lest
next year we have no such material to show you. I am showing
four patients today whose disease is of a simple character, easily
told, and readily recognized.

The first patient is a woman sixty-eight years of age. Her main
complaint is that her eyelids tend to go into a spasm, and in so
doing, shut out her vision. This trouble has been present for at
least three years.

As we see her now, both her eyes are open in a normal fashion.
Suddenly, and without obvious cause, there are premonitory
spasms of the orbicularis oculi muscles, and then a final spasm,
so that the eyes are tightly shut, as if there were an intense irritation of both conjunctival sacs. This is by no means a simple
blink, or ticlike movement, but a savage and ruthless forcible
contraction of both orbicularis oculi muscles. With the spasm,
the patient is blinded, and if it occurs when she is crossing the
street, she has to be led by a friend or relative.

These spasms occur every few minutes in the day, or at somewhat longer intervals. Observers say that they are absent when
she is asleep. She can relieve the spasm by a forced digital
opening of both upper and lower parts of one orbicularis muscle.
Sometimes, the least amount of pressure by her finger is enough
to loosen the muscular spasm.

Emotion, nervousness and tension make this condition worse.

339

She is having these spasms continuously now. You might try to measure what tension there is in these orbicularis muscles, and whether, by forcibly pulling apart both eyelids, you can relieve the spasm. Sometimes this works; at other times, not at all. There are no pathologic changes in the eye itself, internally or externally.

This condition is what is called "*senile blepharospasm.*" It is probably of central origin, and is due to arteriosclerotic changes in the mechanism of eye opening and closure. It is not amenable to treatment. Section of the nerves leading to the orbicularis muscles defeats its own purpose. If too extensive a cutting is done, lagophthalmos ensues, worse than the original trouble, and anyhow, any section of peripheral nerves can only be a temporary measure. Injections of alcohol show the same failure in relief of the spasm. Sometimes an optician can provide a small, curved clip to attach to the patient's spectacles, that will hold up the upper lid, and so enable the patient to get around more easily, without having to resort to the finger-stretching mechanism of defense. These appliances, however, do not always work.

2

THE SECOND patient is one whom I saw for one of my surgical colleagues. The patient was a fat man, with a gallbladder infection, with stones in that organ of an infinite number, and of many shapes and sizes. My surgical friend, successfully, as the French say, tore from him the gallbladder. The operation was a severe one, and resulted in a relatively long period of convalescence, but he is due to leave for his home today.

Because of his illness and the operation, he has lost at least thirty pounds, and is now a mere sylph. He has spent at least three weeks in a room here with two other patients. Naturally, a common topic among them was surgery of the abdomen, before, during and after. He was so weak after surgery that he was well content just to sit all day, and now that he is thin, he likes to do the one thing that he could *not* do before his operation—that is, cross one leg over the other. Being a right-handed man, he crosses the right leg over the left. See, he is doing just this, right now.

And now let us examine the structures so brought into apposition.

The left patella is prominent, its edges sharp and clear-cut. In this position of sitting with his right leg over his left, this sharp patellar edge fits snugly into the area where the common peroneal nerve winds around the neck of the fibula. His muscles are atonic, pads of protective fat are no longer there, and he has sat in this room, with one leg crossed over the other, while the sharp edge of the left patella grinds his right common peroneal nerve into a state of damage that will last for many weeks or months.

Pardon me, but I have not asked what this patient is complaining of, now that his gallbladder has been so successfully removed. Well, since he is sent to me, he must have some disorder of the nervous system. I am inclined to be allergic to gallbladder operations on fat persons. The only thing missing here is that our patient is not the mayor of his town, with due aldermanic pomposity.

Let him walk a few yards! He has a steppage gait on the right. On the examination table, it is found that he has a marked weakness of the anterior tibial muscles and peroneal group. He has some degree of subjective anesthesia on the dorsum of his foot, and lateral aspect of his leg. He can walk on his toes, but not on his heels, but the tendon reflexes are still preserved.

It seems that during the hours of convalescence, while exchanging stories with his boy friends, unconsciously he crushed his common peroneal nerve, while sitting with his legs crossed. He now walks with a right dropped foot that goes flop, flop, as he goes down the corridor. The prognosis is good, since he will doubtless get fat again. His muscles will become hard, and if he sits at all, he will not be so easily able to bring that nerve into jeopardy. He should, however, wear a soft pad over the head of the right fibula, and he should not cross his legs any more. When he becomes fat again, he will not be able to do so. Above all, he should be warned that what he did to himself after surgery will take a long, long time getting over, possibly six months, at the least.

The essential features in these cases of *compression neuropathy of the common peroneal nerve* are: (1) the complete change in habits of the victim; (2) the loss in weight, lack of fat, and atony of the musculature, and (3) the assumption of a certain posture that leads to the damage of an individual nerve which is usually painless and not realized by the patient at the time it is happening.

3

THE THIRD patient, a middle-aged man, comes complaining of deafness, discharge from one ear, and difficulty in swallowing. He has been deaf in the right ear for more than fifteen years, and has had a purulent discharge from the same ear for almost as long. For about five years he has had difficulty in swallowing, so much so that fluids may regurgitate through his nose, on the right, and solid food may strangulate him at meals. He also complains of some weakness when elevating his right arm above his head. Recently his speech has been indistinct, and his tongue feels weak.

Members of the ear, nose and throat department have examined him, and they find perforation of his right eardrum, with copious discharge. In the center of this there is a small vascular tumor. A piece of this tumor was removed for biopsy. Bleeding occurred, and there was some trouble in getting the hemorrhage stopped. As a matter of fact, the bleeding was severe and worrisome.

As we see him this morning, he has a cotton plug in his right ear. His hearing on the left side seems to be normal, since he answers every question rapidly. Stripping him to the waist, we see at once that there is a complete absence of his trapezius and sternocleidomastoid muscles on the right. Examination of his throat shows that the right soft palate and pharyngeal muscles are pulled to the left on phonation. The tongue seems to be partially affected; it is slightly atrophied on the right, there are fibrillary twitchings in it, and on protrusion, it goes definitely to the right. He can not push out the right side of his cheek with his tongue.

We have now, therefore, two sets of lesions that do not seem to correspond. There is an infected right ear, with deafness and discharge, and in the middle of the perforation there is a soft vascular tumor. I should indeed like to know what the character of that tumor is.

From my standpoint, as a neurologist, I have a *Jackson's syndrome* to reckon with, the *syndrome of the jugular foramen,* whereby the ninth, tenth and eleventh cranial nerves are affected. Here, there is something more, in that the twelfth cranial nerve also is involved. What possible connection can these cranial nerve lesions have with the pathologic process in the ear? The petrous portion of the temporal bone should offer a strong barrier posteriorly. Up to a recent moment I was puzzled, befuddled and totally at sea.

The biopsy report has just come in, and it seems to explain our problem. The tumor is a *chemodectoma,* also called an "antichromaffin paraganglioma." This lesion is not so rare as was previously assumed; now we see many which were missed before. These tumors are the same as those arising from the carotid body. Similar cell rests arise at different stages along the internal carotid body. A common source of these tumors is around the bulb of the jugular vein, and the internal carotid artery in the jugular foramen. Closely associated are the ninth, tenth and eleventh cranial nerves. The jugular bulb and internal auditory apparatus are close enough, and the barrier of bone is so slight that the tumor follows a pathway straight into the inner ear, and finally perforates the drum, presenting itself at the external auditory canal. Tinnitus, deafness, suppuration and discharge from the ear follow, and go on for years. It is later that the tumor involves the ninth, tenth and eleventh cranial nerves, and still later that the twelfth becomes involved.

To tackle this tumor, either a brave or reckless disposition is needed. As a warning, the taking of a specimen for biopsy is followed by severe hemorrhage. Exploration through the ear is hazardous, through the posterior fossa of the skull, hopeless, and, generally speaking, both ear and nerve surgeons are thankful to compound for deep roentgen therapy, which, by the way, is no good, since the tumor is sadly insensitive to therapeutic radiation.

From the diagnostic standpoint, however, let you remember this: a long history of deafness and aural suppuration, with a ruptured drum, and a hemorrhagic fleshy tumor protruding through the hole in the drum. Add to this the fact that the taking of a specimen for biopsy was violently bloody and dangerous. Further, add a progressive syndrome of paralysis of the ninth, tenth and eleventh cranial nerves (Jackson's syndrome), and a later and less marked atrophy and paralysis of the corresponding half of the tongue. You will then have the clinical picture of a chemodectoma. There are a slide and section of this tumor here under the microscope, so that you all may see it. It is a rather recent pathologic discovery, so you may be able in the near future to surprise, confuse, malign and stagger one of your superiors! At our age, as teachers, we have a hard time keeping up with what you youngsters discover. Sometimes, nevertheless, we find that these "discoveries" have been described many years ago—and forgotten.

4

LET US GO up now into the children's ward. There is a young damsel there who needs your advice, and who will give you in return certain observations to put in your file of memories.

She is six years of age. She is here because, according to her mother, she is nervous, fidgety and will not stay in bed as her local physician has ordered. At this last sentence, we emit a horse laugh! *Here,* all children stay in bed as required, and Sister sees this is an unbroken rule. In bed, therefore, they stay.

The child has a continuous flow of muscular movement involving all the muscles of her body. These motions have been called "quasi" purposive. This is a lovely word, "quasi"! It means "as if" purposive, whereas the movements are not purposive at all. The child just grimaces, wiggles, fidgets and throws herself around. At one time a group of toes does a jolly old barn dance; at another, her trunk shoots backward and forward on her bottom, and both her arms and her fingers work independently of each other. Her grimaces mean nothing, except that she makes faces, and these and other random gestures are not the results of any emotional stimulus. Note that her elbows, heels and rump are reddened by continuous squirming over coarse, disinfected sheets.

She is a merry little soul, but with each thrill of laughing, her whole body goes into a fresh set of riotous movements. Involvement of her face narrows down her condition to chorea or athetosis. The history is a relatively short one of a few weeks' duration, which fact further increases the probability of her having simple chorea. Let us take the most common disease in childhood, and call her condition *Sydenham's chorea.* This Sydenham is the man who served with the Roundheads, with his Bible in his left hand, and his long steel sword in his right. He probably thought that Oliver Cromwell was one anointed by God, but nevertheless, that did not prevent him from finding that Peruvian bark, containing quinine, is a cure for malaria. He described the children's chorea, and his treatment then was no less worthy than it is today. How he got along with the Cavalier Willis, history does not say, but anyone will swap a describer of chorea of childhood for one who has outlined a vascular circle of anastomosis, and come out even.

Before these choreic movements started in this child, there was a history of a sore throat a few weeks before. There is no record of joint pains, but the child is none the less continually wiggling, and I wish that I could call in, in consultation, Thomas Sydenham. What oratory we should have! He doubtless would be right in every major premise. The only thing is that the Peruvian bark is not helpful in this disease, and he would not get anywhere with the pharmacist of a local drugstore. I do not think, however, that he would go far wrong. He would prescribe some simples, and relaxing warm baths, with gentle massage. The child would sleep magnificently, and awake free from the fidgets. An old practical nurse would be provided then, to carry on to the final cure, which would sooner or later occur. As I have seen, for each generation there is a new cure which works well, except in the more serious forms of the disease.

At the last, I should have asked Thomas Sydenham his final views as to the diagnosis of chorea. Smilingly, he would thrust his hands out, as I can see him do with this child.

"There is a choreic hand," he would say quietly, "and it is flexed at the wrist, and extended at the carpometacarpal joint, and this posture is more marked on the more affected side. You will find it in this child if you look for it here." And there it was.

What mighty ills have not been done by woman!
Who was't betrayed the Capital?—A woman!
Who lost Mark Antony the world?—A woman!
Who was the cause of a long ten years' war,
And laid at last old Troy in ashes?—Woman!
Destructive, damnable, deceitful woman!
                              —THOMAS OTWAY: *The Orphan.*

5

Good morning! This is our next-to-last bedside lecture of the year.
It is fitting that I place before you something that you will all run
into sometime, somewhere, and will blunder hopelessly. It is
usually an episode with a member of the opposite sex. For God's
sake, never, never underestimate the power of a woman! That
is just abject foolishness. Sherlock Holmes admitted that, far
from being omnipotent, he had been beaten at least three times,
and on two of these occasions it was by a woman. In the practice
of clinical medicine, our greatest triumphs are with women, and
they become our most grateful followers. As a contrast, we have
no deadlier enemies than women, or more vicious slanderers. The
poor male struggles along, somewhere in between, but withal he
is decent, kind and not charged with white-hot, sizzling fireworks,
going off at all angles, and at incalculable periods.

This woman, asleep in her bed, is a gift (a doubtfully precious
one) from another hospital. They are glad to be rid of her. At
the same time, let us be fair, just and scientifically accurate. She
is receiving every three hours 1/6 grain of morphine for alleged
severe headaches, and as a result, she is asleep now, and since she
has received other drugs as well, her sensory perception is far from
being accurate. We can, therefore, openly discuss her problem
at the bedside, and without awakening her to full consciousness.

346

Let us call her Mabel. That is not her name, but it does seem to suit her.

Mabel's family life was simple, except in its ultimate emotional revolution. She had a brother who, wise in his time, departed after high school to a distant town, where he was a plumber's apprentice, and later became a fully qualified master plumber—the one who is truly allowed to leave his tools behind. He married his boss's daughter, and to the tune of three children, all has gone merry as a wedding bell.

Mabel, on finishing high school, was urged to take up nursing. The father footed the bill, for the reason that he wanted his daughter to be self-supporting, and not dependent on anyone. The mother had rather mixed feelings. If her daughter became a nurse, she would be no longer dependent on the family. True, but more than that, she might even become an asset, and be able to nurse her father or mother, or both, through their final illnesses, without cost to anyone. A splendid arrangement, no doubt!

A year or so ago, this patient's father dropped dead, thus saving a lot of trouble and expense. It seemed that Mabel's mother was so well equipped in strength and endurance that she was likely to carry on without assistance, forever and a day. Accordingly, Mabel finished her nurses' training, and went into private work, both in the hospital and in the patients' homes. She was gifted with a natural ability in nursing, did well, and was continuously called upon by prominent practitioners to nurse their more important patients. Actually, she was saving money, and becoming rapidly independent of everyone. There was a boy on the side, but he did not count, since financially he was in no way ready for matrimony.

A year ago, like a bomb bursting alongside, she received an urgent letter from her mother's sister, to the effect that she must return immediately, inasmuch as her mother was far from being well. She went home to look over the situation. In spite of the message to the contrary, she found her mother looking astonishingly well. She was not so communicative as usual and talked very little to her daughter, beyond telling her some devious story of a man who had wanted to marry her, and who had discreetly pulled out at the last minute. Her mother had seemed, however, to have lost her incentive to work, had given up a few mildly lucrative posts, and was spending most of her time in bed.

Mabel took the situation in her stride, and "looked after" her mother, which meant running the house, cooking all the meals, and doing plenty of hard and humble work. The mother flourished under this regime, so that she became more and more dependent on her daughter. Characteristically, she became critical, scolding and petulant. She had her days of nagging and of tempers, and contrasting ones of supplication and self-pity, with constant reminders to Mabel that she owed to her mother everything she had obtained as a trained nurse.

One night, after a day of tempers and tantrums, Mabel sat up well into early morning, taking stock of the situation. A strong woman would have cleared out and not bothered about the consequences. Actually, there were several members of the family, aunts and uncles, who would have had to help out, if called upon. A weak woman would have accepted her burden, and carried on until the death of one or both women. . . . Mabel left the next morning, leaving no message.

She returned to Dublin, where she resumed her work as nurse. All the letters she received, and the notes brought by passing travelers, she returned to the sender or destroyed. She read each one first, however, with an unholy sense of guilt, and a vicious joy in giving in to it. To her friends she insisted that no matter what might happen, she would never go back home again.

Her work began to deteriorate, and to cover this up, she complained of severe headaches. At this time she was employed frequently by physicians who specialized in diseases of the ears, nose and throat. One day she asked to have her left ear looked at, since it had become deaf, and there was a copious purulent discharge coming from it. Perforation of the drum was found, with a foul-smelling discharge. There seemed to be no cause for this in her history of infectious diseases. Possibly a "minor cold" was the cause. Instead of abating, the condition became worse. The patient had fever, leukocytosis and chills, and subcutaneous abscesses broke out all over her body. Hospitalization was advised. In the hospital, receiving sulfonamide drugs, and with antiseptic dressings for her abscesses, she improved remarkably. Her temperature went down, her headaches diminished, and the perforation in her eardrum began to heal. She was discharged from the hospital, with some degree of uncertainty on the part of her physicians as to the pathologic course of her infection. Results of culture of a specimen of blood for the various pus-producing organisms were entirely negative.

After being in lodgings in this city for two months, she was readmitted to the hospital by ambulance, even more seriously ill than she had been the first time. Her temperature was at this time 105° F., and her pulse rate one hundred twenty beats per minute. She was sweating profusely, and her mouth was cracked and dry. There was again a profuse purulent discharge from the left ear, and the perforation in her drum, far from being healed, was wide open. She complained bitterly of headache, and continually buried her head in the pillow. In spite of the severe degree of her illness, she was mentally clear, and oriented as to place, circumstance and time.

There was again a new outbreak of subcutaneous abscesses, some of which were discharging, and others that obviously needed surgical incision. These were scattered over various parts of her body. Because of the severe pain in her head, she had been given ¼ grain of morphine, subcutaneously, each four hours. If this was not forthcoming, she cried out with pain and vexation, and made a commotion.

When I saw her yesterday, at the other city hospital, she was relatively free from narcotic drugs, since I had asked that this should be so. She gave a clear story without manifest confusion, as to all that had happened to her. Her main complaint, however, was of constant, severe ache all over her head. Her speech was normal, and the neurologic examination showed no definite signs of involvement of the brain. The optic disks were not swollen. Her pulse was rapid, rather than slowed. She ended the period of history-taking by a querulous demand for morphine to alleviate her headache. I would have you note that this was one time she did *not* get morphine! I examined her most carefully, since my colleagues seemed to be puzzled. Moreover, I had a distinct suspicion that this morning I should find her in a bed in my wards—where she is right now—with all the heavy responsibility of disentangling this mess.

I have a series of charts, with body images printed on them. May I distribute these amongst the members of the class, and will each one of you kindly do as I did yesterday, map out the relative allocation of these subcutaneous abscesses, whether new or old? Mabel is awake by now, and she can be used to perform this piece of clinical research without any hurt to her. Later, we shall adjourn to a vacant room. I am appointing a chairman to sum up the findings on these charts you are going to make.

We are assembled and ready. May I ask, "Mister Chairman, what is your report?"

I gather from you that most of the old and recent abscesses are in the zone of the part of the left thigh, and almost as many are found on the left buttock. There are a few below the knee anteriorly. Relatively few are on the right side of the chest, but the areas of the right shoulder and upper arm are peppered with them. The right part of the abdomen is affected almost as much as the shoulder, but the right lower extremity is singularly free.

"And where," might I ask you, "Mister Chairman, are there no abscesses?"

You hear him answer, like the oracle of Delphi, "The left upper arm, forearm, and hand are free; as are the right buttock, and the back of the right thigh."

Strangely enough, both sides of the face and neck are free from these disfiguring pustules!

I am appointing you students members of a jury, but no trial is as yet under way. Possibly, you are better regarded as members of the grand jury, seeking an indictment.

"Is there," I ask you, "any question you would like to ask, or have you, being clever and quick-witted, observed and detected the answer before the holding of this inquiry?"

I see a small jury member from Ballyjamesduff with his hand up. He asks one simple question, and that is, "Is the patient right-handed or left-handed?"

It is himself that should have settled that question, as I myself had to do in front of all the staff of the hospital from which she came.

I replied, "Of *course*, she is left-handed, and of *course*, these infected abscesses are self-initiated. By the way, a sterilized hairpin was used. Being a nurse, the patient did not want to mix her breed of germs!"

By now you have brought together the head and tail of the problem; one leads imperceptibly on to the other. I had first to find out that these abscesses were self-initiated, later to find out as much as I could of this girl's background. I have made it too easy for you, I fear. Happily, the patient had relatives in the hospital where she had been working, who knew her family problem.

After my examination, I took this girl whom you have seen to-day, a shattered physical and moral wreck, and in a quiet and private room with all kindliness and understanding, I went through her history for the last few years. At first there were blocking and subterfuge, and an all-pervading sense of indifference but finally we rallied to a point of agreement, reached on her part only through a sudden torrent of tears, an emotional breakdown and an abject abnegation.

Had she been strong enough, she would have thrown her mother to the devil; had she been weak enough, she would still be at home, passively agreed to spend all the rest of her life with her mother. Unfortunately, she took a split on the proceedings, and landed herself in a morass of endless sorrow and woe. A career of deception and cheating followed, with no evident surcease of her tremendous sense of guilt. In a sense, her self-mutilation was a punishment, a penance that purged nothing, and her retreat into phantasy had never really reached its complete fulfillment or self-satisfaction. In her consciousness, atonement might be said to have been nonexistent.

I had some curiosity about her self-inflicted wounds, and asked her about them. She used, she told me, a certain hairpin which she sterilized before each proceeding. The most grisly stab of all was the first one, when she ruptured her eardrum with this hairpin, and then infected it with material from a patient in the ward who had chronic otitis media. What agony that must have caused her! The rest followed by degrees, until the serious climax occurred that brought her here.

I discussed with her yesterday her sense of guilt with respect to her mother, and I assured her that it was all wrong; that it was her right and privilege to get away whenever she wished to, and that really she owed nothing, one way or another, to her parents. The hardest core of psychologic difficulty was in regard to her self-inflicted wounds. The feelings of guilt here were equally severe. I think that I shall be able to rationalize this for her, and that she will get over it.

I think that it will be necessary to keep her here for some time. I want to get her off morphine and all habit-forming drugs, and I shall have numerous further interviews with her. Later, she can live outside the hospital, and come to see me in my consulting rooms, until I am satisfied that she is able to take care of herself. My task will then be to clear up her conflicts, and above all, to get her into a state of mind to return to her work.

She will have to make a clean break from here, and let the past bury the past. Again, she must not have the idea of flight from a life that she is too weak to face. She should leave here, determined to make good in another place, without any sense of failure. As the French say, "It is necessary to step back a pace or two to make a better jump."

NOTE: This patient did well in my hospital, as she had done previously in another hospital. The multiple abscesses cleared up, and the ear ceased to drain. The perforation in her eardrum became minimal in size, and she was discharged free of headaches, and seemingly well. She had been free of all drugs for some weeks.

Six months later I heard that she had been admitted to a third hospital, as bad as, if not worse than, before. She had failed to come back to me for guidance and advice. How futile it all seems to be now. These patients are "career" hysterics, and cursed with a *psychopathic personality.* They should be avoided in the same way that the devil shuns holy water! I simply underestimated the terrific power involved here.

From a sudden and unprovided death,
O Lord, deliver us.

—LITANY OF THE SAINTS.

6

Good morning! There is a tragedy in our ward today. (As if such things there were not always a commonplace!) And yet, nothing should be judged so ordinary that all the best skill here should not be used to combat it, in every stage of its evolution.

This young man, aged twenty-eight, is employed by a local furrier in Dame Street. He left home as usual this morning at 7:30, on a bicycle, whistling gaily I suppose, as he went his way. Arriving at his place of business, he started in to stitch some furs he had not finished the night before. He seemed to be well and in the best of spirits, as he talked to his co-workers.

Suddenly, at about 8:30, he gave a tremendous, agonized cry, and clasping his hands to his temples, groaned, "O God, O God, my head!" He fell off the chair to the floor, and had a severe convulsion. An ambulance was called, and this hospital being the nearest, he was admitted here only a few minutes later. It is our business to examine him, find out what is wrong, and apply the necessary treatment. They tell me that his relatives are arriving shortly.

He is lying on his side, in the so-called gun-hammer position. That is, his head is retracted, and his knees are drawn up on his abdomen, which is hollow and sunken. He is comatose; his pulse rate is 120 beats per minute, his respirations about twenty per minute, and his temperature 99.4° Fahrenheit. His blood pressure is normal, being 120 systolic and 95 diastolic.

I wish one of you boys would examine him. Taking his occiput in the palm of your hand, you should try to flex the head on the

353

chest. A few inches of flexion are obtained, and then, as you see, the head comes to a sudden stop. Forcing it induces a groan from the patient, his face becomes contorted, and his knees become even more flexed on the abdomen. Attempts to straighten out his flexed knees, and to extend the lower extremities on the abdomen are frustrated. If you want names, the first sign is Brudzinski's neck-flexing test; the other, Lasègue's straight leg-raising phenomenon, each one indicating severe meningeal irritation present all up and down the neuraxis. I have had you perform these tests so that you will have seen and felt what they are like, and know what they mean.

Will you now kindly open digitally both of this patient's eyelids, one at a time? The left shows nothing abnormal. The right shows a hugely dilated pupil, with divergent strabismus. The right pupil does not react to light; the left does. We can not test reflexes of accommodation when the patient is in this mental state. There are areas of hemorrhage around the right optic disk, but no papilledema. Note that the patient has periods of restlessness in his coma, and that he keeps putting his right hand on his right frontal area, as if there were pain over the eyebrow and brow, up to the hairline. Tendon reflexes, plantar responses and response to abdominal superficial stimulation, all are normal.

Now conditions are rapidly changing: his coma is deepening, his pulse is becoming slow, full and bounding, and Cheyne-Stokes respiration is evident. This is the time for action.

I would call your attention, my dearly belovèd disciple, to the tray alongside the bed, a tray equipped for spinal puncture. It has a hypodermic syringe of procaine hydrochloride (hardly necessary here, in this state of coma), iodine, alcohol, applicator sticks with cotton, and above all, several wicked-looking, large-sized (cisternal) puncture needles. It is for you now to do a spinal puncture. Have you never done one before? All the better, for there is always a first time, and you can not hurt this patient if you follow instructions.

Sister has now brought the patient to the iron edge of the bed, where there is no sag; the patient's back is perfectly perpendicular. Sister has tried to make the lumbar curve convex, rather than concave, but without success. His knees are flexed anyhow. Feel the crest of the ilium, and then drop a line to the spinal column, and next locate the dip between the spine of the second and third lumbar vertebrae. In such an arched back it is hard to find. Where you think it is, inject your procaine hydrochloride, at first intradermally, later subcutaneously and finally, in the deep tissues. Now prepare to be bloody, bold and resolute. Take up the sturdy needle, and with it absolutely perpendicular to the back, start pushing it in. A well-trained rachicentitic expert can tell each tissue the needle goes through, skin, interspinous ligamentous tissue, and finally the dura. There, resistance gives way with a distinct release phenomenon, as if the needle has passed through a taut membrane into a cavity, as of course it has.

Beginner's luck, my young friend! You seem to have hit the subarachnoid space first plunge. Had you not, you would have been ousted, since savaging a patient, and a peculiarly favorite route to get cerebrospinal fluid, are not encouraged.

Let us see if you really have the needle in the spinal subarachnoid space. The stilet is slowly withdrawn from the needle. Immediately a flow of bright red blood comes surging out of the needle, and fills a test tube in a few seconds. A glass manometer is convenient, and is put on the blunt, truncated, silvery end of the needle. A column of blood and fluid comes out, which we measure in the upright glass tube. It reaches the height of 30 cc. of water pressure, and then starts to overflow the manometer. This is removed, and four test tubes are filled with the flow from the needle. The first is pure blood, and the others produce a gradual admixture of blood and cerebrospinal fluid, until the last, which is of a cherry-red color and almost transparent.

This patient has had a sudden **subarachnoid hemorrhage.** At his age, the most likely cause would be rupture of a congenital aneurysm, situated somewhere on the circle of Willis, a common site in younger persons. For later treatment, it will be necessary to localize as far as possible these small aneurysms which have such a deadly effect when they rupture. Further, I do not think that Willis, in his most expansive moments, could have realized that the Supreme Artificer, like a badly trained plumber, could occasionally make a botch of his work at the time it was installed.

Look! Our patient is reviving. His consciousness, breathing and pulse are rapidly improving, and signs of meningeal irritation are lessening. He is beginning to respond to commands, even if in a vague sort of way, as if he were far away mentally, and paying no great attention to a sense of unreality. This is very characteristic of *a rupture of a cerebral aneurysm* in its recovery period. He is now struggling to sit up, and one eye is wide open. The eye on the right, however, shows complete ptosis. Pulling this eyelid upward with my fingers demonstrates, as before, a large, fixed pupil, and an eye diverged far to the right. He has, therefore, what we suspected before, complete paralysis of his right third cranial nerve.

There are, of course, still the peripapillary retinal hemorrhages. His neck is still rigid, and straight leg-raising still hurts him, but neither is so severe as before. His headache, although still present, is not so violent, but he is sensitive over the right forehead to the touch, or the stroking of the right eyebrow.

God knows he needs rest, and we shall let him have it. I am ordering a dose of morphine that will relieve pain, but which will not cover up signs and symptoms. He will sleep, and later we shall decide what is best to be done.

You are fortunate in having seen an incident of, almost from its inception, *rupture of a congenital aneurysm of the circle of Willis.* This morning, a few hours ago, this presumably healthy young man was hit by a stroke that acted with the force of a heavy sledge hammer wielded by a powerful man. He was comatose, and in shock. He had signs of diffuse meningeal irritation, and with his rapid pulse and respiration, as well as the mildly increased temperature, the diagnosis of "meningitis" might have been entertained, especially since the earlier headache was so ferocious in character. Earlier in our medical history, this sort of condition was diagnosed as "acute hemorrhagic meningitis," a complete misnomer.

There were, however, unilaterally localizing signs: (1) the retinal hemorrhage around the optic nerve was mainly on the right side; (2) there was complete paralysis of the third cranial nerve on the right and (3) the pain in his head seemed to be chiefly over the area of supply of the frontal branch of the first division of the fifth nerve. These structures come close together in the anterior portion of the middle cranial fossa, just before the optic nerve enters the optic canal, and the frontal division of the fifth nerve and the third nerve enter the orbit through the superior orbital fissure. Also near by, the internal carotid artery divides into the middle and anterior cerebral arteries, a site of weakness for the three coats of that vessel.

It has been shown that at the various points of junction and bifurcation of these vessels of the circle of Willis, the medial coat of a vessel at its bifurcation may be congenitally absent. It is under these circumstances, then, that at some time during a patient's life there may develop a small aneurysm, usually no larger than a split pea. It may rupture suddenly and death may occur, or it may produce that exquisite mixture between neighborhood signs and diffuse meningeal irritation such as we are seeing this morning, and a temporary recovery from both may ensue.

Rarely does this aneurysm act as a tumor and simulate, without rupture, tumors in the region of the sella turcica. The bold surgeon is doubly cursed who fails to think of this and tries to remove a "tumor" in that region, for he will have a death on the operating table from overwhelming hemorrhage.

Our patient today is kind, in that he shows us by his physical signs where the aneurysm is located. Frequently there are no neighborhood or localizing signs. The patient can be carried through the episode of his rupture, by spinal punctures, rest and general medical care, but the time is bound to come when the question is asked as to just where is this aneurysm located, around that complex little plumber's grief, the circle of Willis.

There is a procedure called "angiography," in which an opaque medium is put in one or both internal carotid arteries, and a rapid series of roentgen-ray exposures are taken to map out the course, outline normality or integrity of the cerebral arteries (or veins). By this means, aneurysms, vascular abnormalities, and the blood supply of tumors can be mapped out, and dealt with accordingly. In this field, angiography is on a par with the introduction of air into the brain by spinal or ventricular routes. I have a series here which you can see afterward, suitably labeled, and on view serially. In the case of this patient, the aneurysm has been localized, but when he has recovered from this rupture, we can get more information from an angiogram, if his condition permits. He may die, while we are waiting. That can not be avoided.

If everything goes well, we can make an angiogram, and immediately after, ligate his common carotid artery in one or more sites. A period of waiting and observation is again necessary. If no untoward results obtain, such as a hemiplegia, a direct attack on the aneurysm can be launched. With the information supplied by the angiograms, the aneurysm is sought by intracranial exploration. Thereafter there must be the most acute surgical judgment as to what to do, in virtue of what is found.

We want to trap that aneurysm, so that no blood, or pressure of blood, ever reaches it. If a sessile small balloon the size of a cherry pit is found, a silver clip may solve the whole problem, so that this weakened blob will never more be a threat to life. All anastomotic channels to that tiny source of sudden death must be put out of commission. We can only go as God directs us, and there is no question that, working inside the skull on these congenitally weak vessels, we need a personal deity who can direct us into the right channels of remedial surgery.

And what of it, if we get patients like our man here, who are so relieved by medical care and spinal puncture that they set their faces against a long series of radical attempts by surgery to cure them? They recover from the immediate rupture, feel well and follow their daily tasks. They know that they have the Sword of Damocles hanging by a mere thread over their uncovered heads. I have seen many such.

After all, life is a gamble, and if they want to play the dice for or against their future, who would blame them? All they can lose is a life, which may indeed be snuffed out by some other, and completely unexpected, tragedy. If our surgical attempts at cure were perfect and easy, *and* without risk, there would be no argument. All we hope for is that in the future this may be so. In the meantime, we must study closely this group of patients, in order to find out what is best for them. If a patient with a ruptured congenital aneurysm of the brain does not die shortly, he may live indefinitely, happily and usefully. In truth, he may have another rupture, and die within a twelvemonth. Nevertheless, these patients, while living, are never human wrecks; they are full of fun, and live to the utmost the precarious life that is given them. They remind me of the sentiment expressed by Horace, "Seize now and here the hour that is, nor trust some later day!"

          ❊   ❊   ❊   ❊   ❊

It has been a very interesting and productive year. I have enjoyed facing you all across a sickbed, wherein a real problem existed. Occasionally the illness we studied was a mild one, and the patient has acted as an interlocutor, entering into the discussion with a keen wit, and has reduced the ceremony to an outburst of gales of laughter. In those instances I have felt that the center of the stage has been stolen from me, that my thunder has been silenced, and that the authority of teaching activity has been grossly challenged. As a contrast today, the discussion was one of solemnity and tragedy. There was no time here for facetiousness or for hilarity. All of our thoughts and judgments have had to be enacted at the highest level. The amenities of teaching over a sickbed must be taken as they exist, and only with respect to their particular degree of emotional tension.

On a given morning, therefore, the physician-teacher, if he is worth his salt, is strung up to concert pitch. He has analyzed the case material, both in depth and breadth, and he has read all he can find up to date in the current scientific books and journals that might be of value. He is loaded, primed, capped and ready to shoot, full of enthusiasm, inspired and exhilarated because he can give to others what he has learned himself, and he rejoices in it. Here there are no dry bones of another age to fling a starving dog. There is no mumbling, didactic, boring routine which is given in exchange for the fees paid by your parents, who hope for an honest return.

The spirit of the lecturer infects the students. After the preliminary pushing around of you students, soothed by a pleasant story, you feel quietude descending on the ward. The class is interested, it mops up, like a parched, sun-scorched earth, the rain, all that is delivered. The patient, too, is on his toes to supply all that is wanted, since he feels that he also is part of this ritual, and he co-operates better than he has ever done. Always the thought comes to the physician-teacher, "Is this all in vain? Will this morning, glowing with new ideas as yet not heard, facts as yet unlearnt, and above all, clinical phenomena as yet unseen, fade within a few hours from the memories of you white-coated boys? Or will it occur, that years later you will remember just such a patient as was shown here this morning, and find a replica in the hospital you are then in—a condition undiagnosed by others—and because of a flash of memory of another sunny morning long before, you will speak up and give a correct opinion?" I sincerely hope that that will be the case.

Clinical teaching is a hard game. It has to be accurate, incisive and stimulating. It should not be attempted unless one has the energy, the fire and the enthusiasm to deliver it. The day one becomes too old or too ill to teach in this manner, it is far better to quit, lest like Socrates, one may corrupt the young, bringing shame on one's own head. It was for that purpose that hemlock was introduced into the pharmacopoeia of the Greeks, precisely to use on doddering teachers of worn-out themes.

I have tried to give you my best in these preceding years. Had I used the question-and-answer method, I might have known the result of the teaching, but this method defeats itself, in that usually the student is too shy to answer in front of his peers, or he may blurt out something that hurts the patient acutely.

I have tried to treat these subjects of our discussions humanely, and as equals. I always assure a patient that he will not be hurt, frightened or shamed, and tell him that the class is for his benefit as well as for ours. I have promised each of them that his feelings will not be disturbed, that his privacy will not be invaded or ravaged, and that a deeply serious and dignified effort will be made on his behalf. For a bad prognosis or a hurtful discussion, you have found that there is always a second room where these discussions take place *in camera*.

Finally, the material has been selected carefully, so that it should be at your level of knowledge. Red herrings across the trail have been discounted, and rarely have I shown an unfinished, undiagnosed problem that would only lead to your ultimate confusion. In my own humble way I hope that I have succeeded; in any case, if the gradual growth of the class of voluntary visitors, to the point of unwieldiness, is any criterion, I must at least have partly succeeded.

In a few days, you will fail or succeed in your final examinations in medicine. I sincerely hope that there will be no failures! You will then become doctors of medicine, with all the privileges and responsibilities pertaining to that state in life. It is not for me to give you a valedictory address. Rather should I be on my knees, praying for you. In your profession, you will receive an infinity of kicks and a minimum of halfpence. In the beginning, your fare will not be chicken and champagne, but the scrag end of a sheep's neck and very small beer. You will have no velvet robes, but instead, tattered, much-mended, shiny breeches. Add a wife, and two or more hungry children, with the ever-pervading stench in the home of boiling diapers, with the worry of a rent unpaid, and a practice that is as full of deadbeats as it is scarce of money, and you have then the full story.

With this grim future in store, you must remember one thing first, second and last, and that is to be kind, both to your patients and to your fellow craftsmen, above you, with you, or beneath you. Do not carry the attitude of the Out-Patient Dispensary with you into the arena of private practice. It is better to learn *first,* in the dispensary, the meaning of charity, and *then* to carry it with you throughout your life, even while dealing with persons who are purse-proud, who, while paying high fees, think a physician is someone to be ordered about.

These same persons may be just as worried as is the poor wreck in the out-patient department of a large hospital. Worry and anxiety alter for the worse our attitude to those around us, and may change a hitherto pleasing personality to an impossible, quarrelsome, querulous and dictatorial being, who is all the worse because of having money and power. I had many fights in my earlier years, and with chagrin found many of these patients drifting to those physicians who were more smooth and far-seeing than I was. As I grew mellow, with age and understanding, the reverse has occurred. By dealing with them honestly, with dignity and kindliness, I have come to find these so-called impossible patients eating out of my hand. I admit that there are a few remaining whom it seems no one can satisfy, but the burden of proof is as to whether the right way has been diligently sought after and religiously tried, so that it may be proved successful in the end.

To be ever-kind should be your principle, from the moment you leave the graduation hall with the parchment in your hand, in a sort of daze that people now call you "Doctor," until your obituary notice appears in your medical journal, noting all the distinguished appointments, degrees, honorary and earned, and your high status in medical politics, which you then can no longer enjoy in the grave. It is *then* that your epitaph should read, in the words of Saint Paul:

Though I speak with the tongues of men and of angels, and have not charity, I am become as sounding brass, or a tinkling cymbal.

INDEX